Intracerebral Hemorrhage

Edited by

Edward Feldmann, MD

Associate Professor
Department of Clinical Neuroscience
Brown University School of Medicine
Director of Neurology, Cerebrovascular Laboratory,
and Division of Cerebrovascular Diseases and Sonography
Rhode Island Hospital
Providence, Rhode Island

**Futura Publishing
Company, Inc.**
Armonk, NY

Library of Congress Cataloging-in-Publication Data

Intracerebral hemorrhage / edited by Edward Feldmann.
     p. cm.
   Includes bibliographical references and index.
   ISBN 0-87-993-575-8
   1. Brain—Hemorrhage. I. Feldmann, Edward.
   [DNLM: 1. Cerebral Hemorrhage. WQL 355 I6085 1994]
  RC394.H37I56 1994
  616.8′1—dc20
  for Library of Congress   93-43785
                                           CIP

Copyright © 1994

Published by
Futura Publishing Company, Inc.
135 Bedford Road
Armonk, New York 10504

LC #: 93-43786
ISBN #: 0-87993-575-8

Printed in the United States of America.

Printed on acid-free paper.

To

Hillary, Jeffrey, and Meggie

Contributors

José Biller, MD
Professor, Department of Neurology, Northwestern University Medical School, Director, Stroke Program, Northwestern Memorial Hospital, Chicago, Illinois

Lawrence M. Brass, MD
Co-Director, Yale Cerebrovascular Center, Associate Professor of Neurology, Yale University School of Medicine, Chief, Neurology Service, West Haven VA Medical Center, New Haven, Connecticut

Lisa M. DeAngelis, MD
Department of Neurology, Memorial Sloan-Kettering Cancer Center, and Department of Neurology and Neuroscience, Cornell University Medical College, New York, New York

Conrado J. Estol, MD
Chief, Cerebrovascular Disease Section, Buenos Aires, Argentina

Edward Feldmann, MD
Associate Professor, Department of Clinical Neuroscience, Brown University School of Medicine, Director of Neurology, Cerebrovascular Laboratory, and Division of Cerebrovascular Diseases and Sonography, Rhode Island Hospital, Providence, Rhode Island

Jeffrey I. Frank, MD
Director, Neuromedical/Neurosurgical Intensive Care, The Cleveland Clinic Foundation, Cleveland, Ohio

Karen Furie, MD
Assistant Instructor, Department of Clinical Neurosciences, Brown University School of Medicine, Providence, Rhode Island

Philip B. Gorelick, MD, MPH, FACP
Associate Professor of Neurology, Director, Cerebrovascular and Neuroepidemiological Sections, Department of Neurological Sciences, Section of Cerebrovascular Disease, Neuroscience Institute, Rush Medical School, Chicago, Illinois

Roger E. Kelley, MD
Associate Professor of Neurology, Department of Neurology, University of Miami, School of Medicine, Miami, Florida

Michael A. Kelly, MD
Associate Professor of Neurology, Cerebrovascular Neuroepidemiological Sections, Department of Neurological Sciences, Section of Cerebrovascular Disease, Neuroscience Institute, Rush Medical School, Chicago, Illinois

Agha Khan, MD
Division of Neurosurgery, Department of Surgery, Sinai Hospital, Baltimore, Maryland

James Kokkinos, MD, FRCAP
Fellow in Cerebrovascular Diseases, Center for Stroke Research, Department of Neurology, Henry Ford Hospital and Health Sciences Center, Detroit, Michigan

Steven R. Levine, MD
Director, Acute Stroke Unit & Clinical Stroke Service Center for Stroke Research, Department of Neurology, Henry Ford Hospital and Health Sciences Center, Detroit, Michigan

Stephan A. Mayer, MD
Fellow in Critical Care Neurology and Cerebrovascular Disease, Neurological Institute of New York, Columbia-Presbyterian Medical Center, New York, New York

Ralph L. Sacco, MS, MD
Assistant Professor of Neurology and Public Health (Epidemiology) in the Sergievsky Center, Neurological Institute of New York, Columbia-Presbyterian Medical Center, New York, New York

Jeffrey L. Saver, MD
Assistant Professor, Department of Neurology, Stroke Program, Northwestern University Medical School, Chicago, Illinois

Michael A. Sloan, MD
Assistant Professor, Departments of Neurology, Radiology, Epidemiology and Preventive Medicine, University of Maryland, School of Medicine, Baltimore, Maryland

Barney J. Stern, MD
Director, Division of Neurology, Department of Medicine, Sinai Hospital, Associate Professor of Neurology, The Johns Hopkins Medical Institutions, Baltimore, Maryland

Stanley Tuhrim, MD
Associate Professor, Department of Neurology, Mount Sinai School of Medicine, New York, New York

Janet L. Wilterdink, MD
Department of Clinical Neurosciences, Brown University and Rhode Island Hospital, Providence, Rhode Island

Preface

A substantial number of strokes are caused by intracerebral hemorrhage. Many of the exciting basic science and clinical advances unfolding in the evaluation and management of ischemic stroke apply as well to hemorrhage, and promising new surgical therapies are on the horizon. Thanks to the declining prevalence of uncontrolled hypertension, the etiologic spectrum of intracranial hemorrhage has become more diverse, reflecting the epidemics of sympathomimetic drug use among our young and vessel weakening amyloid deposition among our elderly.

This book is intended to be a practical aid for neurologists and neurology residents and will also be of value to internists and neurosurgeons as well as any physician who cares for patients with intracerebral hemorrhage. This volume provides an in-depth guide to the epidemiology, pathophysiology, diagnosis, treatment, and prognosis of intracerebral hemorrhage. The contributors are well versed in the clinical and scientific aspects of this disorder. Figures and illustrations cover important diagnostic findings, as do summary tables and flow charts.

We seek to provide a balanced and comprehensive view of the causes and potential treatments of this condition.

Edward Feldmann, MD
Providence, Rhode Island

Contents

Part IV. Management of Intracerebral Hemorrhage

Part V. Prognosis

Part 1

Epidemiology of Intracerebral Hemorrhage

Chapter 1

Epidemiology of Intracerebral Hemorrhage

Ralph L. Sacco, MS, MD and Stephan A. Mayer, MD

Intracerebral hemorrhage (ICH) is bleeding from an arterial source into brain parenchyma, and is widely regarded as the most deadly of stroke subtypes. Recent advances in the medical and surgical management of cerebrovascular disease have failed to significantly improve outcome in patients with ICH. Primary prevention offers the most promise of reducing morbidity and mortality from this disease. A thorough understanding of the epidemiology of ICH can provide important insights into its pathogenesis and guide those public health strategies directed at reducing its incidence.

Epidemiologic Principles

To understand the epidemiology of ICH, the language and methodology that represents the core of epidemiology should be briefly introduced. In contrast to an analysis of a case series, which is a collection of patients with a disease, *descriptive* epidemiology focuses on the study of disease within a defined population. The public health indexes of the impact of a disease are phrased in terms of disease-specific *mortality, incidence,* and *prevalence* as defined in Table 1. The quality of these data depends primarily on the method of *case-ascertainment* and knowledge of the specific study population. For ICH, case-ascertainment depends on the accuracy of diagnosis, which improved dramatically with the introduction of computerized tomographic (CT) scanning in the early 1970s. Accurate measurements of the population size and knowledge of the demographic, socioeconomic, and health indexes of the underlying study population permit calculations of incidence, prevalence, and mortality. These can be compared between different populations and followed over time. Differences in the risk of disease in population subgroups may lead to hypotheses

From Feldmann E (ed). *Intracerebral Hemorrhage.* Armonk, NY: Futura Publishing Company, Inc., © 1994.

Table 1
Common Epidemiologic Indices

Mortality:	The frequency of death within a specific population, calculated over a given time interval. It is often expressed as a *death rate:* deaths from a given disease per 100,000 persons at risk of dying of the disease per year.
Incidence:	The frequency of new cases of a disease within a specific population over a given time interval. It is usually expressed as an *incidence rate:* the number of new cases of a given disease during a specified period (usually 1 year) per 100,000 persons at risk of having the disease for the first time per year.
Prevalence:	The frequency of all current cases of disease within a specific population, calculated for a given time and given place. It is usually expressed as a *prevalence ratio:* the number of persons with a given disease at a specified time per 100,000 persons capable of having the disease at that time.

Reproduced from Reference 89 with permission.

concerning possible *risk factors* defined as variables that increase the probability of disease when an individual is exposed.

Hypotheses regarding causation generated by descriptive studies can in turn be formally tested using the techniques of *analytic* epidemiology. There are two general methods of investigation: *case-control* studies, which compare the frequency of a putative risk factor in persons with and without the disease; and *cohort* studies, prospective and retrospective, which measure disease occurrence over time in patients with or without exposure to the risk factor in question. Most analytic epidemiologic studies report the association between a given risk factor and stroke in terms of *relative rate, relative risk,* or *odds ratio.* These measures of association quantify the relationship between a given factor and the occurrence of ICH. Relative risk is the ratio of incidence among those exposed to those unexposed. The odds ratio represents the ratio of odds of exposure to a factor among cases compared to controls.

A more complete understanding of epidemiologic principles can be acquired through further study of other texts.[1] In this chapter, we review descriptive and analytic epidemiologic data relating to the classification, frequency, and causes of ICH. Epidemiologic study of the natural history of ICH as it applies to prognosis is reviewed in Chapter 15.

Classification of Intracerebral Hemorrhage

Stroke is defined as the abrupt onset of focal or global neurological symptoms caused by ischemia or hemorrhage into the brain resulting from diseases of the cerebral blood vessels. Strokes are classified into infarction or hemorrhage, realizing that overlap occurs in the case of hemorrhagic infarction, in which localized bleeding occurs in association with an ischemic or venous infarct.

Intracranial hemorrhage can be subdivided into two distinct types based on the site and origin of the blood: subarachnoid and intracerebral hemorrhage. Two additional forms of intracranial hemorrhage, *subdural* and *epidural hematoma*, occur outside the brain parenchyma and cerebrospinal fluid (CSF), result almost exclusively from trauma, and are not considered forms of stroke. *Subarachnoid hemorrhage* (SAH) is defined as bleeding into the subarachnoid space and CSF while ICH is characterized by bleeding into the substance of the brain. Both usually occur from arterial bleeding, but the size, type, and distribution of the arterial lesions differ. Subarachnoid hemorrhage is most frequently caused by leakage of blood from a macroscopic cerebral aneurysm located at the base of the brain, particularly at the origin or bifurcation of an artery. Intracerebral hemorrhage usually results from leakage from a smaller, often microscopic, penetrating artery. Intracerebral hemorrhage and SAH may coexist with trauma, when the dome of a ruptured aneurysm is directed into the brain parenchyma, or when blood from ICH extends into the subarachnoid or intraventricular space.

Overall, ICH is much less frequent than cerebral infarction, but the relative frequency depends on the demographic characteristics of the study population. In the Stroke Data Bank (SDB),[2,3] a prospective multicenter study of 1,805 patients admitted for acute stroke, ICH accounted for 13% of all acute hospitalized strokes (Figure 1). This translates into approximately 65,000 new cases of ICH per year in the United States with a significant public health impact measured in terms of disability and health care costs. Computerized tomographic-based stroke registries in both the United States[4] and Europe[5,6] have found similar relative frequencies for ICH, ranging from 8% to 15%. Data from Japan[7] and China,[8,9] however, indicate that ICH represents 20% to 30% of strokes in Asian populations. Descriptive epidemiologic studies have shown that an excess of ICH in Asian populations, rather than fewer ischemic strokes, explains this proportionate increase.

Intracerebral hemorrhage can be further classified according to etiology and location. *Primary* ICH describes spontaneous bleeding in the absence of a readily identifiable precipitant, and is usually attributable to microvascular disease associated with hypertension or aging, such as in amyloid angiopathy. Secondary ICH occurs most often in association with either (1) trauma, (2) impaired coagulation, (3) toxin exposure such as cocaine, or (4) a clinically obvious anatomical lesion (eg, neoplasm, aneurysm, or arteriovenous malformation). Less common causes of secondary ICH include cold exposure,[10] migraine,[11] electroconvulsive therapy,[12] inflammatory vasculitides,[13] and surgical procedures.[14-16] Although the etiologic spectrum of ICH will vary depending on the population studied, data from the Stroke Data Bank (SDB)[2,3] and other large series of CT diagnosed ICH[5,12,17] suggest that 12% to 22% of ICH is related to secondary causes (Table 2). Systematic postmortem examination in patients with fatal ICH may yield a higher percentage of angiographically occult vascular lesions.[18]

Supratentorial ICH (occurring above the cerebellar tentorium) is classified as being either lobar or deep, involving the thalamus, putamen, or caudate

Stroke Subtype Distribution Among 1805 Patients
Stroke Data Bank

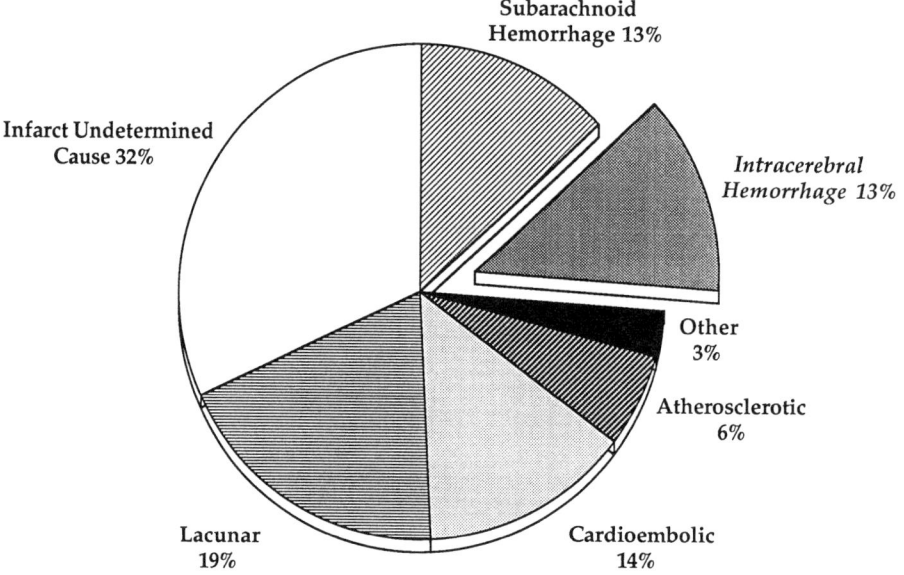

Figure 1. Stroke subtype distribution among 1,805 patients (Stroke Data Bank).

Table 2
Etiology of Nontraumatic CT Diagnosed Intracerebral Hemorrhage in Selected Series

	Stroke Data Bank[2] 1983–86 (n = 237)	Broderick[17] 1988 (n = 184)	Weisberg[12] 1977–79 (n = 277)	Bogousslavsky[5] 1982–87 (n = 109)
	(all figures are percentages)			
Primary ICH	86	88	87	78
Hypertensive	59	64	70	50
Nonhypertensive	27	24	17	28
Secondary ICH	14	12	13	22
Aneurysm/AVM	8	5	6	13
Neoplasm	†	1	2	1
Coagulopathy*	5	5	5	6
Toxin	0	1	0	1
Other	1	0	0	1

* Includes warfarin anticoagulation and thrombolytic therapy.

† Patients with neoplasm were excluded from the Stroke Data Bank.

Table 3
Distribution by Location of CT Diagnosed Primary* Intracerebral Hemorrhage in Selected
Clinical Series

	Stroke Data Bank[2] 1983–86 (n = 203)	Broderick[17] 1988 (n = 162)	Bogousslavsky[5] 1982–87 (n = 85)	Suzuki[7]§ 1983–85 (n = 662)
	(all figures are percentages)			
Supratentorial	85	86	84	88
Lobar	32	38	27	12†
Deep	53	48	57	76
Putamen	25	NS	52††	38
Thalamus	23	NS	5	27
Caudate/Other	5	NS	NS	11
Infratentorial	15	14	16	12
Cerebellum	11	8	7	7
Pons	4	6	9	5

NS: not specified.
* Patients with secondary ICH (due to trauma, coagulopathy, toxin exposure, aneurysm, AVM, or neoplasm), multiple sites of hemorrhage, or primarily intraventricular hemorrhage were excluded from analysis.
§ Includes primary and secondary ICH.
† Includes 3% classified as "other" supratentorial.
†† Described as "lenticular-capsular."

nucleus. *Infratentorial* ICH refers to involvement of either the brainstem, usually the pons, or cerebellum. The distribution by location of CT documented ICH in the SDB[3] and other series[5,17] (Table 3) indicates that in western populations, approximately half of primary ICH are deep, one third are lobar, and one sixth infratentorial. Data from a large series reported by Suzuki[7] indicate that the relative proportion of lobar hemorrhage among Japanese is significantly smaller.

Mortality of Intracerebral Hemorrhage

Stroke is the third leading cause of death worldwide, accounting for 10%–12% of deaths in the United States and other western nations.[19,20] Cerebrovascular disease is the leading cause of death in China and Japan,[21,22] and the second leading cause of death in Taiwan.[23] Intracerebral hemorrhage contributes significantly to stroke-related mortality in Asian countries because of its high incidence and case fatality rate.

International cerebrovascular mortality data from 1968 to 1973 indicated that ICH-specific mortality rates correspond well with geographic differences in ICH incidence.[24] The greatest mortality rate from ICH was reported in Japan

(Table 4). Important methodological issues limit the validity of mortality data obtained from vital statistics. Death certificates may not provide accurate representations of the underlying cause of death, practices in death certification can vary from country to country, and the international coding of diseases has been modified over the years. Despite these potential sources of error, the two-to threefold difference in ICH mortality between Japan and most other western countries is unlikely to be artifactual.

Table 4

Average Annual Age-Adjusted (to 1950 U.S. Population) Mortality Rates for Cerebrovascular Disease in Selected Countries, 1968–1973*

Location	Years	Cerebral Hemorrhage (Deaths/100,000 Per Yr)	Cerebral Embolism And Thrombosis (Deaths/100,000 Per Yr)
Japan	1968, 1970–73	87.4	16.8
Czechoslovakia	1968–73	54.6	21.1
Greece	1968–73	36.9	19.1
Mauritius	1969–73	34.3	26.2
Ireland	1968–72	34.1	44.3
Iceland	1971–73	31.7	18.6
N. Ireland	1968–71, 73	30.0	44.0
Scotland	1968–73	29.2	39.4
Australia	1968–73	28.3	33.8
Finland	1969–73	26.0	43.6
Denmark	1969–73	25.8	10.9
Poland	1970–71	25.2	4.9
Sweden	1969–73	24.0	7.5
England/Wales	1968–73	23.0	35.5
Italy	1968–73	22.3	38.4
France	1968–73	21.8	2.6
Israel	1969, 1970–73	21.3	9.3
United States†	1970	20.0	28.0
New Zealand	1968–72	19.3	29.8
Belgium	1969–72	17.6	36.6
Norway	1969–73	17.4	7.8
Austria	1971–73	12.3	3.9
Netherlands	1969–73	10.8	10.5
Switzerland	1969–73	10.1	4.4
West Germany	1970–73	8.1	N.A.

* Coded according to the 8th revision of the International Classification of Diseases.

† Data for the United States were derived from Baum and Goldstein[26] and age adjusted to 1970 U.S. population.

Adapted from Reference 24 with permission.

In the past 50 years there has been a worldwide decline in mortality due to stroke.[25] A number of studies have suggested that ICH-related mortality has fallen more rapidly than other stroke subtypes. Intracerebral hemorrhage had the largest reduction (50%) in type-specific cerebrovascular mortality rates in the United States from 1968 to 1977.[26] A more pronounced decrease in ICH mortality compared to other stroke subtypes has also been reported in Japan.[27] Although decrements in both ICH incidence and case fatality are presumably responsible for these trends, improved detection by CT of smaller nonlethal hemorrhages may contribute.

Incidence of Intracerebral Hemorrhage

Information concerning the incidence of ICH in geographically defined populations has become clearer only within the last 15 years. Improvements in diagnostic imaging have provided new insight into the effects of temporal trends, geographic variation, and age, gender, and race on ICH incidence.

Impact of Computerized Tomography

Computerized tomography has improved detection of smaller hemorrhages, indicating that ICH is considerably more common and less devastating than had been previously thought. In Rochester, Minnesota, a dramatic increase in both the incidence and 1-month survival rates of ICH between 1975 and 1979 compared to prior years was attributed to the increased use of CT.[28] Based on the larger percentage of patients who were alert at the time of diagnosis (23%) compared with earlier years (4.5%), the authors estimated that nearly one fourth of the cases of ICH in the pre-CT era had been mislabeled as infarctions. However, because CT was performed in only 71% of patients in this study, the true incidence of ICH was still probably underestimated. More recent incidence data from the same area[29] demonstrated a 56% increase in the incidence of ICH between 1965–74 and 1975–84, from 9 to 14 per 100,000 population. This observation either reflects a true increasing incidence, or suggests that up to one third of cases in the pre-CT era may have been misdiagnosed.

Although trends in ICH incidence after the introduction of CT scanning are largely unknown, preliminary data suggest a true increasing incidence that is not solely the result of improved diagnostic accuracy. A significant rise in the incidence of ICH has been reported in New Haven, Connecticut from 1981 to 1989.[30] This trend was accompanied by a fall in ICH related mortality, with stable incidence and mortality rates for stroke of all types. The large proportion of hemorrhages associated with cocaine use in this community led the investigators to conclude that secondary ICH associated with substance abuse may explain these findings.

Geographic Variations

Significant geographic differences exist in the incidence of ICH. Consistently higher rates have been reported in Asian populations compared to western populations (Table 5). For the purposes of comparison, these studies[6,7,31–40] are grouped according to the primary means of diagnosis, CT based or clinical/autopsy based. Variation in stroke incidence rates between studies may result from differences in age distribution, inclusion criteria, diagnostic criteria, and methods of case collection. Regardless of these disparities, the consistently high incidence of ICH in Japanese and Chinese populations compared with North American and European populations is striking. Overall, these studies suggest that ICH occurs two to three times more frequently in Asian populations than in western populations. Incidence rates for ischemic stroke are also higher in

Table 5

Incidence* of Intracerebral Hemorrhage in Selected Studies: Geographic Variation

Location	Time	CT Frequency	Method of Case Collection	Incidence Per 100,000 (Men/Women)	Reference
Clinical/autopsy-based diagnosis:					
Hisayama, Japan†	1974–83	—	Cohort study	140/70[a]	31
Six cities, China†	1982	—	Door-to-door survey	80	32
Shibata, Japan†	1976–78	—	Community registry	61[b]	33
Frederiksberg, Denmark	1971–73	—	Community registry	30	34
Rochester, MN, U.S.A.†	1945–76	—	Records-linkage system	15	35
Framingham, MA, U.S.A.†	1949–75	—	Cohort study	10[c]	36
CT-based diagnosis:					
Akita, Japan	1983–85	100%	Hospital-based	69/41[d]	7
South Alabama, U.S.A.	1980	80%	Hospital-based	23	37
Malmo, Sweden†	1989	51%	Hospital-based	22	38
Oxfordshire, U.K.†	1981–86	80%	Community registry	20	39
Cincinnati, OH, U.S.A.	1988	99%	Hospital-based	15	40
Dijon, France†	1985–89	88%	Community registry	14/12	6

* Incidence rate based on total population at risk except where noted:

  [a] Population age ≥ 40 years.

  [b] Population age ≥ 20 years.

  [c] Population age 20–79 years.

  [d] Population age 30–88 years.

† First-ever strokes only.

China and in Japan than in most other parts of the world, but to a lesser degree,[41] consistent with the large proportion of strokes due to ICH among Asians.

The reasons behind the apparent predisposition of Japanese and Chinese people to ICH are unclear, but genetic influences may be important.[42] Although hypertension is more prevalent in Japan than in the United States,[43] the magnitude of this difference does not fully explain a two- to threefold difference in the incidence of ICH, and the prevalence of hypertension in China is less than in the United States.[42] The possible significance of environmental or dietary factors is suggested by the higher risk for stroke in the northern regions of China and Japan,[32,44] and the lower cerebrovascular mortality rate of Japanese immmigrants to the United States compared to ethnically similar residents of Japan.[45]

Age

The incidence of ICH is low among persons below the age of 45 years, and increases dramatically after the age of 65. This finding has been demonstrated consistently in all studies reporting age-specific ICH incidence rates, and parallels the strong relationship between age and risk of cerebral infarction.[20] In Cincinnati, Ohio,[46] the incidence of ICH doubled with each advancing decade until age 80, after which the incidence became 25 times greater than for the total population, and seven times greater than the preceding decade. Time trend data from Rochester, NY[35] and Hisayama, Japan[31] have demonstrated an increased frequency of elderly persons with ICH. In Rochester, for example, the percentage of patients with ICH over age 75 tripled between 1945–1960 (12%) and 1961–1974 (37%).[35] This may reflect a shift toward nonhypertensive etiologies of ICH, or increased average age of the population.

In contrast with ischemic stroke, many studies[6,31,33,39,40] have shown a plateau or decrease in the incidence of ICH among the very elderly (over 75 years of age) compared with those aged 60–75; in two instances, the finding was limited to women[6] or blacks.[40] The explanation for this finding is unclear. Small numbers of older individuals within a population combined with higher early mortality and lower case detection rates for ICH may result in less reliable data. Competing causes of mortality may account for death prior to manifestation of ICH. Alternatively, this finding may reflect the effect of vascular lesions that place patients at risk for ICH earlier in life, as is the case with aneurysmal SAH.

Gender

Intracerebral hemorrhage tends to occur more frequently in men. Of 11 major incidence studies, men significantly outnumbered women in 6;[7,31,33,36,37,47] rates were equal in 4;[6,38,39,48] and women outnumbered men in 1 study.[46] The largest excesses of male-to-female ICH incidence, ranging from 50% to 100%, have been consistently reported in Japanese populations.[7,31,33,47] The explanation for gender discrepancies is probably related to differences in the prevalence of established ICH risk factors.

Race/Ethnicity

Race/ethnicity is an important determinant of the risk for ICH. As already discussed, the high incidence of ICH in Asians accounts for much of the geographic variation of ICH incidence. In the United States, African-Americans are more likely to have an ICH than whites. This finding mirrors the higher incidence of cerebrovascular disease among African-Americans in general.[4,49,50] Epidemiologic studies of stroke in ethnically diverse communities (southern Alabama,[37] northern Manhattan,[48] and Cincinnati[40,46]) have consistently reported a greater incidence of ICH in blacks compared with whites, particularly in the middle age ranges (Table 6). Hypertension was significantly more frequent among blacks in studies that analyzed risk factors,[37,46] supporting the hypothesis that the high incidence of ICH may be related to the high prevalence of hypertension in African-Americans.[51] Whether other factors may contribute to the excess of ICH among middle-aged blacks remains to be determined.

There are little data concerning the incidence of stroke among Hispanic

Table 6
Incidence of CT-diagnosed Intracerebral Hemorrhage in Selected Studies: Ethnic Variation

Location	Time	Age (Yrs)		Incidence (Per 100,000)		
				Blacks	Whites	Hispanics
Cincinnati[40,46]	1982	All ages		17.5	13.5	
	1988	≤ 34		2	0.5	
		35–54		27	7	
		55–74		58	33	
		≥ 75		36	156	
		All ages		16	15	
Northern Manhattan[48]	1983–86	40–59		31	13	14
		60–79		83	24	32
		≥ 80		152	113	129
		≥ 40*	Men	64	26	24
			Women	60	24	40
South Alabama[37]	1980	All ages	Men	36.6	16.7	
			Women	28.6	7.4	

* Age-adjusted to total northern Manhattan population

Americans. In northern Manhattan,[48] the incidence of ICH in this group was slightly greater than among whites, but less than in African-Americans. The extent to which racial, ethnic, or geographic patterns reflect genetic differences or variations in the prevalence of established or unidentified risk factors is unclear. Further studies are needed to clarify the relationship between race/ethnicity and ICH occurrence.

Risk Factors for Intracerebral Hemorrhage

The three main classes of stroke — cerebral infarction, subarachnoid hemorrhage, and ICH — are distinguished not only by different pathophysiological mechanisms, but by different risk factor profiles. Compared to patients in the Stroke Data Bank with ischemic stroke, ICH patients were younger, but did not differ appreciably with regard to sex or race (Table 7).[2] Although antecedent hypertension occurred with an equally high frequency in both groups, untreated hypertension was more common in patients with ICH. This observation perhaps reflects the importance of the severity of hypertension in the pathogenesis of ICH. In contrast, other well-accepted risk factors for ischemic stroke, such as diabetes, ischemic heart disease, and prior transient ischemic attack, were less frequent in patients with ICH, indicating their relative less of importance in the pathogenesis of cerebral hemorrhage. In the discussion that fol-

Table 7
Selected Descriptive and Clinical Characteristics of Patients in the Stroke Data Bank

	ICH (n = 237)	Infarction (n = 1273)	SAH (n = 243)
Median age	61 yrs	68 yrs	52 yrs
		(all figures are percentages)	
Male	57	47	31
Black	53	58	43
Medical History:			
Hypertension	64	68	42
(% untreated of total)	48	32	43
Diabetes	9	26	5
Myocardial infarction	9	18	3
Angina	5	17	4
*Neurological History:**			
TIA	3	16	1
Prior stroke	13	26	4
Antiplatelet/anticoagulant use	10	13	1

Adapted from Foulkes et al,[2] with permission.
* Complete data not available for all patients.

lows, we review analytic epidemiologic data from case-control and cohort studies pertaining to the relative importance of various risk factors for ICH.

Definite of Risk Factors

Hypertension

Hypertension represents the single most important modifiable risk factor for ICH. In Hisayama, Japan, a direct relationship between the incidence of ICH and blood pressure was documented with no evidence of a threshold or plateau effect.[52] Higher blood pressures were associated with progressively increased ICH incidence. Despite the common belief that hypertension results most frequently in deep or infratentorial ICH,[12] most series indicate that hypertension is an important risk factor for ICH regardless of location.[17] In Cincinnati, Ohio, it was estimated that eliminating hypertension from the population would decrease the incidence of ICH by 49%.[46]

The beneficial impact of antihypertensive treatment on the incidence of ICH was first demonstrated in 1979.[35] In Rochester, Minnesota, using clinical criteria and available autopsy data to confirm the diagnosis, hypertension was found to be a precursor of ICH in 89% of cases. Hypertension was both more frequent and more severe during the earlier years of the study. A steady decline in the incidence of ICH between 1945 and 1976, from 15.7 to 7.3 per 100,000, was found in conjunction with the improved control of hypertension. The authors concluded that the observed decline in the incidence of ICH was attributable to the introduction of effective antihypertensive therapy, thus establishing hypertension as an important modifiable risk factor for ICH.

Similar findings have been reported among residents of Hisayama, Japan.[31] A 47% decrease in the age-adjusted incidence of ICH, from 170 to 90 per 100,000, was documented between cohorts from 1961–1970 and 1974–1983. This trend was accompanied by an increase in mean age (from 63 to 73 years) and a fall in diastolic blood pressure among those with ICH. A concurrent reduction in the prevalence of hypertension in Hisayama was determined to be the most likely explanation for the observed decline in ICH incidence.

More recent series have indicated that approximately 65% of patients with ICH are hypertensive.[2,17] This frequency has declined with improved control of hypertension, resulting in a proportional shift towards nonhypertensive etiologies of ICH.

Ethanol

Excessive use of alcohol has been associated with massive spontaneous ICH.[53] Alcohol has a number of acute and chronic effects that may contribute to hemorrhagic stroke, including acute and chronic hypertension, impaired co-agulation, and direct effects on cerebral vessels.[54]

Epidemiologic support of the association between alcohol consumption and ICH risk comes from both prospective cohort[44,47,55,56] and case-control studies.[57] In the Honolulu Heart Project,[56] the risk of hemorrhagic stroke (including ICH) was directly correlated with both light and heavy alcohol intake. In contrast, a Kaiser-Permanente study[55] reported a "threshold" effect, with higher risks of hemorrhagic stroke only among heavy (≥ 3 drinks per day) drinkers. Although alcohol has been reported as a risk factor for SAH,[58] data from the Kaiser-Permanente study[55] suggested that the magnitude of risk is not as strong as for ICH. The relative risk for intracerebral hemorrhage was 6.82 among heavy drinkers compared to abstainers, whereas the relative risk for SAH (1.62) failed to reach statistical significance. Further discussion of the association between alcohol and ICH is provided in Chapter 9.

Hypocholesterolemia

Low serum cholesterol has been reported as a risk factor for ICH in pro-spective cohort studies from Japan,[47,59] the Honolulu Heart Project,[60–62] and the Multiple Risk Factor Intervention Trial.[63] This finding is in contrast to the inconsistent relationship between elevated cholesterol levels and the risk of ischemic stroke.[63,64] Unlike the situation with alcohol, low cholesterol has not been reported as a risk factor for SAH. The biological explanation for the rela-tionship between low serum cholesterol and ICH risk is unclear. Experimental evidence suggests that very low cholesterol levels may weaken the endothelium of intracerebral arteries and predispose to rupture and bleeding.[63]

Most studies indicate that only persons with very low cholesterol levels ($<$ 160 to 190 mg/dL) are at increased risk for ICH. In the Honolulu Heart Project,[62] the relative risk of ICH among 7,850 Japanese-American men with serum cho-lesterol in the lowest quintile was 2.55 after controlling for age, blood pressure, cigarette smoking, and alcohol consumption. No interaction between blood pressure and serum cholesterol was observed. In contrast, the nonlinear inverse relationship between cholesterol and ICH mortality observed in the Multiple Risk Factor Intervention Trial[63] was confined to hypertensive men.

Anticoagulants

Long-term anticoagulant treatment is associated with a 6- to 11-fold in-creased risk for ICH. In Rochester, Minnesota, anticoagulant treatment pre-ceded ICH in 31% of patients between 1955 and 1969,[35] substantially greater than the 5% to 10% frequency of anticoagulant-associated ICH in more recent series.[11,12,17,46,65] Patients in the older Rochester cohort being treated with antico-agulants were at least six times more likely to develop ICH than untreated individuals. Among patients treated for transient ischemic attacks, long-term oral anticoagulants have been shown to increase the risk of ICH approximately eightfold.[66] Two recent Dutch studies have confirmed the elevated risk of ICH among anticoagulant-treated persons. A population based study from 1970–1979 in Leiden, The Netherlands, reported a relative risk of 11 for ICH among individuals being treated with anticoagulants.[67] Among patients receiving anticoagulants, ICH was found to be associated with hypertension, but not with age or sex. A subsequent study[68] demonstrated similar results, with patients being treated with anticoagulants eight times more likely to develop ICH.

Many patients with anticoagulant-associated ICH are also hypertensive.[65] Thus, the extent to which anticoagulation independently increases the risk of hemorrhage is unknown. The degree to which varying levels of anticoagulation affect the risk of ICH is also unclear. More recent use of lower dose warfarin should result in lower risk of ICH. Finally, the relationship between ICH and reduced hemostasis is not limited to warfarin, but also includes thrombolytics[69] and aspirin.[70]

Drug Abuse

Cocaine and amphetamine use is widely acknowledged as an important cause of ICH.[71] The risks associated with this and other forms of recreational drug use were determined in case series and are the subject of ongoing epidemiologic studies. Further discussion of this topic is provided in Chapter 4.

Possible Risk Factors

Other various factors have been associated with ICH. Liver disease was highly represented (15.5%) in an autopsy series of ICH[72] and was significantly associated with ICH in a case-control study.[57] Other epidemiologic studies, however, have failed to support the association between liver disease and ICH.[73,74] Thrombocytopenia, clotting abnormalities, and alcohol use in some patients with liver disease may predispose to ICH.

Seasonal variations in the incidence of ICH has been observed in Japan,[7,75] Minnesota,[76] Britain,[77] Iowa,[78] and Brussels,[79] with peak rates in late fall and winter. This phenomenon has also been recognized anecdotally in China as "Spring Festival Stroke," which occurs annually in January or February.[42] However, seasonal variations have not been substantiated in studies from Boston and Chicago,[10] the Lehigh Valley,[80] and Dijon.[81] The proposed mechanism is an elevation of blood pressure in cold ambient temperatures.

Cigarette smoking bears a strong relationship to the risk for SAH,[36,82–85] and in recent years has become increasingly recognized as a risk factor for ischemic stroke.[83,86,87] The role of smoking as a risk factor for ICH is less clear,

Table 8
Strength of Association of Currently Recognized Risk Factors For Subtypes of
Cerebrovascular Disease

	ICH	Infarction	SAH
Hypertension	++	++	+
Age	++	++	+
Anticoagulants	++	0	±
Alcohol	++	±	+
Hypocholesterolemia	++	0	0
Cigarettes	±	+	++
Hypercholesterolemia	0	±	0
Diabetes	0	++	0
Heart disease	0	++	0
TIA	0	++	0
Estrogens	0	+	±

++: strong association demonstrated
+: moderate association demonstrated
±: equivocal
0: no relationship
Synthesized from Schoenberg et al.[89] Longstreth et al.[82] Marmot et al.[83] and Davis et al.[86]

but is suggested by the results of the Multiple Risk Factor Intervention Trial.[83] In this prospective study of 350,977 men, smoking was related to death from ICH, but to a lesser degree than for SAH or cerebral infarction. In contrast, a number of studies have failed to demonstrate an association between smoking and ICH, while at the same time confirming the association with SAH.[36,85,88]

Prior ischemic stroke emerged as an important risk factor for ICH in one case-control study.[46] However, this study failed to control for the possible confounding effects of hypertension, age, and anticoagulant treatment. Confirmation of this finding with multivariate techniques is required before prior stroke can be considered an independent risk factor for ICH.

Well-established risk factors for ischemic stroke that have not been identified as strong risk factors for ICH include: diabetes mellitus; heart disease; transient ischemic attack; and oral estrogens. Table 8 shows the strength of association of some currently recognized risk factors for stroke by subtype, as synthesized from recent reviews of stroke epidemiology.[2,82,83,86,89] More recent studies have identified other potential risk factors for ischemic stroke that have not been included in the table, including fibrinogen, obesity, sickle cell anemia, antiphospholipid antibodies, mitral valve prolapse, patent foramen ovale, and polycythemia.

Relative Importance of Intracerebral Hemorrhage Risk Factors

Analytic epidemiologic studies of multiple risk factors for ICH are summarized in Table 9. These investigations vary considerably with regard to method-

Table 9
Selected Studies of Multiple Risk Factors for Intracerebral Hemorrhage

	Definite Risk Factors				Possible Risk Factors			
	Age	HTN	ETOH	HypoChol	Cigs	DM*	CHD	CI
Case-Control Studies								
Cincinnati, OH[46]	+	+				+	+	+
Madrid, Spain[57]		+	+	−	−			
Cohort Studies								
Hawaii†[60–62,87]	−	+	+	+	+	−	−	
Taisho, Japan[33]	−	+	+	+	−	−		
Hisayama, Japan[52]	−	+	−	−	−			
Akita, Japan[59]	−	+		+		−		
MRFIT[63]	+	+		+	+			
Oakland, CA†[55]	+	+	+		−			

+: statistically significant association found
−: no significant association found.
HTN: hypertension; DM: diabetes mellitus; CI: cerebral infarction; CHD: coronary heart disease; ETOH: ethanol; Cigs: cigarettes; HypoChol: hypocholesterolemia; MRFIT: Multiple Risk Factor Intervention Trial.
* Presence of glycosuria in Taisho and Akita studies.
† Analysis applies to hemorrhagic stroke (ICH and subarachnoid hemorrhage).

ology (case-control versus prospective cohort), means of diagnosis (clinical versus CT based), statistical analysis (univariate versus multivariate), and the population studied. Nonetheless, they provide information regarding the relative importance of various risk factors for ICH. As mentioned previously, ICH incidence increases significantly beyond age 45. The lack of a significant age effect in many of the cohort studies[33,52,59,60] is misleading, since only subjects over 40 were generally included. Hypertension was the only risk factor found to be associated with ICH in all of the studies. Alcohol consumption and hypocholesterolemia were risk factors for ICH in the majority of studies, while less convincing findings exists for smoking, diabetes, coronary artery disease, or prior ischemic stroke. Liver disease and coagulopathy are also probable risk factors, but much less prevalent.

Data from two recent case-control studies of CT diagnosed ICH included in Table 9[46,57] provide specific information regarding the magnitude of the relative risk (RR). In Cincinnati,[46] the greatest relative risk of ICH was associated with age (RR = 25 for those age 80 or more). The other significant factors were prior ischemic stroke (RR = 22), coronary artery disease (RR = 8), hypertension (RR = 4), and diabetes (RR = 3). In the study from Spain,[57] the significant factors were alcoholism (RR = 7), hypertension (RR = 5), liver disease (RR = 5), electrocardiogram abnormalities (RR = 3), and elevated hematocrit (no RR given). Because neither study used multivariate techniques, the degree to which these risk factors were independently associated with ICH could not be determined.

Future Directions

Intracerebral hemorrhage has diverse etiologies and complex pathogenesis. Although hypertension remains the dominant risk factor, emerging epidemiologic data indicate that aging, toxin exposure, and coagulation disorders contribute to the causation. Improved control of hypertension and the aging of the population are likely to result in a continued shift of the etiologic spectrum of ICH toward nonhypertensive causes. Age-related vascular degenerative processes, including but not limited to amyloid angiopathy, may play an important role in the pathogenesis of nonhypertensive ICH. Major challenges for the future include the delineation of age-dependent mechanisms that predispose to ICH, and the elucidation of possible genetic or environmental factors that explain the high frequency of ICH in specific ethnic and geographic subgroups. Improved understanding of these mechanisms may eventually lead to the discovery of currently unidentified risk factors. The successful implementation of public health measures directed at the control and elimination of these risk factors will decrease the great burden currently attributed to ICH.

References

1. Kelsey J, Thompson W, Evans AS: *Methods in Observational Epidemiology.* New York, NY: Oxford University Press, 1986.
2. Foulkes MA, Wolf PA, Price TR, et al: The Stroke Data Bank: design, methods, and baseline characteristics. *Stroke* 1988;19:547.
3. Massaro AR, Sacco RL, Mohr JP, et al: Clinical discriminators of lobar and deep hemorrhages: the Stroke Data Bank. *Neurology* 1991;41:1881.
4. Friday G, Lai SM, Alter M, et al: Stroke in the Lehigh Valley: racial/ethnic differences. *Neurology* 1989;39:1165.
5. Bogousslavsky J, Van Melle G, Regli F: The Lausanne Stroke Registry: analysis of 1000 consecutive patients with first stroke. *Stroke* 1988;19:1083.
6. Giroud M, Gras P, Chadan N, et al: Cerebral hemorrhage in a French prospective population study. *J Neurol Neurosurg Psychiatr* 1991;54:595.
7. Suzuki K, Kutsuzawa T, Takita K, et al: Clinico-epidemiologic study of stroke in Akita, Japan. *Stroke* 1987;18:402.
8. Huang CY, Chan FL, Yu YL, et al: Cerebrovascular disease in Hong Kong Chinese. *Stroke* 1990;21:230.
9. Kay R, Woo J, Kreel L, et al: Stroke subtypes among Chinese living in Hong Kong: the Shatin Stroke Registry. *Neurology* 1992;42:985.
10. Caplan LR, Neely S, Gorelick P: Cold-related intracerebral hemorrhage. *Arch Neurol* 1984;41:227.
11. Cole A, Aube M: Late-onset migraine with intracranial hemorrhage (abstract). *Neurology* 1987;37(Suppl):238.

12. Weisberg LA, Stazio A, Shamsina M, et al: Nontraumatic parenchymal brain hemorrhages. *Medicine* 1990;69:277.
13. Picard L, Levesque M, Crouzet G, et al: The moya-moya syndrome. *J Neuroradiol* 1974:1:47.
14. Barbas N, Caplan L, Baquis G: Dental chair intracerebral hemorrhage. *Neurology* 1987;37:511.
15. Hanes S, Maroom J, Janetta P: Supratentorial intracerebral hemorrhage following posterior fossa surgery. *J Neurosurg* 1978;49:881.
16. Humphreys RP, Hoffman HJ, Mustard WT: Cerebral hemorrhage following heart surgery. *J Neurosurg* 1975;43:671.
17. Broderick J, Brott T, Tomsick T, et al: Importance of hypertension in lobar hemorrhages (abstract). *Neurology* 1992;42(suppl 3):181.
18. McCormick WF, Rosenfield DB: Massive brain hemorrhage: a review of 144 cases and an examination of their causes. *Stroke* 1973;4:946.
19. National Center for Health Statistics (U.S.): *Vital Statistics of the United States, 1987, Vol. II. Mortality, part A*. Washington, DC: Public Health Service, 1990.
20. Bonita R: Epidemiology of stroke. *Lancet* 1992;339:342.
21. Owada K, Tanaka H, Ueda Y, et al: Epidemiology of cerebrovascular disease in Japan. *Osaka City Med J* 1973;19:37.
22. Li SC, Cheng XM: Epidemiology of cerebrovascular disease: a general review. *Chin J Nervous Mental Dis* 1982;8:50.
23. Hu HH, Chu FL, Wong WJ, et al: Trends in mortality from cerebrovascular disease in Taiwan. *Stroke* 1989;17:1121.
24. Frataglioni L, Massey EW, Schoenberg DG, et al: Mortality from cerebrovascular disease. International comparisons and temporal trends. *Neuroepidemiology* 1983;2:101.
25. Bonita R, Stewart A, Beaglehole R: International trends in stroke mortality: 1970–1985. *Stroke* 1990;21:989.
26. Baum HM, Goldstein M: Cerebrovascular disease type-specific mortality: 1968–1977. *Stroke* 1982;13:810.
27. Omae T: Prevention of stroke. *Am J Stroke* 1981;3:97.
28. Drury I, Whisnant JP, Garraway WM: Primary intracerebral hemorrhage: impact of CT on incidence. *Neurology* 1984;34:653.
29. Broderick JP, Phillips SJ, Whisnant JP, et al: Incidence rates of stroke in the eighties: the end of the decline in stroke? *Stroke* 1989;20:577.
30. Chyatte D, Nolte KB, Chen TL, et al: Changes in the incidence and mortality of ICH. *Stroke* 1992;23(suppl 1):2.
31. Ueda K, Hasuo Y, Kiyohara Y, et al: Intracerebral hemorrhage in a Japanese community, Hisayama: incidence, changing pattern during long term follow-up, and related factors. *Stroke* 1988;19:48.
32. Li S, Schoenberg BS, Wang C, et al: Cerebrovascular disease in the People's Republic of China: epidemiologic and clinical features. *Neurology* 1985;35:1708.
33. Tanaka H, Ueda Y, Date C, et al: Incidence of stroke in Shibata, Japan: 1976–1978. *Stroke* 1981;12:460.

34. Stensgaarg Hansen B, Marquardsen J: Incidence of stroke in Frederiksberg, Denmark. *Stroke* 1977;8:663.
35. Furlan AJ, Whisnant JP, Elveback LR: The decreasing incidence of primary intracerebral hemorrhage: a population study. *Ann Neurol* 1979;5: 367.
36. Sacco RL, Wolf PA, Bharucha NE, et al: Subarachnoid and intra-cerebral hemorrhage: natural history, prognosis, and precursive factors in the Framingham study. *Neurology* 1984;34:847.
37. Gross CR, Kase CS, Mohr JP, et al: Stroke in south Alabama: incidence and diagnostic features—a population based study. *Stroke* 1984;15:249.
38. Jentorp P, Berglund G: Stroke registry in Malmö, Sweden. *Stroke* 1992; 23:357.
39. Bamford J, Sandercock P, Dennis M, et al: A prospective study of acute cerebrovascular disease in the community: the Oxfordshire Community Stroke Project—1981–86. 2. Incidence, case fatality rates and overall outcome at one year of cerebral infarction, primary intracerebral and subarachnoid hemorrhage. *J Neurol Neurosurg Psychiatr* 1990;53:16.
40. Broderick JP, Brott T, Tomsick T, et al: The risk of subarachnoid and intracerebral hemorrhages in blacks as compared to whites. *N Engl J Med* 1992;326:733.
41. Aho K, Harmsen P, Hatano S, et al: Cerebrovascular disease in the community: results of a WHO collaborative study. *Bull WHO* 1980;58:113.
42. Shi F, Hart RG, Sherman DG, et al: Stroke in the People's Republic of China. *Stroke* 1989;20:1581.
43. Baba S, Pan WH, Ueshima H, et al: Blood pressure levels, related factors, and hypertension control status of Japanese and Americans. *J Hum Hypertens* 1991;5:317.
44. Kuller LH: Epidemiology of stroke. In: Schoenberg BS, ed: *Neurologic Epidemiology: Principles and Applications*. New York, NY: Raven Press, 1978: 281.
45. Worth RM, Kato H, Rhoads GG, et al: Epidemiologic studies of coronary heart disease and stroke in Japanese men living in Japan, Hawaii and California: mortality. *Am J Epidemiol* 1975;102:481.
46. Brott T, Thalinger K, Hertzberg V: Hypertension as a risk factor for spontaneous intracerebral hemorrhage. *Stroke* 1986;17:1078.
47. Tanaka H, Ueda Y, Hayashi M, et al: Risk factors for cerebral hemorrhage and cerebral infarction in a Japanese rural community. *Stroke* 1982;13: 62.
48. Sacco RL, Hauser WA, Mohr JP: Hospitalized stroke in blacks and hispanics in northern Manhattan. *Stroke* 1991;22:1491.
49. Caplan LR: Strokes in African-Americans. *Circulation* 1991;83:1469.
50. Schoenberg BS, Anderson DW, Harer AF: Racial differentials in the prevalence of stroke: Copiah County, Mississippi. *Arch Neurol* 1986;43:565.
51. Saunders E: Hypertension in African-Americans. *Circulation* 1991;83: 1465.
52. Omae T, Ueda K: Risk factors of cerebral stroke in Japan: prospective

epidemiologic study in Hisayama community. In: Katsuki S, Tsubaki T, Toyokura Y, eds: *Proceedings of the 12th World Congress of Neurology*. Amsterdam: Excerpta Medica, 1982:119.

53. Weisberg LA: Alcoholic intracerebral hemorrhage. *Stroke* 1988;19:1565.

54. Gorelick PB: Alcohol and stroke. *Stroke* 1987;18:268.

55. Klatsky AL, Armstrong MA, Friedman GD: Alcohol use and subsequent cerebrovascular disease hospitalizations. *Stroke* 1989;20:741.

56. Donohue RP, Abbot RD, Reed DM, et al: Alcohol and hemorrhagic stroke: the Honolulu Heart Program. *JAMA* 1986;255:2311.

57. Calandre L, Arnal C, Ortega JF, et al: Risk factors for spontaneous cerebral hematomas. Case-control study. *Stroke* 1986;17:1126.

58. Hillbom M, Kaste M: Alcohol intoxication: a risk factor for primary subarachnoid hemorrhage. *Neurology* 1982;32:706.

59. Ueshima H, Iida M, Shimamoto T, et al: Multivariate analysis of risk factor for stroke: eight-year follow-up study of farming villages in Aikita, Japan. *Prev Med* 1980;9:722.

60. Kagan A, Popper JS, Rhoads GG: Factors related to stroke incidence in Hawaii Japanese men: the Honolulu Heart Study. *Stroke* 1980;11:14.

61. Kagan A, Popper JS, Rhoads GG, et al: Dietary and other risk factors for stroke in Hawaiian Japanese men. *Stroke* 1985;16:390.

62. Yano K, Reed DM, MacLean CJ: Serum cholesterol and hemorrhagic stroke in the Honolulu Heart Program. *Stroke* 1989;20:1460.

63. Iso H, Jacobs DR, Wentworth D, et al: Serum cholesterol levels and six-year mortality from stroke in 350,977 men screened for the multiple risk factor intervention trial. *N Engl J Med* 1989;320:904.

64. Tell GS, Crouse JR, Furberg CR: Relation between blood lipids, lipoproteins, and cerebrovascular atherosclerosis: a review. *Stroke* 1988;19:423.

65. Kase CS, Robinson RK, Stein RW, et al: Anticoagulant-related intracerebral hemorrhage. *Neurology* 1985;35:943.

66. Whisnant JP, Niall EF, Cartlidge MB, et al: Carotid and vertebral-basilar transient ischemic attacks: effect of anticoagulants, hypertension and cardiac disorders on survival and stroke occurence — a population study. *Ann Neurol* 1978;3:107.

67. Wintzen AR, de Jonge H, Loeliger EA, et al: The risk of intracerebral hemorrhage during oral anticoagulant treatment: a population-based study. *Ann Neurol* 1984;16:553.

68. Franke CL, de Jonge J, van Sweiten JC, et al: Intracerebral hematomas during anticoagulant treatment. *Stroke* 1990;21:726.

69. Maggioni AP, Franzosi MG, Santoro E, et al: The risk of stroke in patients with acute myocardial infarction after thrombolytic and antithrombotic treatment. *N Engl J Med* 1992;327:1.

70. The Steering Committee of the Physician's Health Study Research Group: Preliminary report: findings from the aspirin component of the ongoing Physician's Health Study. *New Engl J Med* 1988;318:262.

71. Feldmann E. Intracerebral hemorrhage. *Stroke* 1991;22:684.

72. Boudouresques G, Hauw JJ, Meininger V, et al: Etude neuropathologique des hemorrhagies intracraniennes de l'adulte. *Rev Neurol* 1979;135:197.

73. Abu-Zeid HAH, Choi NW, Maini KK, et al: Relative role of factors associated with cerebral infarction and cerebral hemorrhage. *Stroke* 1977;8:106.

74. Wolf PA, Dawber TR, Thomas HE, et al: Epidemiology of stroke. In: Thompsen RA, Green JR, eds: *Advances in Neurology*. Volume 16. New York: Raven Press, 1977:5.

75. Shinkawa A, Ueda K, Hasuo Y, et al: Seasonal variation in stroke incidence in Hisayama, Japan. *Stroke* 1990;21:1262.

76. Ramirez-Lassepas M, Haus E, Lakatua DJ, et al: Seasonal (circannual) periodicity of spontaneous intracerebral hemorrhage in Minnesota. *Ann Neurol* 1980;8:539.

77. Haberman S, Capildeo R, Clifford Rose F: The seasonal variation in mortality from cerebrovascular disease. *J Neurol Sci* 1981;52:25.

78. Biller J, Jones MP, Bruno A, et al: Seasonal variation of stroke: does it exist? *Neuroepidemiology* 1988;7:89.

79. Capon A, Demeurisse G, Zheng L: Seasonal variation of cerebral hemorrhage in 236 cases in Brussels. *Stroke* 1992;23:24.

80. Sobel E, Zhang Z, Alter M, et al: Stroke in the Lehigh Valley: seasonal variation in incidence rates. *Stroke* 1987;18:38.

81. Giroud M, Beuriat P, Vion PH, et al: Les accidents vasculaires cerebrax dans la population Dijonnaise: incidence, repartition, mortalitie. *Rev Neurol* 1989;145:221.

82. Longstreth WT, Koepsell TD, Yerby YS, et al: Risk factors for subarachnoid hemorrhage. *Stroke* 1985;16:377.

83. Marmot MG, Poulter NR: Primary prevention of stroke. *Lancet* 1992;339:344.

84. Bonita R: Cigarette smoking, hypertension and the risk of subarachnoid hemorrhage: a population-based case-control study. *Stroke* 1986;17:831.

85. Colditz GA, Bonita R, Stampfer MJ, et al: Cigarette smoking and risk of stroke in middle-aged women. *N Engl J Med* 1988;318:937.

86. Davis PH, Hachinski V: Epidemiology of cerebrovascular disease. In: Anderson DW, ed: *Neuroepidemiology: A Tribute to Bruce Schoenberg*. Boca Raton: CRC Press, 1991:27.

87. Abbot RD, Yin Y, Reed DM, et al: Risk of stroke in male cigarette smokers. *New Engl J Med* 1986;315:717.

88. Shinton R, Beevers G: Meta-analysis of relation between cigarette smoking and stroke. *Br Med J* 1989;298:789.

89. Schoenberg BS, Schulte BPM: Cerebrovascular disease: epidemiology and geopathology. In: Vinken PJ, Bruyn GW, Klawans HL, et al., eds: *Handbook of Clinical Neurology. Vascular Diseases*. Part I, Vol. 53. Amsterdam: Elsevier, 1988:1.

Part II

Etiology of Intracerebral Hemorrhage

Chapter 2

Hypertensive Intracerebral Hemorrhage

Janet L. Wilterdink, MD

Hypertension is the most common cause of spontaneous intracerebral hemorrhage (ICH). Yet, its exact role in the pathogenesis of ICH remains difficult to define. This chapter focuses on the changing epidemiologic features of hypertensive intracerebral hemorrhage (HIH), the current understanding of cerebrovascular physiology in hypertension, pathologic features of hypertensive cerebrovascular disease, especially those that relate to HIH, and the pathogenesis of HIH. Brief discussions of the clinical features of HIH and the management of hypertension in HIH are also included.

Epidemiology

Epidemiologic data provide much of the basis for linking hypertension and ICH. However, different methods of identifying hypertension have led to inconsistencies among published studies. Early studies defined hypertension as systolic blood pressure greater than 190 mm Hg and diastolic pressure greater than 110 mm Hg,[1,2] while more recent studies use pressures of 140 to 160 mm Hg systolic and 90 to 95 mm Hg diastolic to define hypertension.[3-5] Also, certain studies used the admission blood pressure to diagnose hypertension, reporting a 70% to 80% association with ICH.[3,6,7] An elevated blood pressure at the time of hemorrhage, however, is an unreliable method of diagnosing hypertension, because many patients with ICH have a transient rise in blood pressure in response either to increased intracranial pressure (Cushing's response) or to an acute catecholamine release.[3,8,9] A premorbid diagnosis of hypertension is more specific and is found in fewer (40% to 50%) patients with ICH, but requires a previous medical evaluation.[3,5,9] Electrocardiographic or post mortem diagnosis of left ventricular hypertrophy is also found in slightly less than half of

From Feldmann E (ed). *Intracerebral Hemorrhage*. Armonk, NY: Futura Publishing Company, Inc., © 1994.

patients with ICH.[10,11] This is a relatively insensitive index of hypertension, since hypertensive cerebrovascular disease may precede other clinically measurable end organ injury.[12] A combination of these criteria, that is, a history of hypertension, left ventricular hypertrophy, or sustained elevated blood pressure after hemorrhage is probably the best available means of identifying hypertension. This approach establishes a 60% overall incidence of hypertension in ICH (56% to 62%).[3,13,14] Other sources of variability in the reported prevalence of hypertension among causes of ICH include patient selection bias and the stringency by which other etiologies are excluded.

Because the prevalence of hypertension in the general population is so high, the coexistence of hypertension and ICH in any individual does not define HIH. Approximately one third of white American males aged 18 to 74 years have hypertension, the prevalence of which steadily increases with age, from 16% in 18 to 24 year olds to 59% in 65 to 74 year olds.[15] A significant percentage of patients with ICH and hypertension have another etiology for ICH. In an autopsy study, 58 of 144 patients with massive spontaneous ICH also had hypertension. In only 21, however, was hypertension the only identified etiology. Other coexisting causes included saccular aneurysm, tumor, angioma, and bleeding diathesis. Some, but not all, hemorrhage sites were multiple or in locations considered atypical for HIH.[10] Hypertension may be a risk factor for ICH when other causes are present, but this is not well defined.

Improved treatment of hypertension is credited with the reduction in the incidence of and mortality from ICH. The incidence of ICH declined in Rochester, MN, from 15.7 per 100,000 in 1945 through 1952 to 7.3 per 100,000 in 1969 through 1976.[16] The frequency and severity of hypertension declined concomitantly. In 1950 through 1954, hypertension was almost universally present in patients with ICH, and more than half of these had a mean arterial pressure greater than 150 mm Hg. Twenty-five years later, only 48% of patients with ICH were hypertensive, and none had a mean arterial pressure greater than 130 mm Hg.[17] These trends, while less marked, are also seen in the United States as a whole.[18] In Finland, a decrease in the annual rate of ICH from 26.2 per 100,000 to 15.4 per 100,000 between 1970 and 1979 was also attributed to more aggressive treatment of hypertension.[19] A slight increase in the incidence of ICH after 1975 is believed to be an artifact of the advent of computed tomography (CT), which has increased the diagnosis of small ICH previously misclassified as infarction.[20] An apparent decline in the case fatality rate of ICH may also be explained by improved diagnosis of smaller ICHs which have a better prognosis. Thus, one study reported a mortality decrease from 22% in 1968 to 13% in 1977, but this may not reflect an actual improvement in the outcome of ICH.[17,21]

Certain epidemiologic features specific to HIH are noteworthy. Patients with HIH are approximately 10 years younger than stroke patients overall, with a mean age in the late 50s to early 60s. While the overall age range is 21 to 87 years, the majority of HIH occur in the sixth and seventh decades.[13,22] There is no striking male or female predominance.[6,23,24] The incidence of HIH is significantly higher in the black than white population.[3,4,25] In one study, for example, the incidence of ICH in black males was 36.6 per 100,000 versus 16.7 per 100,000 in white males.[4] Black patients with HIH are younger than white patients.[22] This reflects the epidemiology of hypertension in the black population, where it is more prevalent and occurs at a younger age.[15,22,23,25]

Pathophysiology

Our current understanding of the pathophysiology of HIH comes from human studies and animal models, particularly a genetic strain of spontaneously hypertensive rats (SHR) and a variant which are stroke prone (SHRSP). These studies have advanced our understanding of cerebrovascular physiology in normotensive and hypertensive individuals and, with extensive micropathologic data, have provided some insight into the pathogenesis of HIH.

Hypertension and Cerebrovascular Physiology

The regulation of cerebral blood flow is complex, involving several different mechanisms. Locally produced metabolites such as hydrogen and potassium ions and adenosine adjust local cerebral blood flow to match the local metabolic need. Neurotransmitters (acetylcholine, histamine, and norepinephrine), circulating substances (pCO_2, pO_2, hormones, hemoglobin concentration, and platelet products), and hemodynamic parameters also influence blood flow. Some of these have a direct action on vascular smooth muscle, others act indirectly through the release of endothelium-derived constricting and relaxing factors.[26-28]

In normal individuals, cerebral blood flow remains constant over a range of mean arterial pressures between 60 and 150 mm Hg. This autoregulation is achieved by vasoconstriction or vasodilation of cerebral resistance vessels, predominantly small cerebral arteries and arterioles, and, to a lesser extent, larger cerebral vessels. Vasoconstriction and vasodilation occur largely as a direct myogenic response of medial smooth muscle to intraluminal pressure. Metabolic mediators may also play a role. The autoregulatory response is not fixed but is modulated by pCO_2 and by the sympathetic nervous and renin-angiotensin systems.[26,29] Hypercapnia and hypocapnia shorten and widen the range of autoregulation, respectively. α Adrenergic activation extends the upward arterial pressure limit of autoregulation. Angiotensin converting enzyme inhibition shifts the autoregulatory curve downward to lower blood pressures (Figure 1).[26]

In hypertensive individuals, the autoregulatory curve is shifted to higher arterial pressures by physiologic and structural adaptations of the vessel wall. Tonic α adrenergic sympathetic and renin-angiotensin stimulation produce an increase in vascular motor tone, extending the upward limit of the autoregula-

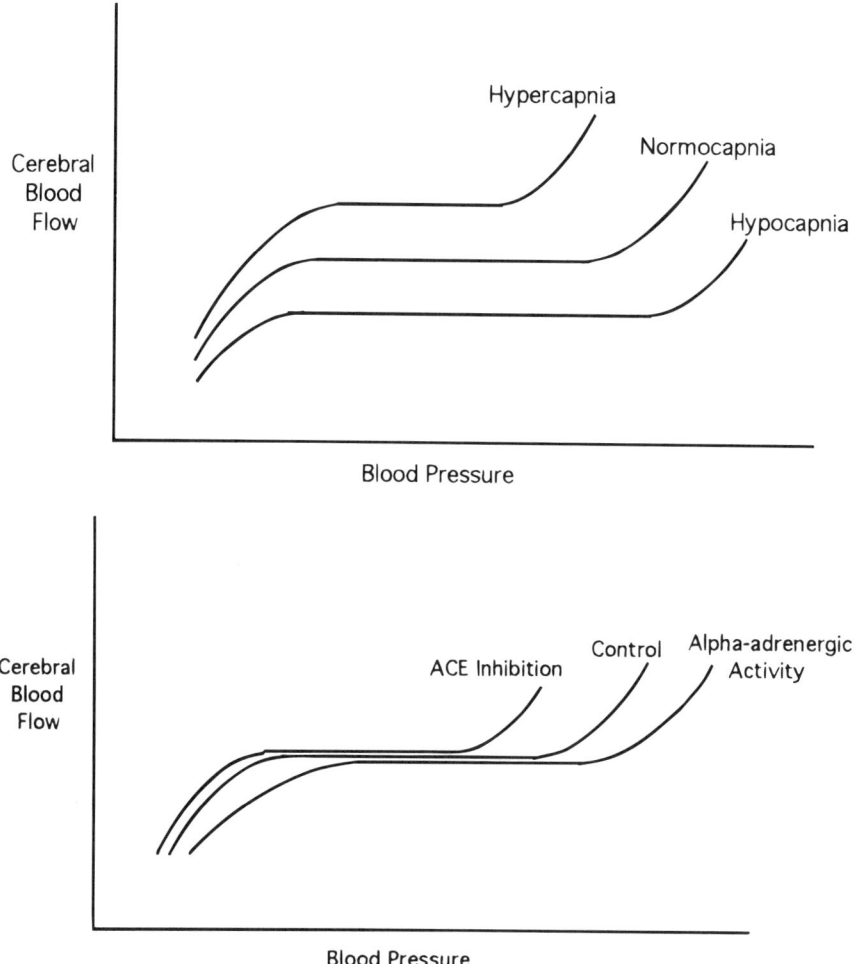

Figure 1: Schematic diagrams showing autoregulation of cerebral blood flow under normal conditions and during hyper- and hypocapnia (top), and in response to ACE (angiotensin converting enzyme) inhibition, and alpha adrenergic stimulation (bottom). Adapted, with permission from Strandgaard S, Paulson OB, Hypertensive disease and the cerebral circulation. In Laragh JH, Brenner BM eds: *Hypertension: Pathophysiology, Diagnosis and Management*. New York: Raven Press; 1990:399.

tion. When this is prolonged, medial smooth muscle hypertrophies, narrowing the vessel lumen, increasing vascular resistance, and contributing to the upward shift of the autoregulatory curve.[26,30,31]

These changes have some advantages. Increased wall thickness and decreased lumen diameter reduce arterial wall tension, allowing it to withstand higher pressures. The increase in vascular resistance in arteries upstream increases the vasoconstricting power of the smaller resistance vessels and also protects them from the deleterious effects of hypertension.[26,32] This benefit has been shown in SHR, in which sympathetic denervation by superior cervical sympathetic ganglionectomy attenuates the structural changes, limits the upward shift in the autoregulatory curve, and increases the incidence of hemorrhagic stroke.[32]

These adaptations have negative consequences as well. Structurally narrowed arteries have an impaired capacity to vasodilate, thus raising the lower as well as the upper limit of autoregulation. As a consequence, cerebral blood flow in hypertensive individuals is more sensitive to small decreases in systolic pressure. Studies suggest that hypertensive humans as well as SHR are more susceptible to cerebral ischemia during systemic hypotension.[31,33] Impaired vasodilation is seen in response to hypercapnia and other metabolic and humoral factors, as well as to decreased arterial pressure.[34] Endothelium dependent mechanisms appear to be particularly affected.[27] Other negative consequences of hypertension may include decreased responsiveness of cerebral blood flow to local metabolic stimuli and impaired collateral formation.[32]

Recently, it has been shown that impaired vasodilation may be specific to larger resistance vessels, and that small arterioles (less than 20 μm) develop an increase in distensibility during chronic hypertension. Some authors speculate that while this may serve to preserve cerebral blood flow somewhat during hypotension, it may decrease the tensile strength of arteriolar walls, making them more susceptible to rupture during acute severe increases in systolic arterial pressures.[32]

Physiologic changes in chronic hypertension may be partially reversible. With antihypertensive therapy in SHR, vascular tone and medial muscular hypertrophy decrease, and the autoregulatory curve readapts toward normal. However, in humans, especially those who are elderly or who have long-standing hypertension, readaptation is less likely because permanent structural changes such as muscular hyperplasia and degenerative change have taken place.[26]

Micropathology of Hypertensive Cerebrovascular Disease

Histopathologic changes in the cerebral microvasculature of hypertensive individuals have been extensively described over the past 50 years. The large number of descriptive terms, including lipohyalinosis, segmental fibrinoid degeneration, angionecrosis, plasmatic arterionecrosis, moth eaten change, and more represent a spectrum of histopathologic changes resulting from acute or chronic hypertension. These changes are seen in small cerebral arteries and arterioles, are more severe in the small penetrating vessels in the deep white matter than in cortical vessels of similar size, are more severe distally than proximally, and are most prominent at sites of arterial branching. They are believed to represent a progressive replacement of smooth muscle cells by collagen (hyalinization), altered permeability of the vessel wall to circulating proteins leading to an accumulation of proteinaceous material (fibrinoid change),

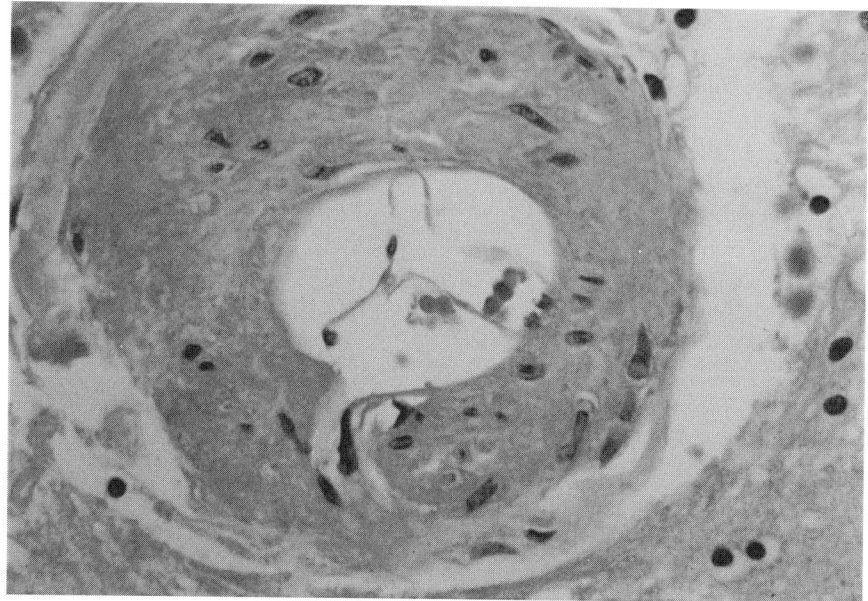

Figure 2: A penetrating artery in a hypertensive patient. The vascular wall is thickened. Much of the media is replaced by hyaline and proteinaceous deposit. (H&E, provided by MW Ambler, MD)

and subintimal fat deposition (Figure 2). This process may alternately lead to lumenal occlusion or to structural weakening, with or without dilatation and microaneurysm formation.[29]

Of all the described pathologic changes occurring in hypertension, microaneurysms have historically received the greatest attention and controversy, especially regarding the pathogenesis of HIH. The first description of microaneurysms by Charcot and Bouchard in 1868[35] lacked microscopic technical detail, leading later authors to believe that Charcot and Bouchard were describing pseudoaneurysms. The latter, also called bleeding globes, were described by Cole and Yates[36] and Fisher,[37] who found them at margins of ICH of all types. These are actually small blood clots loosely attached to the arterial wall at sites of microrupture and bleeding. Recently, electron microscopy has also demonstrated small cavities that are attached to blood vessels and are formed by the resorption of small hemorrhages.[38]

True microaneurysms have also been described by many authors, and likely by Charcot and Bouchard as well. These may be saccular or fusiform. Saccular microaneurysms arise often, but not exclusively, at the sites of arterial bifurcations (Figure 3). They are between 300 to 2,000 μm in diameter and arise from parent vessels between 40 to 300 μm in diameter. Electron microscopy demonstrates that medial smooth muscle and the internal elastic lamina taper on entering the sac, eventually disappearing in the aneurysmal sac wall, which lacks muscle or elastic tissue as well as a definite endothelial lining. The outer

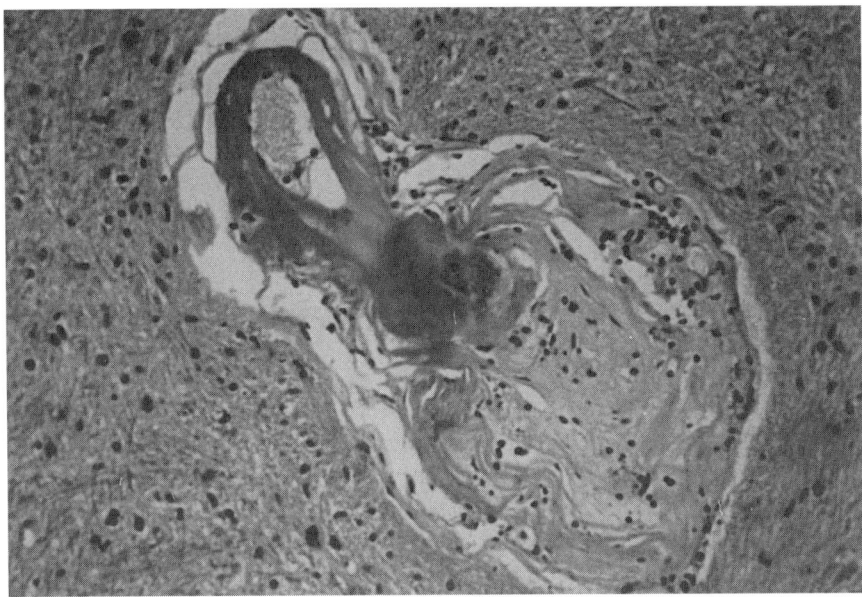

Figure 3: A saccular microaneurysm arising from a small penetrating artery showing typical hypertensive vascular changes. (H&E, provided by MW Ambler, MD)

collagenous layer is continuous with the adventitia of the parent vessel. The fibrin lined aneurysm may contain organized mural thrombi. The parent artery may or may not have other pathologic evidence of hypertensive degeneration.[1,2,37–40] Based on this distinction, Fisher identified two subtypes, saccular microaneurysms and lipohyalinotic aneurysms.[37] Fusiform aneurysms are often asymmetric, arising from vessels 80 to 300 mm in diameter. At the site of fusiform enlargement, the elastica and media are lost, the vessel wall containing fibrin and fat-filled macrophages is less compact, and the lumen is often occluded. Extravasated red blood cells, hemosiderin-filled macrophages, and astroglial proliferation representing microperivascular hemorrhage frequently surround all types of microaneurysms.[1,2,37–39]

The association of microaneurysms with hypertension was recognized early. In a pathologic examination of 54 brains, Russell found saccular microaneurysms in 15 of 16 hypertensive individuals and in only 10 of 38 normotensives.[2] These findings were confirmed by Cole and Yates in a larger series in which microaneurysms were found in 46% of 100 hypertensive patients and in 7% of 100 age and sex matched controls.[1] Later authors believed that these data underestimated the association with hypertension, because their definition of hypertension included a diastolic blood pressure of greater than 110 mm Hg and cardiac hypertrophy, which would reclassify some individuals as hypertensive rather than normotensive.[41] Both studies found that microaneurysms occur in multiples and in a distinctive anatomic distribution. Most were found in the putamen, pallidum, and thalamus, with a smaller number in the internal capsule and centrum semiovale and the cortical gray matter. More recently, electron microscopy of 98 brains revealed microaneurysms in 3 of 20 normotensives, in 25 of 53 asymptomatic hypertensives, and in 38 of 38 patients with HIH.[40]

More recent evidence suggests that other hypertensive vascular pathologic changes may be important in producing HIH. For example, quantification of medial smooth muscle mass by electron microscopic ultrastructural morphometry in cerebral vessels was used to compare nonhypertensive controls with hypertensive patients with or without HIH. Hypertensive patients had substantial reduction in the percentage of smooth muscle per whole media area. Loss of smooth muscle was most marked in the distal lenticulostriate artery, but was also seen in the proximal lenticulostriate artery, and, to a lesser extent, in the cortical circumflex artery.[42] A similar loss of smooth muscle was quantified by other authors who counted smooth muscle nuclei.[40] The authors postulated that decreased medial muscle mass represented structural weakening of vessels that rupture and bleed.

In addition to quantification of smooth muscle degeneration, electron microscopy has also clarified the spectrum of hypertensive vascular wall degeneration. In hypertensive patients, focal cytoplasmic necrosis of smooth muscle cells appears first in the outer layers of the media in mildly affected arteries. In more diseased arteries, the outer, then the inner muscle layer, and, ultimately, the intima become necrotic. Severely injured arterial walls contain an accumulation of plasma contents and granular and vesicular debris. Fragmentation of the elastic lamina, intimal thickening, and irregular atrophy of the smooth muscle cells give the vessel wall a characteristic moth-eaten appearance. In the most severely affected arteries, insudation of plasma contents into the vessel wall presumably results from increased permeability of the endothelium, in which intracellular junctions are disrupted, and enlarged pinocytotic vesicles containing plasma proteins and lipoproteins are seen.[38,40,43] An electron microscopic study of SHRSP demonstrated that this spectrum of cerebrovascular pathologic change follows a temporal sequence. The less severe pathologic changes are seen first at 16 weeks and progress through the stages described to severely damaged arterial walls at 28 weeks of life. The authors noted, additionally, the presence of monocytes adhering to the endothelium and in the subintimal space of highly damaged vessels.[44]

A variety of schema have been proposed to explain the mechanism by which hypertension produces the histopathologic changes described. Some theories, such as microdissection of the vessel wall, have no histopathologic corroboration. Another theory proposes that the changes are due to vessel ischemia. Because small vessels lack vasa vasora, they rely on intraluminal blood flow for energy.[40,44] When small blood vessels develop medial smooth muscle hypertrophy in response to chronic hypertension, regional blood flow is diminished, and blood borne oxygen and nutrients must diffuse across a greater wall thickness. At the same time, the hypertrophied muscle has an increased metabolic requirement.[45] In this setting, a disparity between metabolic supply and demand may lead to ischemia and necrosis of smooth muscle cells. This theory seems compatible with the finding of focal cytoplasmic necrosis in smooth muscle cells appearing first in the outermost part of the media where nutrient and oxygen concentration are likely in least supply.[44] Other authors propose that vascular wall degeneration is brought about by increased endothelial permeability. Plasma contents then leak into the vessel wall, and monocytes and platelets adhere to the disrupted endothelium and release hydrolytic enzymes such as elastase and collagenase which destroy smooth muscle cells.[40,43,44] The cause of this increased endothelial permeability is unclear. It may be secondary to mechanical disruption during acute blood pressure elevations.[43] Lysosomal enzymes produced during smooth muscle cell injury may play a role.[40] Alternatively, Yamori et al propose that biomembrane abnormalities and altered permeability are intrinsic to hypertensive individuals.[46]

The roles of age and acute versus chronic hypertension in producing hypertensive vascular change and HIH are debated. Some suggest that hyalinization results from chronically elevated blood pressure, while muscle degeneration and fibrinoid change may occur after acute increases in blood pressure.[37] An autopsy study in pregnancy-induced hypertension reported typical fibrinoid necrosis in small cerebral arteries in three of seven patients. These patients were young, and did not have pre-existent hypertension.[47] Other studies report that microaneurysms and hyalinization are seen in both young and old hypertensive patients, but also less commonly in normotensive individuals who are elderly.[1,2,40] It is likely that the duration and severity of hypertension and the patient's age each contribute to pathologic vascular abnormalities.[1,2,16,40,42]

Despite careful pathologic studies, there is no consensus regarding which specific pathologic entity is responsible for producing HIH. The actual bleeding site, let alone its underlying vascular structural pathology, is difficult to accurately identify due to the destruction produced by the hemorrhage. Although Cole and Yates found microaneurysms in 18 of 21 patients with massive HIH and in 13 of 13 patients with small HIH, they could not be identified as the source of hemorrhage.[1] Electron microscopy in 27 surgical and autopsy cases of HIH identified 61 sites of arterial rupture. Only two of these occurred at microaneurysms. The remainder occurred at or near arterial bifurcations in parent arteries, which, at the site of rupture, showed typical hypertensive pathologic changes.[38] While Russell believed that if a microaneurysm ruptured early in its development it produced HIH, or otherwise went on to occlude and produce infarction,[2] other authors believe that microaneurysms are the source of limited, subclinical bleeding or extravasation only, and that other underlying vascular changes are sufficient to weaken the vessel wall and produce HIH.[37-39]

The observation of multiple sites of small artery or arteriolar rupture in HIH have been interpreted differently by different investigators. It is not always possible to distinguish between primary and secondary sites of rupture. An early theory proposed that angionecrosis produced vascular disease in multiple sites, which simultaneously ruptured and produced a large hemorrhage.[37,38,48] This seems unlikely since HIH is rarely, if ever, multifocal.[49] Some believe that rupture of a single artery causes an expanding hematoma which exerts traction on other small arteries, causing them to rupture in an avalanche fashion, contributing to the growth of the hematoma.[38,39] Others, however, believe that this secondary rupture is unlikely to be significant.[36,47] In experimentally simulated ICH, intracerebral injections of blood or other substances produce only small amounts of secondary bleeding at the periphery of the "clot."[50] Moreover, when angiographic studies in patients with HIH demonstrate a bleeding site (dye extravasation), it appears to originate from a single source.[48]

Gross Pathologic Features and Pathogenesis of HIH

The anatomic distribution of HIH (Table 1)[6] correlates with the sites of the most severe microvascular pathologic changes seen in hypertensive cerebrovascular disease — the small penetrating arteries supplying the centrencephalon, the basal ganglia, thalamus, cerebellum, and pons. Possible explanations for this distribution of vascular pathology include the lack of collateralization of these vessels with other end arteries such as in the leptomeningeal circulation,[45,51] and that these vessels, arising directly from the main arterial trunks, are subject to greater arterial pressure.[2,29] Also, anatomic variability in the neural innervation of cerebral blood vessels may be the cause of their divergent response to hypertension.[28,52] While the small vessels of the cerebral cortex are less affected in hypertension than those of the deep white and gray matter, they are not immune. Therefore, while the cerebral cortex is considered to be an infrequent site of HIH, many believe that hypertension does cause a significant number, about 30%, of the hemorrhages that occur there.[5,14,53]

It is not clear whether a precipitant such as acute hypertension is required to produce HIH in a susceptible individual. Some evidence suggests that an acute rise in blood pressure precedes some, if not all, HIH. In SHRSP, but not normal rats, a small injection of norepinephrine produced an increase in blood pressure and HIH.[46] In an editorial, Caplan reviewed cases of ICH in unusual settings, such as sympathomimetic use, cold exposure, and acute dental or other pain, and proposed that an acute rise in blood pressure and cerebral blood flow was a common and likely etiologic denominator.[54] Other anecdotes report ICH in the setting of acute stress, such as running from a burning building or narrowly missing a motor vehicle accident, but these are exceptional.[22,24] In a series of 393 patients, 10 occurred during some form of emotional excitement,

Table 1
Anatomic Distribution of Hypertensive Intracerebral Hemorrhage[6]

Putamen	53%
Thalamus	13%
Pons	5%
Cerebellum	10%
Other	19%

and only 14.5% occurred during sleep when blood pressure is relatively low.[25] Similarly, other authors have found a circadian rhythmicity of ICH onset that correlated with diurnal variation in blood pressure.[55]

In contrast to other etiologies of ICH, HIH is usually a brief monophasic event lasting 1 to 2 hours, with subsequent clinical deterioration associated with edema formation, rather than extension of hemorrhage.[6,56] Eleven patients injected with chromium CR-51-labeled erythrocytes within 4 hours of hemorrhage onset did not subsequently show significant radioactivity within the hemorrhage, while the opposite was true for hemorrhages due to arteriovenous malformation or aneurysm.[57]

Continued or recurrent bleeding from the hemorrhage site does occur in some situations. Serial angiography in seven patients with hypertensive putamenal hemorrhages performed between 30 minutes to 7 hours after hemorrhage onset showed progressive extravasation of dye from the peripheral lateral lenticulostriate artery in all cases.[48] Another study showed continued bleeding in 5 of 12 patients in the first 5 hours.[58] Finally, three studies report a total of 18 patients with HIH and evidence of progression by serial CT examination. In 15 of these patients, the blood pressure was persistently elevated, with a systolic blood pressure greater than 195 mm Hg. Intraventricular extension was also a risk factor for progressive bleeding on CT. It was postulated that intraventricular rupture decompresses the hematoma, lowering local tissue pressure and decreasing its tamponade effect on the bleeding vessel, promoting further bleeding.[8,59,60]

When hemorrhage occurs it spreads along a path of least resistance, primarily following the fiber tracts of the white matter. Gray matter, with its dense neuropil, is more resistant to the shearing forces of the growing hematoma and is more likely than white matter to be compressed rather than infiltrated by the spreading hematoma.[45,61,62] Intraventricular extension is not infrequent when subjacent structures are involved. Cytotoxic and vasogenic edema develops in the parenchyma surrounding the hematoma, generally reaching a maximum in 3 to 5 days. Resorption of blood by macrophages at the periphery of the hemorrhage takes place over weeks to months leaving a cavity lined by hemosiderin-laden macrophages and surrounded by an area of necrotic tissue.[61,62]

While there may be many mechanisms by which HIH produces tissue injury and destruction, perihemorrhage ischemic injury appears to be important. The local microcirculation is interrupted by the mass effect produced by the sudden introduction of the clot volume into a closed intracranial space. The development of edema may exacerbate this and the resulting ischemia.[50,62–64] Stereotactic injections of blood or inert material in animal models of ICH are accompanied by decreases in regional cerebral blood flow in the immediate clot penumbra within minutes after clot formation.[50,62,64,65] Pathologic studies demonstrate an area of ischemic necrosis around the hemorrhage, the severity and extent of which depends on the size of the hemorrhage.[50,66] Injection of blood affects regional cerebral blood flow differently than injection of inert material, suggesting that chemical as well as mechanical effects of the clot may be important.[65,67] Pretreatment with the calcium channel blocker nimodipine partially limits secondary perilesional ischemia in experimental models of ICH.[66]

Clinical Features of HIH

The clinical course of HIH reflects the pathologic features described above. Neurologic symptoms usually have a smooth onset, over 1 to 2 hours, reflecting the expansion of the hematoma. However, the onset may be stroke-like with maximal severity at onset in about one-third of patients.[56] Subsequent worsening over the following 3 to 5 days occurs with the development of edema. Stabilization and slow recovery of neurologic deficits occur over the next days to months, paralleling the resorption of the hematoma.[56,68]

The variety of sites and syndromes of HIH have been better appreciated in the CT era.

Putamen

The putamen is the most frequent site of HIH (50% to 80%), commonly arising posterolaterally and enlarging in an ovoid fashion, displacing the insula laterally and the internal capsule and thalamus medially. When very large, these extend into the lateral and medial structures and, about 30% of the time, into the ventricles.[5,23,45,61] All patients have a contralateral motor-sensory deficit of varying severity. Other signs are less universal, their presence depending on the extent of the hemorrhage. A large percentage have cortical signs appropriate to side. Neurophthamologic signs, such as pupillary abnormalities, visual field deficit, eye deviation, or other oculomotor deficit are seen in more than half of patients. Nonspecific symptoms such as headache occur in 30% to 65% and vomiting in about 40% of patients.[6,23,56]

Thalamus

Thalamic hemorrhages have been better distinguished from basal ganglia hemorrhages in the CT era. They may extend laterally into the posterior limb of the internal capsule, medially into the third ventricle, and caudally into the rostral mesencephalon.[61] Intraventricular extension is more common than in putamenal hemorrhages, occurring in 50% to 70% of patients.[69,70] Profound primary modality sensory loss is universal and is usually accompanied by some degree of motor deficit secondary to internal capsular involvement. Oculomotor signs are quite frequent secondary to tegmental spread or compression, and cortical signs may also be seen. Less specific signs such as headache, nausea and vomiting, and alteration of consciousness are seen in approximately equal frequency as in putamenal hemorrhage.[6,56,69–71]

Cerebellum

Cerebellar hemorrhages usually arise in the dentate nucleus, extend laterally into the white matter, and often rupture into the fourth ventricle.[24,61,72] Ventromedial extension into the pontine tegmentum occurs in a smaller percentage of patients (24% to 30%). Nausea, vomiting, and ataxia occur in more than 95%. More than half complain of dizziness, and almost three fourths of headache. Immediate alteration of consciousness is not common but often follows, sometimes precipitously. This is an ominous sign, reflecting compression of the fourth ventricle and acute obstructive hydrocephalus or compression of the pontine reticular activating formation. Cerebellar signs and symptoms, axial ataxia, nystagmus, vertigo, and dysarthria are prominent. Limb ataxia occurs with involvement of the cerebellar hemisphere or pontine tracts. Other brainstem signs, such as facial paresis or extraocular muscle paresis occur with brainstem involvement.[6,24,73–76]

Pons

Brainstem hemorrhages commonly arise in the midline of the basis pontis, dissecting symmetrically laterally and rostrally, often into the tegmentum, but usually not caudally, producing the classic tetrad of coma, quadriparesis, small unreactive pupils, and absent horizontal eye movements.[6,24,61,77] They may rupture into the fourth ventricle. A syndrome of restricted lateral pontine tegmentum hemorrhage has been recently described. These arise from the lateral portion of the pons and mesencephalic tegmentum and produce extraocular movement deficits, contralateral sensory and motor symptoms, and ipsilateral cerebellar signs.[78]

Caudate

Caudate hemorrhages arise in the head of the caudate and rupture into the ventricles early. Thus, a subarachnoid hemorrhage-like presentation may occur with headache and vomiting, meningismus, and transient or prolonged loss of consciousness. About half have lateralizing motor-sensory signs or symptoms that indicate internal capsule involvement.[79–81]

Internal Capsule

Recently, small internal capsular hemorrhages have been described, arising in the posterior limb or genu. These produce fairly typical lacunar syndromes. Pure motor stroke, pure sensory stroke, sensorimotor stroke and ataxic-hemiparesis secondary to HIH in the internal capsule have all been described.[82–85]

Lobar

Lobar hematomas secondary to HIH are round or oval and are centered in the immediate subcortical white matter.[61] The clinical spectrum of neurologic deficits is large and site specific. Headache and vomiting occur commonly, as in other sites. Seizures are more common in lobar than deep hemorrhages.[53,86,87] One study attempted to separate the clinical syndromes of lobar HIH versus lobar ICH of other etiologies and found that lobar HIH were larger and more often associated with intraventricular extension, altered consciousness, and seizures.[86]

Diagnosis

The advent of CT has changed our understanding of ICH, better defining its epidemiology and spectrum of clinical symptomatology. It remains the most sensitive test for the diagnosis of acute ICH, but less reliably determines its etiology.

There are few guidelines for the diagnostic evaluation of patients with presumed HIH, but there are data that argue against making this diagnosis presumptively. Because the prevalence of hypertension is high, its presence in any given patient with ICH may be incidental or contributory, rather than causal. Various studies estimate that hypertension is the etiology in roughly 50% to 80% of putamenal,[3,5,13,14] 80% to 100% of thalamic,[5,13] 50% to 70% of caudate,[79–81] 90% to 100% of capsular,[83] 60% to 75% of cerebellar,[3,5,73,74,76] 55% to 70% of pontine,[3,5,13,77] and 20% to 40% of lobar[3,5,13,51,86–88] hemorrhages. Therefore, a significant number of patients with hypertension and typically located hypertensive hemorrhage will have another etiology when other diagnoses are pursued.[10,88]

Therefore, it is appropriate for all patients with presumed HIH to be screened for other causes such as bleeding diathesis or structural etiology with a complete blood count, platelet count and coagulation times, and an imaging study (CT or magnetic resonance imaging [MRI]) 4 to 6 weeks after hemorrhage onset. Patients with atypical features for HIH should be evaluated aggressively for other causes. Atypical features may include location (including lobar), a poorly documented history of hypertension, or multifocal hemorrhage.[68]

Treatment

The management of patients with ICH is largely supportive. However, there are many controversial treatment issues, such as the management of intracranial hypertension, the use of steroids and prophylactic anticonvulsants, and the indications for surgical intervention. While these issues are discussed elsewhere in this volume, the management of hypertension is this setting will be discussed.

Treatment of elevated blood pressure in the setting of ICH is a complex and unresolved issue. The potential deleterious effect of elevated blood pressure in this setting is controversial. Some authors state there is no conclusive evidence that high blood pressure contributes to continued bleeding,[89] but some studies show hematoma progression occurring primarily in the setting of persistently elevated blood pressure.[8,59,60] Elevated blood pressure is also believed to exacerbate the vasogenic edema associated with acute ICH.[51,89]

On the other hand, treatment of elevated blood pressure in this setting has potential hazards that may worsen outcome. Abrupt lowering of blood pressure in chronic hypertensives in whom the lower limit of autoregulation is elevated may cause diffuse cerebral hypoperfusion and watershed infarction.[51,90] Autoregulation is particularly disrupted in areas of acute brain injury. Cerebral blood flow in these regions passively follows changes in systolic blood pressure.[26] Therefore, when systolic arterial pressure is lowered, arteries in the normal but not the injured brain parenchyma respond by vasodilation, thereby "stealing" blood away from the already vulnerable area. Finally, when intracranial pressure is elevated, maintenance of cerebral blood flow requires a concomitant increase in cerebral perfusion pressure, that is, a higher systemic arterial pressure. In this setting, vasodilating agents may both exacerbate increased intracranial pressure and diminish cerebral perfusion pressure, worsening cerebral ischemia.[26,51,91]

Based on these considerations, some guidelines can be provided. Most authors recommend that only very high, sustained blood pressures should be treated, such as systolic blood pressures greater than 195 mm Hg or diastolic pressures greater than 130 mm Hg. Blood pressure should be corrected gradually. An acute decrement of 25% in mean arterial pressures is considered to be safe. Precipitous drops in blood pressure should be avoided and quickly reversed. Vasodilators such as dihydralazine and sodium nitroprusside should be avoided, particularly when increased intracranial pressure is suspected. In theory, better choices include short-acting α adrenergic blockers (chlorpromazine or labetalol) or angiotensin converting enzyme inhibitors, both of which may shift the autoregulatory curve and, therefore, have a less deleterious effect on cerebral blood flow.[26]

Chronic treatment of hypertension in patients who have had HIH is strongly recommended. Untreated hypertension probably increases the risk of HIH recurrence as well as the risk of ischemic stroke. Animal studies suggest that some regression of structural vascular hypertensive changes and re-adaptation of the autoregulatory curve toward normal occurs over several months. In humans, this is less well documented and may take longer. The choice of drug to use is less clear. In elderly patients and in chronically hypertensive individuals, it is recommended that blood pressure lowering be gradual and that the target blood pressure be somewhat higher than "normal."[26,49]

Prognosis

The most important predictor for mortality is hemorrhage size.[6,23] While overall mortality for ICH is approximately 40%,[13,14,25,92] the subset of patients with hematomas greater than 5 cm in diameter on CT or with an estimated volume greater than 1,000 mm^3 have a mortality greater than 60%.[14,25] The age of the patient also impacts negatively,[13,14] but other factors associated with high mortality may simply reflect hemorrhage size. For example, patients who are comatose on admission or who have a wider spectrum of neurologic deficits have a very high mortality, while those who are alert with isolated neurologic signs fare better.[14,56] Clinical or radiographic evidence of continued bleeding is a poor prognostic sign.[45] Intraventricular hemorrhage also has a higher mortality rate, increasing the mortality for deep hemorrhages from 20% to 40% to 60% to 70%.[7,23,25] The higher mortality with intraventricular extension may reflect its association with a larger hematoma size and risk of continued bleeding. While some authors found that neither a history of hypertension nor admission blood pressure affected prognosis,[14,23] Weisberg found a worse prognosis for lobar hemorrhages associated with hypertension compared with those in nor-motensive individuals.[86]

Outcome is somewhat different for hemorrhages in the posterior fossa, where location rather than size is critical. Classic midline pontine hemorrhages causing coma and quadriplegia are small, but nearly universally fatal.[22,24] Re-stricted lateral tegmental pontine hemorrhages have a much better prognosis.[78] Cerebellar hemorrhages are reported to have a 50% to 64% mortality overall. If the patient develops stupor, coma, or brainstem signs, mortality approaches 100%.[24,72]

While the overall mortality from ICH is quite high, functional recovery among survivors is good, with approximately 75% having a good to excellent neurologic outcome.[14,25] Predicting functional recovery, however, is difficult. In basal ganglia and thalamic hemorrhages, direct corticospinal tract involvement correlates with motor disability,[93] but this may be difficult to predict on initial clinical and radiologic evaluation. The size of the hematoma and severity of initial neurologic deficits are likely to correlate with functional recovery.[6]

Recurrence of HIH is quite rare and is usually associated with untreated hypertension. In one study, only 2 of 82 patients with hypertensive cerebellar or pontine hemorrhage had a previous hypertensive hemorrhage.[24] Similarly, in a series of 518 patients with HIH, 14 were recurrent, all in a different site from the first, with a mean interval of about 13 months. These patients had not received regular antihypertensive treatment after the initial hemorrhage.[94] The rarity of recurrent HIH in prospectively followed patients may reflect aggressive treatment of their hypertension.[14,25]

References

1. Cole FM, Yates P: Intracerebral microaneurysms and small cerebrovascular lesions. *Brain* 1967;90:759.

2. Russell RWR: Observations on intracerebral aneurysms. *Brain* 1963;86:425.

3. Brott T, Thalinger K, Hertzberg V: Hypertension as a risk factor for spontaneous intracerebral hemorrhage. *Stroke* 1986;17:1078.

4. Gross CR, Kase CS, Mohr JP, et al: Stroke in South Alabama: incidence and diagnostic features — a population based study. *Stroke* 1984;15:249.

5. Bogousslavsky J, Van Melle G, Regli F: The Lausanne stroke registry: analysis of 100 consecutive patients with first stroke. *Stroke* 1988;19:1083.

6. Ojemann RG, Mohr JP: Hypertensive brain hemorrhage. *Clin Neurosurg* 1975;23:220.

7. Weisberg LA: Computerized tomography in intracranial hemorrhage. *Arch Neurol* 1979;36:422.

8. Chen ST, Chen SD, Hsu CY, et al: Progression of hypertensive intracerebral hemorrhagé. *Neurology* 1989;39:1509.

9. Calandre L, Arnal C, Fernandez Ortega J, et al: Risk factors for spontaneous cerebral hematomas. Case-control study. *Stroke* 1986;17:1126.

10. McCoemick WF, Rosenfield DB: Massive brain hemorrhage: a review of 144 cases and an examination of their causes. *Stroke* 1973;4:946.

11. Bahemuka M: Primary intracerebral hemorrhage and heart weight: a clinicopathologic case-control review of 281 patients. *Stroke* 1987;18:5311.

12. Okazaki H, Whisnant JP: Clinical pathology of hypertensive intracerebral hemorrhage. In: Mizukami M, Kogure K, Kanaya H, et al., eds: *Hypertensive Intracerebral Hemorrhage*. New York: Raven Press, 1983:177.

13. Schutz J, Bodeker RH, Damian M, et al: Age-related spontaneous intracerebral hematoma in a German community. *Stroke* 1990;21:1412.

14. Fieshi C, Carolei A, Fiorelli M, et al: Changing prognosis of primary intracerebral hemorrhage: results of a clinical and computed tomographic follow-up study of 104 patients. *Stroke* 1988;19:192.

15. Lew EA: Hypertension and longevity. In: Laragh JH, Brenner BM, eds: *Hypertension: Pathophysiology, Diagnosis and Management*. New York: Raven Press, 1990:175.

16. Furlan AJ, Whisnant JP, Elveback LR: The decreasing incidence of primary intracerebral hemorrhage: a population study. *Ann Neurol* 1979;5:367.

17. Drury I, Whisnant JP, Garraway WM: Primary intracerebral hemorrhage: impact of CT on incidence. *Neurology* 1984;34:653.

18. Anderson GL, Whisnant JP: A comparison of trends in mortality from stroke in the United States and Rochester, Minnesota. *Stroke* 1982;13:804.

19. Kotila M: Declining incidence and mortality of stroke? *Stroke* 1984;15:255.

20. Broderick JP, Phillips SJ, Whisnant JP, et al: Incidence rates of stroke in the eighties: the end of the decline in stroke? *Stroke* 1989;20:577.

21. Baum HM, Goldstein M: Cerebrovascular disease type specific mortality: 1968–1977. *Stroke* 1982;13:810.

22. Freytag E: Fatal hypertensive intracerebral haematomas: a survey of the pathological anatomy of 393 cases. *JNNP* 1968;31:616.

23. Hier DB, Davis KR, Richardson EP, et al: Hypertensive putaminal hemorrhage. *Ann Neurol* 1977;1:152.

24. Dinsdale HB: Spontaneous hemorrhage in the posterior fossa. *Arch Neurol* 1964;10:200.

25. Douglas MA, Haerer AF: Long-term prognosis of hypertensive intracerebral hemorrhage. *Stroke* 1982;13:488.

26. Strandgaard S, Paulson OB: Hypertensive disease and the cerebral circulation. In: Laragh JH, Brenner BM, eds: *Hypertension: Pathophysiology, Diagnosis and Management.* New York: Raven Press, 1990:399.

27. Mayhan WG, Faraci FM, Heistad DD: Impairment of endothelium-dependent responses of cerebral arterioles in chronic hypertension. *Am J Physiol* 1987;253:H1435.

28. Hamel E, Edvinsson L, MacKenzie ET: Heterogenous vasomotor responses of anatomically distinct feline cerebral arteries. *Br J Pharmacol* 1988;94:423.

29. Gauthier JC: Cerebral ischaemia in hypertension. In: Russell RWR, ed: *Vascular Diseases of the Central Nervous System.* New York: Churchill Livingstone, 1983:224.

30. Werber AH, Heistad DD: Effects of chronic hypertension and sympathetic nerves on the cerebral microvasculature of stroke-prone spontaneously hypertensive rats. *Circ Res* 1984;55:286.

31. Barry DI, Strandgaard S, Graham DI, et al: Cerebral blood flow in rats with renal and spontaneous hypertension. *J Cereb Blood Flow Metab* 1982; 2:347.

32. Baumbach GL, Heistad DD: Cerebral circulation in chronic arterial hypertension. *Hypertension* 1988;12:89.

33. Meyer JS, Shiazu K, Fukuuchi Y, et al: Impaired neurogenic cerebrovascular control and dysautoregulation after stroke. *Stroke* 1972;4:169.

34. Yamori Y, Oorie R: Developmental course of hypertension and regional cerebral blood flow in stroke prone spontaneously hypertensive rats. *Stroke* 1977;8:456.

35. Charcot JM, Bouchard C: Nouvelles recherches sur la pathogenie de l'hemorrhagie. *Arch Physiol Norm Path* 1868;1:110.

36. Cole FM, Yates PO: Pseudo-aneurysms in relationship to massive cerebral haemorrhage. *JNNP* 1967;30:61.

37. Fisher CM: Cerebral miliary aneurysms in hypertension. *Am J Pathol* 1972;66:313.
38. Takebayashi S, Kaneko M: Electron microscopic studies of ruptured arteries in hypertensive intracerebral hemorrhage. *Stroke* 1984;14:28.
39. Fisher CM: Pathological observations in hypertensive cerebral hemorrhage. *J Neuropathol Exp Neurol* 1971;30:536.
40. Yoshida Y, Shinkai H, Ooneda G: Morphogenesis of microaneurysm and plasmatic arterionecrosis in hypertensive cerebral hemorrhage. In: Mizukami M, Kogure K, Kanaya H, et al. eds: *Hypertensive Intracerebral Hemorrhage*. New York: Raven Press, 1983:181.
41. Rosenblum WI: Miliary aneurysms and "fibrinoid" degeneration of cerebral blood vessels. *Hum Pathol* 1977;8:133.
42. Takebayashi S: Ultrastructural morphometry of hypertensive medial damage in lenticulostriate and other arteries. *Stroke* 1985;16:449.
43. Frediksson K, Nordborg C, Kalimo H et al: Cerebral microangiopathy in stroke-prone spontaneously hypertensive rats. An immunohistochemical and ultrastructural study. *Acta Neuropathol* 1988;75:241.
44. Tagami M, Nara Y, Kubota A, et al: Ultrastructural characteristics of occluded perforating arteries in stroke-prone spontaneously hypertensive rats. *Stroke* 1987;18:733.
45. Huckman MS, Weinberg PE, Kim KS, et al: Angiographic and clinicopathologic correlates in basal ganglionic hemorrhage. *Radiology* 1970;95:79.
46. Yamori Y, Horie R, Nara Y, et al: Experimental pathology of hypertensive intracerebral hemorrhage: studies on the pathogenesis and prevention in the stroke-prone spontaneously hypertensive rat. In: Mizukami M, Kogure K, Kanaya H, et al., eds: *Hypertensive Intracerebral Hemorrhage*. New York: Raven Press, 1983:191.
47. Richards A, Graham D, Bullock R: Clinicopathological study of neurological complications due to hypertensive disorders of pregnancy. *JNNP* 1988;51:416.
48. Mizukami M, Araki G, Mihara H, et al: Arteriographically visualized extravasation in hypertensive intracerebral hemorrhage. Report of seven cases. *Stroke* 1972;3:527.
49. Weisberg L: Multiple spontaneous intracerebral hematomas: clinical and computed tomographic correlations. *Neurology* 1981;31:897.
50. Kingman TA, Mendelow AD, Graham DI, et al: Experimental intracerebral mass: description of model, intracranial pressure changes and neuropathology. *J Neuropathol Exp Neurol* 1988;47:128.
51. Phillips SJ, Whisnant JP: Hypertension and Stroke. In: Laragh JH, Brenner BM, eds: *Hypertension: Pathophysiology, Diagnosis and Management*. New York: Raven Press, 1990:417.
52. Sato S, Suzuki J: Anatomical mapping of the cerebral nervi vasorum in the human brain. *J Neurosurg* 1975;43:559.
53. Ropper AH, Davis KR: Lobar cerebral hemorrhages: acute clinical syndromes in 26 cases. *Ann Neurol* 1980;8:141.
54. Caplan L: Intracerebral hemorrhage revisited. *Neurology* 1988;38:624.

55. Sloan MA, Price TR, Foulkes MA, et al: Circadian rhythmicity of stroke onset. Intracerebral and subarachnoid hemorrhage. *Stroke* 1992;23:1420.

56. Mohr JP, Caplan LR, Melski JW, et al: The Harvard Coooperative Stroke Registry: a prospective registry. *Neurology* 1978;28:754.

57. Herbstein DJ, Schaumburg HH: Hypertensive intracerebral hematoma. An investigation of the initial hemorrhage and rebleeding using chromium CR 51-labeled erythrocytes. *Arch Neurol* 1974;30:412.

58. Kowada M, Yamaguchi K, Matsuoka S, et al: Extravasation of angiographic contrast material in hypertensive intracerebral hemorrhage. *J Neurosurg* 1972;36:471.

59. Kelley RE, Berger JR, Scheinberg P, et al: Active bleeding in hypertensive intracerebral hemorrhage: computed tomography. *Neurology* 1982;32:852.

60. Broderick J, Brott T, Tomsick T: Ultra-early evaluation of intracerebral hemorrhage (ICH). *Stroke* 1989;20:158.

61. Kaufman HH, Schochet SS: Pathology, pathophysiology, and modeling. In: Kaufman HH, ed: *Intracerebral Hematomas*. New York: Raven Press, 1992: 13.

62. Bullock R, Brock-Utne J, van Dellen J, et al: Intracerebral hemorrhage in a primate model: effect on regional cerebral blood flow. *Surg Neurol* 1988; 29:101.

63. Mendelow AD: Spontaneous intracerebral haemorrhage. *JNNP* 1991;54: 193.

64. Nath FP, Jenkins A, Mendelow AD, et al: Early hemodynamic changes in experimental intracerebral hemorrhage. *J Neurosurg* 1986;65:697.

65. Nehls DG, Mendelow AD, Graham DI, et al: Experimental intracerebral hemorrhage: progression of hemodynamic changes after production of a spontaneous mass lesion. *Neurosurgery* 1988;23:439.

66. Sinar EJ, Mendelow AD, Graham DI, et al: Experimental intracerebral haemorrhage: the effect of nimodipine pretreatment. *JNNP* 1988;51:651.

67. Ropper AH, Zervas NT: Cerebral blood flow after experimental basal ganglia hemorrhage. *Ann Neurol* 1982;11:266.

68. Ojemann RG, Heros RC: Spontaneous brain hemorrhage. *Stroke* 1983;14: 468.

69. Walshe TM, Davis KR, Fisher CM: Thalamic hemorrhage: a computed tomographic-clinical correlation. *Neurology* 1977;27:217.

70. Barraquer-Bordas L, Illa I, Escartin A, et al: Thalamic hemorrhage. A study of 23 patients with diagnosis by computed tomography. *Stroke* 1981; 12:524.

71. Kawahara N, Sato K, Muraki M, et al: CT classification of small thalamic hemorrhages and their clinical implications. *Neurology* 1986;36:165.

72. Heros RC: Cerebellar hemorrhage and infarction. *Stroke* 1982;13:106.

73. Ott KH, Kase CS, Ojemann RG, et al: Cerebellar hemorrhage: diagnosis and treatment. A review of 56 cases. *Arch Neurol* 1974;31:160.

74. Brennan RW, Bergland RM: Acute cerebellar hemorrhage. Analysis of clinical findings and outcome in 12 cases. *Neurology* 1977;27:527.

75. Melamed N, Satya-Murti S: Cerebellar hemorrhage. A review and reappraisal of benign cases. *Arch Neurol* 1984;41:425.
76. Little JR, Tubman DE, Ethier R: Cerebellar hemorrhage in adults. Diagnosis by computerized tomography. *J Neurosurg* 1978;48:575.
77. Goto N, Kaneko M, Hosaka Y, et al: Primary pontine hemorrhage: clinicopathological correlations. *Stroke* 1980;11:84.
78. Caplan LR, Goodwin JA: Lateral tegmental brainstem hemorrhages. *Neurology* 1982;32:252.
79. Weisberg LA: Caudate hemorrhage. *Arch Neurol* 1984;41:971.
80. Waga S, Fujimoto K, Okada M, et al: Caudate hemorrhage. *Neurosurgery* 1986;18:445.
81. Stein RW, Kase CS, Hier DB, et al: Caudate hemorrhage. *Neurology* 1984; 34:1549.
82. Weisberg LA, Wall M: Small capsular hemorrhages. Clinical-computed tomographic correlations. *Arch Neurol* 1984;41:1255.
83. Mori E, Yamadori A, Kudo Y, et al: Ataxic hemiparesis from small capsular hemorrhage. Computed tomography and somatosensory evoked potentials. *Arch Neurol* 1984;41:1050.
84. Groothuis DR, Duncan GW, Fisher CM: The human thalamocortical sensory path in the internal capsule: evidence from a small capsular hemorrhage causing a pure sensory stroke. *Ann Neurol* 1977;2:328.
85. Mori E, Tabuchi M, Yamadori A: Lacunar syndrome due to intracerebral hemorrhage. *Stroke* 1985;16:454.
86. Weisberg LA: Subcortical lobar intracerebral haemorrhage: clinical-computed tomographic correlations. *JNNP* 1985;48:1078.
87. Kase CS, Williams JP, Wyatt DA, et al: Lobar intracerebral hematomas. Clinical and CT analysis of 22 cases. *Neurology* 1982;32:1146.
88. Inzitari D, Giordano GP, Ancona AL, et al: Leukoaraiosis, intracerebral hemorrhage, and arterial hypertension. *Stroke* 1990;21:1419.
89. Lavin P: Management of hypertension in patients with acute stroke. *Arch Intern Med* 1986;146:66.
90. Ledingham JGG, Rajagopalan: Cerebral complications in the treatment of accelerated hypertension. *Q J Med* 1979;189:25.
91. Hayashi M, Kobayashi H, Kawano H, et al: Treatment of systemic hypertension and intracranial hypertension in cases of brain hemorrhage. *Stroke* 1988;19:314.
92. Wiggins WS, Moody DM, Toole JF, et al: Clinical and computerized tomographic study of hypertensive intracerebral hemorrhage. *Arch Neurol* 1978;35:832.
93. Mizukami M, Nishijima M, Kin H: Computed tomographic findings of good prognosis for hemiplegia in hypertensive putaminal hemorrhage. *Stroke* 1981;12:648.
94. Lee KS, Bae HG, Yun HG: Recurrent intracerebral hemorrhage due to hypertension. *Neurosurgery* 1990;26:586.

Chapter 3

Cerebral Amyloid Angiopathy

Karen Furie, MD, Edward Feldmann, MD

Cerebral amyloid angiopathy (CAA) is believed to account for approximately 10% of intracerebral hemorrhages.[1] It is characterized pathologically by homogeneous eosinophilic deposits of β amyloid protein fibrils in the media and adventitia of arterioles and small caliber cerebral and leptomeningeal arteries. Cerebral amyloid angiopathy has also been demonstrated in the brains of the normal elderly population and in patients with assorted neurologic disorders: Alzheimer's disease, diffuse Lewy body disease, hereditary cerebral hemorrhage, arteriovenous malformations, radiation necrosis, demyelinating syndromes, cerebral infarction, vasculitis, dementia pugilistica, hereditary ataxia, and the spongiform encephalopathies.[2-6]

Epidemiology

It is difficult to define the epidemiology of CAA because of bias in the available retrospective data, which are based on hospital and autopsy-based populations rather than community studies.[7] Another element which confounds efforts to characterize the prevalence of CAA is the failure of many studies to control for age and coexistent pathology. Center-to-center variability in the technique of pathologically identifying CAA could also significantly affect the reported prevalence.[4]

In the normal population, the prevalence of CAA increases with age.[7-11] In one autopsy study of 84 normal individuals aged 60 to 97, CAA was found in 36% of brains. The percentage of persons with CAA increased linearly with age: 8% in the seventh decade, 20% in the eighth decade, 37% in the ninth decade, and 58% in the tenth decade.[9] The extent of involvement does not necessarily correlate with symptoms. Three percent of individuals with CAA have severe amyloid deposition but remain asymptomatic.[8]

Sporadic CAA has been implicated as a cause of lobar intracerebral hemor-

From Feldmann E (ed). *Intracerebral Hemorrhage.* Armonk, NY: Futura Publishing Company, Inc., © 1994.

rhages seen in the elderly. In one retrospective series, approximately 12% of intracerebral hemorrhages were due to CAA, and all were lobar in location.[12] Another retrospective study compared the histologic appearance of brains with CAA and intracerebral hemorrhage to those of patients with neuropsychiatric disease and a control elderly population. They found a prevalence of vascular amyloid of 45% in the control group and 54% in the neuropsychiatric population. The patients with intracerebral hemorrhage were found to have more severe CAA, as well as fibrinoid necrosis and microaneurysms.[13] In patients treated surgically for intracerebral hemorrhage, approximately 8% were found to have CAA by biopsy.[13] At autopsy, however, CAA was found in 7 of these 41 brains, giving a prevalence of 17.1%.[14] Clearly, the diligence with which CAA is sought and the sampling techniques used affect the reported prevalence of the disorder.

Familial CAA

Hereditary cerebral hemorrhage in association with amyloid deposition (HCHWA) was first described in unrelated Icelandic (HCHWA-I) and Dutch (HCHWA-D) families.[15] A cluster of patients with HCHWA with a natural history similar to HCHWA-I has been reported in Japan.[16] Other dominantly inherited HCHWA variants have been described. These may present with cerebral ischemic events, early onset dementia, corticospinal tract signs, and cerebellar signs, but no intracerebral hemorrhage.[17] Alternatively, HCHWA may present with myelopathy, peripheral neuropathy, psychosis, coma, seizures, visual impairment, and deafness in association with intracerebral hemorrhage.[18]

Hereditary Cerebral Hemorrhage with Amyloid Deposition—Dutch Type

Hereditary cerebral hemorrhage with amyloidosis of the Dutch type (HCHWA-D) is an autosomal dominant form of CAA which has been described in four families from two coastal villages in the Netherlands. All HCHWA-D patients have abnormalities on neuropsychiatric testing, and 50% to 75% of patients become demented at some point in their illness.[19]

Stroke was the initial presentation in all 24 patients described by Haan et al, with age of stroke onset between 43 and 66 years. The strokes are hemorrhagic in 87% and ischemic in 13%.[20] Transient neurologic events may precede the initial intracerebral hemorrhage by 3 to 8 years. There are several characteristic features of these hemorrhages. Typically irregular in shape, they are situated in the parietal lobe, have an acute onset, and often progress.[20] Recurrent intracerebral hemorrhage is seen in one third of patients. Rebleeding has been reported to occur anywhere from 3 weeks to 14 years after the initial hemorrhage.[21] The mortality after the initial hemorrhage approaches 70%.[19]

Hereditary Cerebral Hemorrhage with Amyloid—Icelandic Type

While HCHWA-I and HCHWA-D are similar syndromes, HCHWA-I has a considerably earlier age of onset and has none of the intraparenchymal amyloid plaques seen in HCHWA-D. HCHWA-I is transmitted in an autosomal dominant fashion and is associated with lethal intracerebral hemorrhage by age 50.[20,21] Dementia was a feature at the time of presentation in approximately 10% of patients with HCHWA-I. However, progressive dementia was demonstrable by neuropsychiatric testing in 74% of 52 patients with HCHWA-I.[22] Patients with HCHWA-I averaged 3.2 vascular events in their lives, and the events may have been hemorrhagic or ischemic.[22] Survival ranged from 10 to 23 years.[22]

Molecular Biology of CAA

Amyloid is formed as a by-product of aberrant protein synthesis, resulting either from mutated protein precursors or dysfunctional synthetic enzymes. The product of such errors is a β pleated protein, which is deposited in normal tissue.[23] Three types of cerebral amyloid have been identified: β-protein, cystatin C, and PrP.

The β-protein precursor, amyloid precursor protein (APP), is encoded on chromosome 21. The β-protein is a 40 amino acid residue of the cleavage of the 751-770 amino acid APP. Neurons and systemic tissues contain mRNA encoding the β-protein, but they do not normally express it.[24] In the normal processing of APP, the amino terminal of the protein is cleaved to form a protease inhibitor, protease nexin II. If this protein is synthesized in vitro, the β-protein is not formed.[25] In HCHWA-D, a point mutation at position 22 in the APP gene, substituting glutamine for glutamic acid, results in a structural abnormality of the β-protein.[26] The proximity between the mutation site and the usual APP cleavage point may alter normal cleavage, resulting in the production and deposition of β-protein.[25-27]

Other mechanisms involved in the processing of the APP may be implicated in amyloid deposition. β-Protein has been detected in the vessels of patients with sporadic CAA, Down's syndrome, normal aging, and Alzheimer's disease, but the APP sequence is not mutated.[1,11,28–31] One possible mechanism is phosphorylation of APP by protein kinase C causing abnormal cleavage sites and the resultant formation of amyloid.[32] Although chromosome 21 encodes both APP and familial Alzheimer's disease, there is no linkage between them.[26]

The HCHWA-I cerebral vessels do not contain β amyloid protein.[15,33] An aberrant cystatin C, an inhibitor of cysteine proteinases, is deposited in vessels.[26] In these patients, the gene sequence for cystatin C contains a point mutation resulting in the substitution of glutamine for leucine. As a result, proteolytic cleavage of the precursor protein is altered, and the abnormal cystatin C accumulates in vessels as amyloid.[26,34] The concentration of cystatin C in the cerebral spinal fluid of HCHWA-I patients is lowered. This may relate to fragility imparted with the point mutation causing enhanced degradation.[35] Carrier states of the genetic defect have been identified, but their natural history remains unknown.[36]

Histopathology

Vascular Pathology

Amyloid replaces smooth muscle in the media of small and medium sized arteries, separating the internal elastic and external basement membranes. Amyloid stains with Congo red and produces yellow-green birefringence under polarized light (Figure 1). On electron microscopy, amyloid fibrils appear as 5- to 10-nm straight fibrils. The vessels affected by amyloid deposition are small leptomeningeal and cortical arteries. The distribution is multifocal. The topographic predominance is variable and may be frontal, temporal, parietal, or occipital.[9,37] This lack of concordance across studies is believed to reflect disparate study populations.[1,14,38-40] The hippocampus and subcortical white matter are usually spared.[41] It has been postulated that the parieto-occipital cortex is mainly affected in HCHWA, whereas sporadic CAA involves the frontotemporal cortex.[20] One autopsy series reported a distribution of hemorrhages, in decreasing frequency, as frontal,[42] parietal,[33] occipital,[43] temporal,[44] and hippocampal.[7,37]

In addition to the deposition of amyloid, arteries in the brains of patients with CAA exhibit other pathologic changes. This amyloid vasculopathy, which primarily involves leptomeningeal vessels, is characterized by chronic perivascular or transmural lymphocytic infiltrates, hyaline arteriolar degeneration, and fibrinoid necrosis. There may be multiple arteriolar glomerular formations or aneurysms. Deposition of amyloid within the vessel wall is believed to cause these vascular abnormalities directly.[37] In patients with CAA and Alzheimer's disease, affected vessels have intense acetylcholinesterase and butyrylcholinesterase activity identical to that seen in neurofibrillary tangles and senile plaques.[45] These enzymes may contribute to aberrant protein synthesis, thus leading to further amyloid production. Alternatively, they may weaken the blood-brain barrier, and thus be involved in the pathophysiology of the intracerebral hemorrhages.

There are several mechanisms proposed to explain the relationship between amyloid deposition and intracerebral hemorrhage. Replacement of contractile elements of the vasculature with amyloid is believed to cause loss of

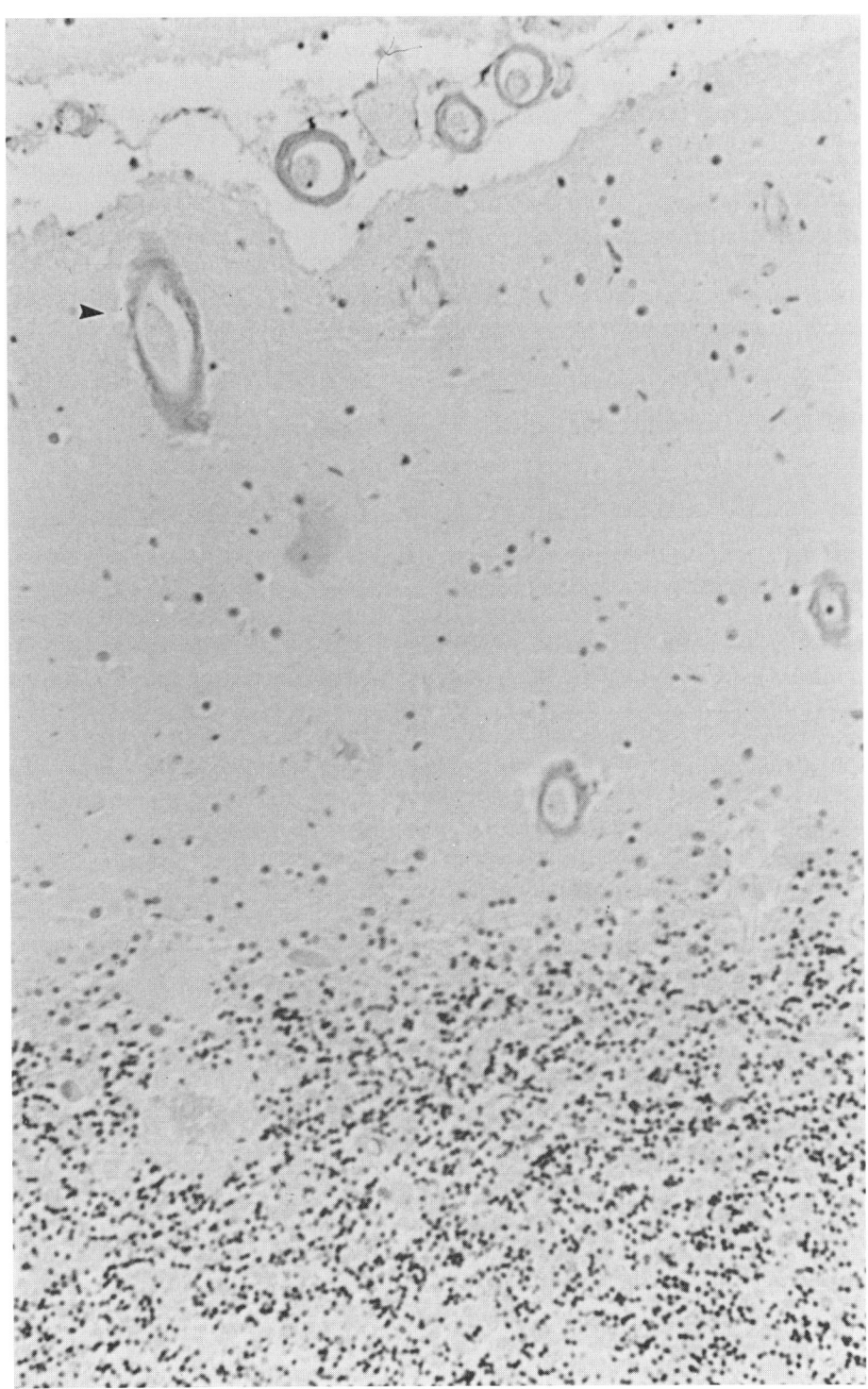

Figure 1: Granular layer of the cerebellum with amyloid deposition in medium sized vessels.

hemostasis.[46] Increased fragility of these vessels, fibrinoid degeneration, and microaneurysm formation have also been postulated as mechanisms. One study found that fibrinoid necrosis was present in 72% of patients with CAA and intracerebral hemorrhage, but in none of the patients with CAA without intracerebral hemorrhage.[8] However, in another small group of patients with lobar hemorrhage and CAA, fewer than half of the patients had vasculopathic changes. Investigators have not been able to correlate CAA vasculopathy with intracerebral hemorrhage in the majority of patients.[7] Although it has been postulated that fibrinoid necrosis leads to aneurysm formation and subsequent hemorrhage, these studies failed to consistently reveal direct evidence implicating CAA-affected vessels in the hemorrhage.

Parenchymal Pathology

The parenchymal changes seen in CAA reflect the consequences of the vascular pathology and direct deposition of amyloid in the brain tissue. Autopsy study of patients with severe CAA reveal large lobar hematomas, small cortical infarcts, multiple petechial hemorrhages, and senile plaques and neurofibrillary tangles. Cortical infarcts correlated with thrombosis of CAA-laden cortical vessels. All patients had ventricular enlargement secondary to atrophy or leukomalacia. The white matter of the semiovale was frequently vacuolated with swollen oligodendrocytes. Perivascular spaces were enlarged and contained mononuclear cells and hemosiderin-laden macrophages.[47]

Amyloid plaques are found in patients with sporadic CAA and HCHWA-D, but not HCHWA-I.[21,48,49] Unlike the senile plaques seen in Alzheimer's disease, these are larger, lack a central, strongly congophilic core, are not surrounded by neurites, and have a variable shape.[17]

CAA brains frequently demonstrate periventricular demyelination, believed to be due to ischemia caused by amyloid deposition in vessels supplying the deep white matter. The demyelination spares the U-fibers and axons. There may also be swollen oligodendrocytes and astrocytic gliosis.[47]

Signs and Symptoms

Intracerebral Hemorrhage

CAA usually manifests clinically with intracerebral hemorrhage. In the elderly, it accounts for up to 17% of intracerebral hemorrhages.[50] The hemorrhages are lobar, sparing the brainstem, cerebellum, and basal ganglia.[1] The hemorrhage may extend into the ventricles and subarachnoid space.[14,39] At autopsy, there are commonly multiple hemorrhages in various stages of resolution.[14] Presenting features include headache, nausea and vomiting, loss of consciousness, and focal neurologic deficits. Headache is the most common feature, present in nearly 70% of cases. Factors which have been documented to precipitate bleeding include minor head trauma, anticoagulation, antiplatelet therapy, and thrombolytic therapy.[14,38,51–54] There have been reports of CAA-induced intracerebral hemorrhage after minor neurosurgical procedures.[55] A recent retrospective series shows a low rate of bleeding complications in patients with CAA undergoing brain biopsy.[44,56] Hypertension coexists with CAA in 30% of patients, but it is not believed to be a major risk factor for bleeding.[1,7] Recurrent hemorrhages are common. In one small study, 20% of patients with sporadic CAA had recurrent bleeds within weeks of the initial hemorrhage.[14]

The prognosis for a meaningful recovery in patients with intracerebral hemorrhage is poor. There is a high rate of mortality after the initial hemorrhage. Those who do survive often have significant neurologic deficits.[1,14,39,48,57,58] One study reported 100% mortality within 4 months of intracerebral hemorrhage.[12] Despite therapeutic intervention, two other series reported a high mortality within weeks of the initial hemorrhage.[14,57] More advanced age and larger, multifocal, and recurrent hemorrhages herald a poor outcome.

Transient Ischemia and Infarction

Patients with CAA often experience transient ischemic attacks (TIAs) or infarcts. These symptoms were reported by 13 of 23 patients with sporadic CAA.[59] However, not all patients experience ischemic episodes. Patients with intracerebral hemorrhage in one small study were found to have no ischemic lesions at pathologic examination.[12] Cortical infarcts in patients with CAA are superficial. The responsible amyloid-laden obliterated arterioles can be identified.[37] Other evidence of CAA-associated vasculopathy may be present. The infarcts are usually multiple but may occur in isolation.[14] Petechial hemorrhages are commonly found in close proximity to the small cortical infarcts.[12,47] Radiographically, the infarcts do not conform to the wedge-shaped lesions typically seen with cortical infarcts due to other vascular abnormalities.[21]

Dementia

The dementia seen in patients with CAA is often attributed to recurrent ischemic and hemorrhagic events. There have been reports of cognitive decline occurring without new demonstrable lesions.[19] It is also possible that demyelination associated with the CAA vasculopathy or intraparenchymal CAA may be contributing to the dementing process. CAA is commonly found in patients with Alzheimer's disease.[23,43] The reported prevalence of CAA in Alzheimer's disease ranges from 48% to 100%. However, less than one third of these patients have severe amyloid deposition in the brain.[23,37,42,60]

Subarachnoid Hemorrhage

Secondary subarachnoid hemorrhage in association with an intracerebral hemorrhage is common in patients with CAA. There has been a report of primary subarachnoid hemorrhage due to CAA. At autopsy, no aneurysm, arteriovenous malformation, or intracerebral hemorrhage was detected. However, there was heavy amyloid infiltration of meningeal vessels.[48] CAA should be considered as a possible etiology of subarachnoid hemorrhage in the 5% to 10% of all patients with subarachnoid hemorrhage who have no underlying lesion detected on angiogram, particularly the elderly.

Differential Diagnosis

Hypertensive hemorrhages are common in the elderly population. These patients typically have a history of longstanding hypertension, and they may have other vascular risk factors as well. The hemorrhages are located in the basal ganglia, caudate, thalamus, cerebellum, and pons. This contrasts with the lobar hemorrhages which typify CAA. Hypertensive hemorrhage has an acute onset and rarely progresses. Multifocal or recurrent hemorrhages are rare. Cerebral amyloid angiopathy-associated intracerebral hemorrhages more often progress after an acute onset.[20] Extension of the hemorrhage into the subarachnoid space occurs in CAA but is extremely rare in hypertensive intracerebral hemorrhage.[8] Radiographically, hypertensive hemorrhages appear round, whereas those of CAA are often irregular. Arteriovenous malformations may also cause simultaneous lobar and subarachnoid hemorrhage. They generally present earlier in life than CAA. Arteriovenous malformations and aneurysms usually present with subarachnoid hemorrhage, although there may be a coexisting intraparenchymal hematoma. These diagnoses can be excluded by performing an angiogram. Trauma and coagulopathies may lead to intracerebral hemorrhage. A history and admission laboratory data (prothrombin time, partial prothrombin time, platelet count, bleeding time) are helpful in establishing either of these diagnoses. Cerebral vasculitis is a cause of hemorrhage in younger patients and may be associated with classic angiographic findings. It is very rare in the population at risk for CAA.

Laboratory Features

Cerebrospinal Fluid

There are no pathognomonic cerebrospinal fluid (CSF) abnormalities in HCHWA-D and sporadic CAA.[36] Patients with HCHWA-I and their asymptomatic first-degree relatives have low CSF levels of cystatin C. Asymptomatic carriers of the disease may be identified by this CSF abnormality.[35,36] Using an enzyme-linked immunosorbent assay in patients with intracerebral hemorrhage, low CSF cystatin levels have been shown to correlate with pathologically proven CAA.[61] Patients with HCHWA-D and Alzheimer's disease have been found to have a decreased level of amyloid precursor protein in the CSF.[62]

Neuroradiologic Findings

A noncontrast head CT scan is a sensitive study for detecting acute hemorrhage. Findings suggestive of CAA hemorrhage include the lobar location and intraventricular of subarachnoid extension.[39] Periventricular hypodensities have also been noted.[47]

The magnetic resonance imaging (MRI) features of CAA are multiple, punctate hemorrhagic lesions in association with periventricular leukoencephalopathy (Figure 2). The multiple nonspecific white matter signal hyperintensities

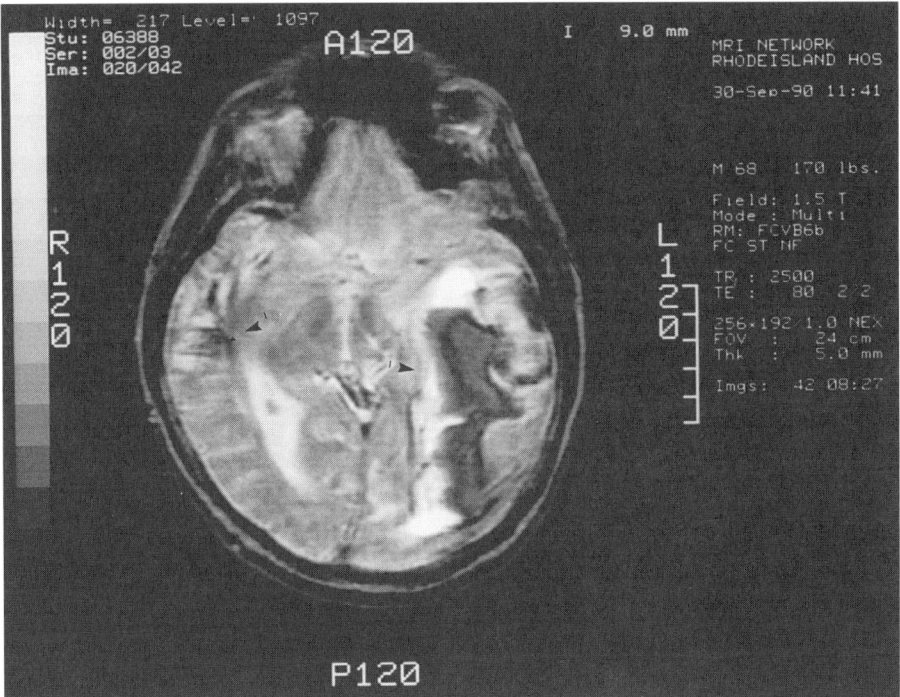

Figure 2: MRI appearance of amyloid angiopathy. *A:* T$_2$ weighted MRI image demonstrating hemorrhages of different ages. The left tempero-parietal hemorrhage is subacute with surrounding edema and mass effect. A right temporal older, resolving hemorrhage with hemosiderin and gliosis is also shown. *B:* Proton density MRI showing a chronic right parietal hemorrhage and the characteristic periventricular leukoencephalopathy.

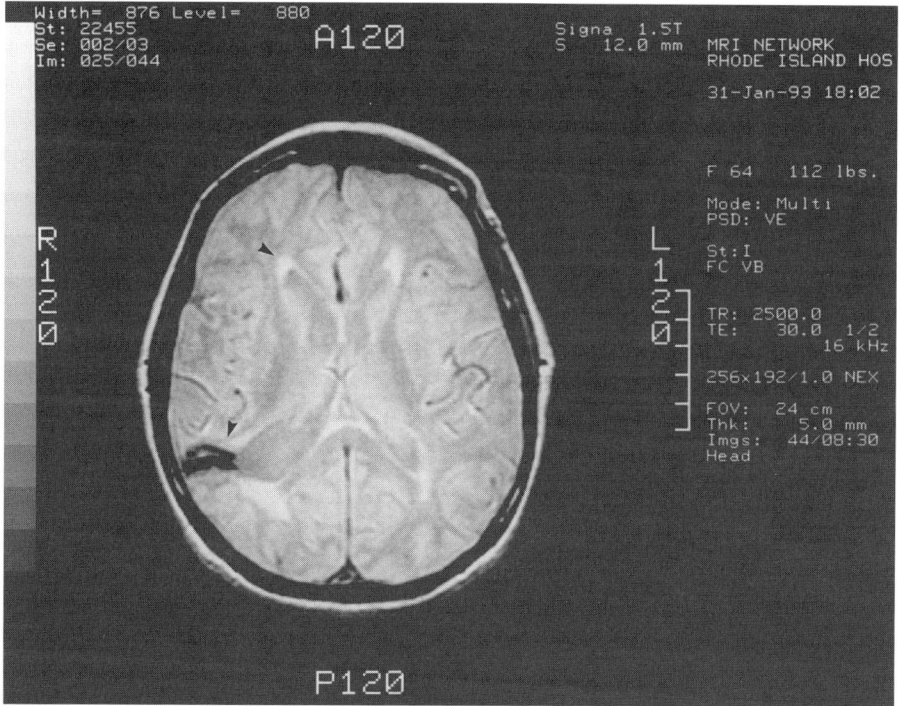

Figure 2: (*continued*)

on T$_2$ weighted spin-echo pulse sequences are believed to represent small vessel infarcts.[63,64]

There are no CAA-specific abnormalities on angiography. However, it is the definitive study to exclude an underlying vascular anomaly as a cause of intracerebral hemorrhage.[65] Occasionally the hemorrhage itself may produce a mass effect demonstrable on angiography.[8,38,66]

Neuropathology

Definitive diagnosis of CAA is made by demonstrating the presence of congo-red staining, birefringent material in the walls of arterioles, and small to medium sized arteries obtained in a biopsy specimen.[35] Immunohistochemical methods can further classify the subtype of amyloid protein involved. A study of 46 patients with CAA showed that all had immunoreactivity with β amyloid monoclonal antibodies. Nine cases also reacted to cystatin C antibodies.[46] More than seven of these nine cases had very heavy amyloid infiltration and massive fatal intracerebral hemorrhages. The presence of CAA-associated vasculopathy in biopsy specimens taken from areas of lobar hemorrhage provides indirect evidence for the mechanism of bleeding.[37]

Treatment

The presence of *known* CAA in elderly patients may affect clinical decisions regarding acute thrombolytic therapy, acute and chronic anticoagulation, antiplatelet therapy, and neurosurgery. In one series of 13 patients with CAA and ischemic symptoms, intracerebral hemorrhage occurred in three patients after the administration of anticoagulation for the treatment of TIA.[59] Known CAA should be viewed as a contraindication to anticoagulation. The use of thrombolytic therapy in a patient with known CAA in the setting of acute myocardial infarction is questionable, given the significant risk of inducing an intracerebral hemorrhage. There is insufficient evidence that aspirin significantly increases the risk of hemorrhage in patients with CAA to warrant cessation of antiplatelet therapy. However, aspirin has been believed to precipitate hemorrhage in case reports. Cautious and judicious use of antiplatelet agents in patients with CAA may be used to reduce the risk of myocardial infarction and stroke. The obvious difficulty with these recommendations is that most physicians are unaware that patients harbor clinically important CAA until after intracerebral hemorrhage has occurred, possibly as a complication of thrombolytic, antiplatelet, or anticoagulant therapy.

Surgical management of intracerebral hemorrhage is directed at evacuating the hematoma. A retrospective series of 12 patients who underwent evacuation of intracerebral hemorrhage due to CAA revealed a poor outcome.[44] One third of the patients died as a result of the hemorrhage or its complications, and one quarter were neurologically disabled. Of the five patients who were well enough to leave the hospital, all with moderately severe hemorrhages, one had recurrent hemorrhages and died. Surgery had been performed 11 to 21 days after the ictus. Another retrospective study of nine patients revealed a 22% surgical mortality, but six of the patients displayed neurologic improvement postoperatively.[67] In both studies, a separate group of patients with CAA without intracerebral hemorrhage who underwent brain biopsy in order to diagnose Alzheimer's disease had no increased bleeding complications.

Acute medical therapy of CAA-associated lobar hemorrhage consists of monitoring blood pressure, administering prophylactic anticonvulsants, and aggressively managing significant elevations in blood pressure.[8] In cases with severe cerebral edema and impending herniation, hyperventilation and mannitol can be used. The chronic management of patients after CAA-associated intracerebral hemorrhage should be directed at minimizing factors which predispose to hemorrhage.

References

1. Vinters HV: Cerebral amyloid angiopathy. A critical review. *Stroke* 1987; 18:311.

2. Feldmann E, Tornabene J: The diagnosis and management of cerebral amyloid angiopathy. *Clin Geriatr Med* 1991;7:617.

3. Coria F, Castano EM, Frangione F: Brain amyloid in normal aging and cerebral amyloid angiopathy is antigenically related to Alzheimer's beta-protein. *Am J Pathol* 1987;129:422.

4. Esiri MM, Wilcock GK: Cerebral amyloid angiopathy in dementia and old age. *J Neurol Neurosurg Psych* 1986;49:1221.

5. Wu E, Lipton RB, Dickson DW: Amyloid angiopathy in diffuse Lewy body disease. *Neurology* 1992;42:2131.

6. Akiyama H, Yamada T, Kawamata T, et al: Association of amyloid P component with complement proteins in neurologically diseased brain tissue. *Brain Res* 1991;548:349.

7. Masuda J, Tanaka K, Ueda K, et al: Autopsy study of incidence and distribution of cerebral amyloid angiopathy in Hisayama, Japan. *Stroke* 1988; 19:205.

8. Case Records of the Massachusetts General Hospital (Case 10-1988). *N Engl J Med* 1988;318:623.

9. Tomonago M: Cerebral amyloid angiopathy in the elderly. *J Am Geriatric Soc* 1981;29:151.

10. Wright JR, Calkins E: Relationship of amyloid deposits in the human aorta to aortic sclerosis. A post-mortem study of individuals over sixty years of age. *Lab Invest* 1974;30:766.

11. Yamada M, Tsukagoshi H, Otomo E, et al: Systemic amyloid deposition in old age and dementia of Alzheimer type: the relationship of brain amyloid to other amyloid. *Acta Neuropathol* 1988;77:136.

12. Ishii N, Nishihara Y, Horie A: Amyloid angiopathy and lobar cerebral haemorrhage. *J Neurol Neurosurg Psych* 1984;47:1203.

13. Vonsattel JPG, Myers RH, Hedley-White T, et al: Cerebral amyloid angiopathy without and with cerebral hemorrhages: a comparative histological study. *Ann Neurol* 1991;30:637.

14. Kalyan-Raman UP, Kalyan-Raman K: Cerebral amyloid angiopathy causing intracranial hemorrhage. *Ann Neurol* 1984;16:321.

15. Van Duinen SG, Castano EM, Prelli F, et al: Hereditary cerebral hemorrhage with amyloidosis in patients of Dutch origin is related to Alzheimer disease. *Proc Natl Acad Sci* 1987;84:5991.

16. Fujihara S, Shimode K, Nakamura M, et al: Cerebral amyloid angiopathy with the deposition of cystatin C (gamma-trace) and beta-protein. *Prog Clin Biol Res* 1989;317:939.

17. Plant GT, Revesz T, Barnard RO, et al: Familial cerebral amyloid angiopathy with nonneuritic amyloid plaque formation. *Brain* 1990;113:721.

18. Uitti RJ, Donat JR, Rozdilsky B, et al: Familial oculoleptomeningeal amyloidosis. Report of a new family with unusual features. *Arch Neurol* 1988; 45:1118.

19. Haan J, Lanser JBK, Zijderveld I, et al: Dementia in hereditary cerebral hemorrhage with amyloidosis-Dutch type. *Arch Neurol* 1990;47:965.

20. Haan R, Algra PR, Roos RAC: Hereditary cerebral hemorrhage with amy-

loidosis-Dutch type. Clinical and computed tomographic analysis of 24 cases. *Arch Neurol* 1990;47:649.

21. Luyendijk W, Bots GTAM, Vegter-van der Vlis, et al: Hereditary cerebral hemorrhage caused by cortical amyloid angiopathy. *J Neurol Sci* 1988;85: 267.

22. Blondal H, Benedikz E: Dementia in hereditary cystatin C amyloidosis. *Prog Clin Biol Res* 1989;317:157.

23. Vinters HV, Miller BL, Pardridge WM: Brain amyloid and Alzheimer disease. *Ann Intern Med* 1988;109:41.

24. Miller DL, Currie JR, Iqbal K, et al: Relationships among the cerebral amyloid peptides and their precursors. *Ann Med* 1989;21:83.

25. Selkoe DJ: Deciphering Alzheimer's disease: the amyloid precursor protein yields new clues. *Science* 1990;248:1048.

26. Levy E, Carman MD, Fernendez-Madrid IJ, et al: Mutation of the Alzheimer's disease amyloid gene in hereditary cerebral hemorrhage, Dutch type. *Science* 1990;248:1124.

27. Tabaton M, Cammarata S, Mandybur T, et al: Senile plaques in cerebral amyloid angiopathy show accumulation of amyloid precursor protein without cytoskeletal abnormalities. *Brain Res* 1992;593:299.

28. Case Records of the Massachusetts General Hospital (Case 49-1982). *N Engl J Med* 1982;307:1507.

29. Coria F, Prelli F, Castano EM, et al: Beta-protein deposition: a pathogenetic link between Alzheimer's disease and cerebral amyloid angiopathies. *Brain Res* 1988;463:187.

30. Fernandez-Madrid I, Levy E, Marder K, et al: Codon 618 variant of Alzheimer amyloid gene associated with cerebral hemorrhage. *Ann Neurol* 1991; 30:730.

31. Karlinsky H, Vaula G, Haines JL, et al: Molecular and prospective phenotypic characterization of a pedigree with familial Alzheimer's disease and a missense mutation in codon 717 of the β-amyloid precursor protein gene. *Neurology* 1992;42:1445.

32. Buxbaum JD, Gandy SE, Cichetti P, et al: Processing of Alzheimer beta/A4 amyloid precursor protein: modulation by agents that regulate protein phosphorylation. *Proc Natl Acad Sci* 1990;87:6003.

33. Yamada M, Tsukagoshi H, Wada Y, et al: Absence of the cystatin C amyloid in the cerebral amyloid angiopathy, senile plaque, and extra-CNS amyloid deposits, of aged Japanese. *Acta Neurol Scand* 1989;79:504.

34. Van Broeckhoven C, Haan J, Bakker E, et al: Amyloid beta protein precursor gene and hereditary cerebral hemorrhage with amyloidosis (Dutch). *Science* 1990;248:1120.

35. Lofberg H, Grubb AO, Nilsson EK, et al: Immunohistochemical characterization of the amyloid deposits and quantitation of pertinent cerebrospinal fluid proteins in hereditary cerebral hemorrhage with amyloidosis. *Stroke* 1987;18:431.

36. Jensson O, Gudmundsson G, Arnason A, et al: Hereditary cystatin (gam-

ma-trace) amyloid angiopathy of the CNS causing cerebral hemorrhage. *Acta Neurol Scand* 1987;76:102.

37. Mandybur TI: The incidence of cerebral amyloid angiopathy in Alzheimer's disease. *Neurology* 1975;25:120.

38. Gilbert JJ, Vinters HV: Cerebral amyloid angiopathy: incidence and complications in the aging brain I. Cerebral hemorrhage. *Stroke* 1983;14:914.

39. Gilles C, Brucher JM, Khoubsserian P, et al: Cerebral amyloid angiopathy as a cause of multiple intracranial hemorrhages. *Neurology* 1984;43:730.

40. Mandybur TI: Cerebral amyloid angiopathy: the vascular pathology and complications. *J Neuropathol Exper Neurol* 1986;45:79.

41. Vinters HV, Gilbert JJ: Cerebral amyloid angiopathy: incidence and complications in the aging brain II. The distribution of amyloid vascular changes. *Stroke* 1983;14:924.

42. Yankner BA, Mesulam MM: β-Amyloid and the pathogenesis of Alzheimer's disease. *N Engl J Med* 1991;26:1849.

43. Mountjoy CQ, Tomlinson BE, Gibson PH: Amyloid and senile plaques and cerebral blood vessels: a semi-quantitative investigation of a possible relationship. *J Neuro Sci* 1982;57:89.

44. Leblanc R, Preul M, Robitaille Y, et al: Surgical considerations in cerebral amyloid angiopathy. *Neurosurgery* 1991;29:712.

45. Mesulam M, Carson K, Price B, et al: Cholinesterases in the amyloid angiopathy of Alzheimer's disease. *Ann Neurol* 1992;31:565.

46. Maruyama K, Ikeda S, Ishihara T, et al: Immunohistochemical characterization of cerebrovascular amyloid in 46 autopsied cases using antibodies to beta protein and cystatin C. *Stroke* 1990;21:397.

47. Gray F, Dubas F, Roullet E, et al: Leukoencephalopathy in diffuse cerebral amyloid angiopathy. *Ann Neurol* 1985;18:54.

48. Ohshima T, Endo T, Nukui H, et al: Cerebral amyloid angiopathy as a cause of subarachnoid hemorrhage. *Stroke* 1990;21:480.

49. Thorsteinsson L, Georgsson G, Asgeirsson B, et al: On the role of monocytes/macrophages in the pathogenesis of central nervous system lesions in hereditary cystatin C amyloid angiopathy. *J Neurol Sci* 1992;108:121.

50. Feldmann E. Intracerebral hemorrhage. I. Etiologies. Current concepts of cerebrovascular disease and stroke. *J Neurol* 1990;25:1.

51. Pendlebury WW, Iole ED, Tracy RP, et al: Intracerebral hemorrhage related to cerebral amyloid angiopathy and t-PA treatment. *Ann Neurol* 1991;29:210.

52. Smith DB, Hitchcock M, Philpott PJ: Cerebral amyloid angiopathy presenting as transient ischemic attacks. *J Neurosurg* 1985;63:963.

53. Leblanc R, Haddad G, Robitaille Y: Cerebral hemorrhage from amyloid angiopathy and coronary thrombolysis. *Neurosurgery* 1992;31:586.

54. Yong WH, Robert ME, Secor DL, et al: Cerebral hemorrhage with biopsy-proved amyloid angiopathy. *Arch Neurol* 1992;49:51.

55. Torack RM: Congophilic angiopathy complicated by surgery and massive

hemorrhage. A light and electron microscopy study. *Am J Pathol* 1975;81: 349.

56. Matkovic Z, Davis S, Gonzales M, et al: Surgical risk of hemorrhage in cerebral amyloid angiopathy. *Stroke* 1991;22:456.

57. Cosgrove CR, Leblanc R, Meagher-Villemure K, et al: Cerebral amyloid angiopathy. *Neurology* 1985;35:625.

58. Hendricks HT, Franke CL, Theunissen PH: Cerebral amyloid anngiopathy: diagnosis by MRI and brain biopsy. *Neurology* 1990;40:1308.

59. Okazaki H, Reagan TJ, Campbell RJ: Clinicopathologic studies of primary cerebral amyloid angiopathy. *Mayo Clin Proc* 1979;54:22.

60. Ulrich J, Probst A, Wuest M: The brain diseases causing senile dementia. A morphological study on 54 consecutive autopsy cases. *J Neurol* 1986; 233:118.

61. Shimode K, Fujihara S, Makamura M, et al: Diagnosis of cerebral amyloid angiopathy by enzyme-linked immunosorbent assay of cystatin C in cerebrospinal fluid. *Stroke* 1991;22:860.

62. Van Nostrand WE, Wagner SL, Haan J, et al: Alzheimer's disease and hereditary cerebral hemorrhage with amyloidosis—Dutch type share a decrease in cerebrospinal fluid levels of amyloid β-protein precursor. *Ann Neurol* 1992;32:215.

63. Haan J, Roos RAC, Algra PR, et al: Hereditary cerebral hemorrhage with amyloidosis—Dutch type. Magnetic resonance imaging findings in 7 cases. *Brain* 1990;113:1251.

64. Loes DJ, Biller J, Yuh WTC, et al: Leukoencephalopathy in cerebral amyloid angiopathy: MR imaging in four cases. *AJNR* 1990;11:485.

65. Roosen N, Martin JJ, De La Porte C, et al: Intracerebral hemorrhage due to cerebral amyloid angiopathy. *J Neurosurg* 1985;63:965.

66. Patel DV, Hier DB, Thomas CM, et al: Intracerebral hemorrhage secondary to cerebral amyloid angiopathy. *Radiology* 1984;151:397.

67. Greene GM, Godesky JC, Biller J, et al: Surgical experience with intracranial hemorrhage secondary to cerebral amyloid angiopathy. *Stroke* 1990; 21:170.

Chapter 4

Recreational Drug Abuse

James Kokkinos, MD, Steven R. Levine, MD

Those who use or abuse illicit drugs, diet pills, and other sympathomimetics place themselves at increased relative risk for stroke and intracerebral hemorrhage (ICH).[1] The absolute risk is probably quite low: of 216,189 prescriptions for phenylpropanolamine-containing cough and cold remedies there was 1 ICH[2]; of 3,712 substance abusers admitted to hospital for reasons other than for rehabilitation, 3 had cocaine related ICH.[3] From the perspective of the doctor faced with a patient with ICH, however, illicit drugs and over-the-counter sympathomimetic drugs are often found to have played a role in the hemorrhage. For example, cocaine use had risen from approximately 10% of people aged 18 to 25 in the 1970s to 25% in the 1980s. As can be seen from Table 1, the proportion of cases of ICH that are due to drugs varies across studies and depends on the prevalence of drug abuse in the community and the age of the patient. Table 2 lists the drugs that have been reported as being associated with ICH. Each drug will be discussed individually later in this chapter. The mechanisms by which these drugs can be associated with ICH are listed in Table 3 and discussed individually in the next section.

About 85% to 90% of reported drug-associated strokes occur in the third or fourth decade, although the age range is perinatal to 63 years. The "1960s generation," however, has aged, so more and more patients from the fifth and sixth decades are being seen with strokes secondary to drug abuse.[4]

Most drug-related ICHs occur either immediately after or within a few hours of drug administration.[1] No consistent relationship has emerged between the site of ICH and drug abuse. Kaku and Lowenstein[1] found that 73% of their 24 patients with drug-related ICH had a peripheral (lobar) location, while 37% of their 49 patients with ICH not associated with drugs had lobar ICHs. Toffol et al[5] found lobar ICHs in 38 of their 67 (57%) young patients with nondrug-related ICH. Of their 5 patients with drug-related ICH, 3 (60%) had lobar locations and 2 had putaminal bleeds. Sloan et al[4] found 1 lobar and 1 basal ganglia drug-related ICH.

Supported in part by NIH grant NS23393 and the American Heart Association, Michigan Affiliate.

From Feldmann E (ed). *Intracerebral Hemorrhage*. Armonk, NY: Futura Publishing Company, Inc., © 1994.

Table 1

Drug-Related Intracerebral Hemorrhage in a Series of Intracerebral Hemorrhage of All Causes

Ages Screened	Number With ICH	Number Due to Drugs	Drugs Abused	Reference
15–44	73	24 (33%)	Mostly cocaine and amphetamines, occasionally heroin, methylphenidate	Kaku and Lowenstein[1]
15–45	72	5 (7%)	Amphetamines and phenylpropanolamine	Toffol et al[5]
any age	28	2 (7%)	Over-the-counter sympathomimetics	Sloan et al[4]
17–44	8	1 (12%)	Sympathomimetics	Lacey et al[6]

Table 2

Drugs That Have Been Associated with Intracerebral Hemorrhage

1. Cocaine
2. Amphetamines
3. Phenylpropanolamine
4. Other amphetamine-like sympathomimetics: ephedrine, pseudoephedrine
5. Heroin
6. Pentazocine and Tripelennamine (Ts and Blues)
7. Phencyclidine

Table 3

Mechanisms of Drug-Related Intracerebral Hemorrhage

1. Acute hypertension
2. Vasoconstriction
3. Infective endocarditis
4. Vasculitis
5. Human immunodeficiency virus infection
6. Thrombocytopenia or qualitative platelet defects
7. Hepatitis and bleeding diathesis
8. Nephropathy and hypertension
9. Tablet filler emboli
10. Underlying cerebral vascular malformation

Mechanisms

In individual patients with drug-related ICH, multiple mechanisms often coexist. For example, a patient may have had an arteriovenous malformation since birth or vasculitis secondary to chronic drug addiction. The patient's ICH, however, occurs very soon after drug administration because of acute severe hypertension secondary to the drug's pharmacologic action. Vascular malformations are uncommonly found in amphetamine abusers with ICH, while they are more common in cocaine abusers with ICH. Vasculitis, on the other hand, has been clearly shown to follow amphetamine abuse, whereas it is rare with cocaine.

Acute Hypertension, Vasoconstriction, and Nephropathy

All the drugs listed in Table 2 can cause acute hypertension and vessel constriction except for the opioids, heroin, and pentazocine. Heroin can cause a nephropathy, which in turn can result in hypertension.

Experimentally, an extremely high blood pressure is required to rupture a normal artery. Consequently, most ICHs following acute hypertension probably occur where vessels have already been damaged. Vessels may be damaged by chronic hypertension, amyloid angiopathy, in vascular malformations and aneurysms, by vasculitis, or from recent ischemia of both brain and vessels. The drug that caused acute hypertension may also cause the vascular damage, as seen in vasculitis secondary to amphetamines or drug-induced vasoconstriction resulting in ischemia. Caplan[7] has postulated that acute hypertension is an underemphasized mechanism of ICH, playing a role in ICHs that follow exposure to drugs, extreme cold, or dental pain. Another possible mechanism may occur during migraine attacks, where migraine putatively causes intense and prolonged vasoconstriction, followed by reperfusion of ischemic capillaries resulting in their rupture. A similar mechanism is postulated to exist with drugs that cause vasoconstriction.

Infective Endocarditis

Infective endocarditis with *Staphylococcus aureus* and *Candida albicans* is a common complication of parenteral drug abuse. The mitral, aortic, and tricuspid valves are involved with equal frequency. In most patients, these valves were previously normal. Patients present with constitutional symptoms or embolic phenomena. Fever and murmur are common, as are petechiae, Roth spots in their retinae, Janeway lesions in the pulps of their fingers, hematuria, or proteinuria. Leukocytosis, neutrophilia, raised sedimentation rate, positive rheumatoid factor, and raised immune complexes are typically seen. A transthoracic two-dimensional echocardiogram will reveal vegetations in about half of the cases, while transesophageal echocardiography is considerably more sensitive for left-sided valvular vegetations. Management involves blood cultures and prompt antibiotic administration. Valve replacement may be required. Stroke is not an indication for valve replacement or anticoagulation, since recurrent stroke is uncommon once the patient has been treated with appropriate antibiotics.[8]

Intracranial hemorrhage is a well-known complication of infective endocarditis. Hart et al[8] found intracranial hemorrhages in 9 (7%) of 133 episodes of native valve endocarditis. This figure rose to 17% in patients with *Staphylococcus aureus* infection of native mitral or aortic valves, and to 30% in patients who were intravenous drug abusers with *Staphylococcus aureus* infection. No patient was receiving anticoagulants. Among patients with infective endocarditis and intracranial hemorrhage, *Staphylococcus aureus* was the infecting organism in 53%, *Staphylococcus epidermidis* in 12%, and streptococci in 18%.[9] Another report included one ICH due to *Candida albicans* infection.[10]

Staphylococcus aureus is not only the commonest organism involved, it also tends to be associated with intracranial hemorrhage early in the course.[9] Among 15 patients with infective endocarditis from various organisms and intracranial hemorrhage, the hemorrhage occurred within 48 hours of admission in 9 patients (60%), and after hospital discharge in 3 (20%).[9]

Endocarditis-associated ICHs tend to be lobar hematomas. In one report, of nine endocarditis-associated intracranial hemorrhages, eight were lobar and one was primarily subarachnoid. Another report found lobar hematomas in 12 of 16 cases, hemorrhagic infarcts in 4 of 16 cases, and subarachnoid hemorrhage in 2 cases.[10]

Many patients with endocarditis-associated intracranial hemorrhage have associated cerebral ischemia. Of 16 patients, 4 had hemorrhagic infarcts, while in 5 others their ICH was preceded by ischemic episodes.[10] The mortality of infective endocarditis-associated intracranial hemorrhage is high, approaching 59% (10 of 17).[9]

The mechanism of intracranial hemorrhage in patients with infective endocarditis involves septic embolization to the brain. Thus, patients with tricuspid valve endocarditis are not at risk. Septic emboli of the arterial wall may be associated with a well-delineated "mycotic" aneurysm. If no aneurysm can be discerned by angiography, pyogenic arteritis is the presumptive arterial pathology. The distinction is important as only mycotic aneurysms are amenable to surgery. Pyogenic arteritis, however, more often leads to ICH. In one pathologic study of 16 patients with intracranial hemorrhage complicating infective endocarditis, 10 had pyogenic arteritis while only 5 had mycotic aneurysms. As previously mentioned, another important mechanism is hemorrhagic transformation of cerebral infarction due to septic embolization.

Mycotic aneurysms may result in subarachnoid hemorrhage or ICH. Usually, they are associated with embolic infarction or meningitis, or are asymptomatic. They may be the presenting feature of endocarditis, or may develop during antibiotic treatment.[11]

Preventing intracranial hemorrhage by searching angiographically or mycotic aneurysm in all patients with infective endocarditis may not be effective. Hart[9] argues that the number of patients who would actually benefit is small, 1.1% of his patients. Mycotic aneurysms have been variably reported in 2% to 10% of patients with infective endocarditis. A proportion of these patients will not be medically fit for surgery, or they will have surgically inaccessible or multiple mycotic aneurysms.

Surgical treatment appears more attractive from the perspective of a patient with a known mycotic aneurysm. Frazee et al[12] analyzed 13 such patients. All were treated with appropriate antibiotics and five underwent surgery. Six of the eight nonsurgically treated patients died, compared to none of the surgically treated patients. Brust et al[11] analyzed 17 patients with 28 documented mycotic aneurysms. Five patients experienced aneurysm rupture during or at the conclusion of antibiotic treatment, and two of these five died. All four patients who had surgery on unruptured aneurysms made uneventful recoveries. Of 20 aneurysms that were treated only with antibiotics, 10 became smaller or disappeared, but 10 became larger or remained the same. Based on this experience, Brust et al recommended prompt four-vessel angiography in any patient with infective endocarditis and neurologic abnormalities not attributable to systemic toxicity, including asymptomatic computed tomography findings or spinal fluid pleocytosis. Early surgery was recommended for medically stable patients if single, accessible, distal mycotic aneurysms were found. With multiple or proximal aneurysms, the decision needs to be individualized.

Vasculitis

Vasculitis secondary to drug abuse is a well-established pathologic entity. ICH is a more common complication of drug-related vasculitis than cerebral infarction, while the opposite is true with other forms of vasculitis. In 1970 Citron et al[13] reported 14 young drug abusers with necrotizing angiitis of multiple organs, indistinguishable from polyarteritis nodosa by clinical, angiographic, and histologic criteria. These patients abused multiple drugs, most often methamphetamine, heroin, and LSD; the most commonly abused drug was methamphetamine. At autopsy, one patient had cerebellar hemorrhage, cerebral and pontine infarcts, and changes typical of polyarteritis nodosa in her cerebral vessels. In two other studies, amphetamine, heroin, and cocaine abusers were found to have angiographic and histologic evidence of cerebral necrotizing vasculitis.[14,15] Rumbaugh et al[16,17] gave monkeys amphetamines and found that this produced histologic and angiographic evidence of cerebral vasculitis. One patient who took only phenylpropanolamine had an ICH evacuated, and histopathologic examination revealed necrotizing vasculitis.[18] Another patient[19] who abused only heroin had no cerebral pathology, but spinal cord biopsy revealed necrotizing vasculitis. Three patients have been reported[20,21] who took only cocaine and had acute and chronic inflammatory cells within their small cerebral arteries; other features of classic vasculitis such as fibrinoid necrosis and fragmentation of the elastic lamina were lacking.

Unfortunately, many reports in the literature allege that methylphenidate,[22] ephedrine,[23,24] pseudoephedrine,[25] or "Ts and Blues"[26] caused vasculitis, but they provide no histologic evidence. The diagnosis of vasculitis was made on the basis of angiographic findings including segmental narrowing and dilatation or "beading" of distal cerebral arteries. While this angiographic finding is seen with cerebral vasculitis, it is also found in many other conditions, such as vasospasm secondary to subarachnoid hemorrhage or to the drugs themselves, fibromuscular dysplasia, atherosclerosis, and multiple cerebral emboli. Two phenylpropanolamine users with ICH and beading on angiogram had biopsies that were negative for vasculitis.[27,28] Conclusive evidence for drug-related cerebral vasculitis has been shown only for amphetamines and phenylpropanolamine, and possibly for heroin and cocaine. Only a small proportion of those who abuse these drugs actually develop vasculitis.

Neurologists differ in how aggressively to pursue proof for vasculitis. Because some patients have histologic evidence for vasculitis with negative angiograms, meningeal biopsy is required to definitely exclude the diagnosis.[4,20–33] Furthermore, as already stressed, beading on angiogram may not be due to vasculitis, and the underlying etiology may be an infection or an unrelated disease. This strengthens the support for leptomeningeal biopsy, if no other tissue can be biopsied. Specimens should be sent to histology and microbiology. Neurologists opposing this approach argue that if the patient can abstain from drugs, the prognosis is good even without treatment, so perhaps no invasive investigations need to be performed.

The type of vasculitis following drug abuse has important therapeutic implications. True polyarteritis nodosa and isolated cerebral nervous system angiitis require corticosteroid and cyclophosphamide treatment. For polyarteritis nodosa, 5-year survival untreated is 13%, with corticosteroids it is 48%, and with corticosteroids plus cyclophosphamide it is 80%. However, different types of vasculitis exist in different patients. The 14 patients reported by Citron et al[13] had true polyarteritis nodosa. The patient with vasculitis secondary to phenylpropanolamine[18] had vasculitis confined to her central nervous system, but Glick et al[18] cite histologic evidence for an entity distinct from "isolated central nervous system angiitis." An amphetamine abuser with mononeuritis multiplex but no central nervous system involvement had a sural nerve biopsy that revealed hypersensitivity angiitis,[29] a type of vasculitis in which involvement of the central nervous system is rare. An abuser of amphetamines, heroin, and cocaine was found to have histologic evidence of vasculitis involving not only medium and small arteritis, but also elastic arteries.[15] The latter should be spared in true polyarteritis nodosa.

Data do not exist on how to treat patients with drug-induced cerebral vasculitis. Some neurologists have used no specific treatment. One patient was doing well after 6 months of no treatment.[14] Some have used corticosteroids only. One such patient who had a persistent fever became afebrile 48 hours after commencing steroids.[13] Some patients deteriorated despite steroids.[28,30,31]

However, deterioration occurred several days after initial intracranial hemorrhage and may have been due to cerebral edema. Some neurologists empirically use high-dose corticosteroids, such as prednisone 60 mg/day, plus cyclophosphamide, 2 mg/kg per day, for weeks to months.[18,32] Two such patients improved by clinical and angiographic criteria.

Long-term outcome of patients with drug-induced vasculitis has not been systematically reported. Many neurologists believe that if these patients abstain from drugs, their prognosis for recurrent stroke is excellent.

Human Immunodeficiency Virus Infection

Parenteral drug abusers are clearly at risk for developing human immunodeficiency virus (HIV) infection and the acquired immune deficiency syndrome (AIDS). Between 0.8% and 15% of patients with AIDS have developed ICH, the proportion being higher in autopsy than in clinical studies. HIV infection may present with stroke.[34]

The cause of stroke in HIV infection is often not found,[34] but many potential mechanisms may be responsible. The most common finding in AIDS patients with ICH is thrombocytopenia.[35] An illness akin to autoimmune thrombocytopenic purpura is often seen in patients with AIDS or in HIV-seropositive patients.[36] Thrombocytopenia may also be secondary to the drug abuse that led to AIDS. Patients with AIDS also may develop disseminated intravascular coagulation which, in conjunction with nonbacterial thrombotic endocarditis, can produce thrombotic or hemorrhagic strokes.[37] Patients with AIDS may develop hemorrhage into brain tumors, or ICH may follow a neurosurgical procedure. Vasculitis and other vasculopathies occur with HIV infection, as HIV can directly infect vascular endothelial cells.[35] Vasculopathies may also follow other AIDS-related infections, such as syphilis, aspergillus, tuberculosis, herpes zoster, toxoplasmosis, cytomegalovirus, or cryptococcus.

Platelet Abnormalities

Thrombocytopenia in association with drug abuse was first reported in 1978, when five heroin users presented with a syndrome resembling autoimmune thrombocytopenic purpura.[38] Since then, many abusers of heroin or cocaine have been reported with thrombocytopenia and a syndrome indistinguishable from autoimmune thrombocytopenic purpura with increased megakaryocytes in the bone marrow, peripheral destruction of antibody coated platelets, negative antinuclear antibody, and a therapeutic response to prednisone or splenectomy. These patients typically present with petechiae, bruising, epistaxis, and gastrointestinal or genitourinary bleeding. ICH is uncommon, but does occur. Most of these patients either had AIDS or were found to be HIV-seropositive. In one series of 15 patients with narcotic-related immunopathic thrombocytopenic purpura, 13 were HIV-seropositive.[39] More recently, however, six habitual cocaine users were reported[40] with immunopathic thrombocytopenic purpura, and they were all HIV-seronegative.

The natural history of this illness is unpredictable[40] and it may remit spontaneously. Of 79 HIV-seropositive homosexuals without AIDS, with autoimmune thrombocytopenic purpura, 9 spontaneously reverted to normal platelet counts 5 to 27 months after the diagnosis, without splenectomy or corticosteroids. When treated, these patients generally receive prednisone, 30 to 40 mg/day for 1 to 2 weeks and then are rapidly tapered to a maintenance dose of 10 to 15 mg/day.[39] The aim is to use the lowest corticosteroid dose that will result in a platelet count over 25,000/μl, without significant purpura. The patient is then observed for 10 months. If the patient requires more than 10 to 15 mg of prednisone/day at this stage, splenectomy is advised. Of 22 narcotic addicts treated in this way,[39] 6 had a complete response to corticosteroids, 13 a moderate response (platelets rose to over 50,000/μl), and 3 did not respond. Two patients responded to splenectomy, one completely and the other partially. Of six patients with cocaine-related thrombocytopenia who were HIV-seronegative,[40] five achieved normal platelet counts within 10 days of starting prednisone. The dose was tapered over 4 weeks without relapse. The one remaining patient had a partial response and, after 7 weeks, and had a splenectomy with subsequent normalization of platelet counts.

Animal studies illustrate that cocaine can result in qualitative, as well as quantitative, platelet defects. High, but not low, doses of cocaine were found to block the aggregating effects of collagen and ADP on platelets in rabbit platelet-rich plasma.[41]

Hepatitis

Drug addicts who share "dirty" needles often become infected with hepatitis B. This may result in massive hepatic necrosis or chronic active hepatitis and cirrhosis. Drug addicts may also develop δ hepatitis, which only occurs in patients also infected with hepatitis B. δ Hepatitis increases the likelihood of developing massive hepatic necrosis, and may contribute to the severity of chronic hepatitis B. Hepatitis C is usually due to blood transfusion and not parenteral drug abuse, and often leads to chronic active hepatitis and, occasionally, cirrhosis.

Patients with massive hepatic necrosis or significant chronic liver disease have a bleeding diathesis which may contribute to the development of ICH. Patients with chronic active hepatitis, cirrhosis, or massive hepatic necrosis have dysfibrinogenemia and decreased coagulation factors, and those with hypersplenism may also have thrombocytopenia. Massive hepatic necrosis may also result in disseminated intravascular coagulation. Rarely, patients with hepatitis B develop polyarteritis nodosa or glomerulonephritis.

Tablet Filler Emboli

Drug abusers who dissolve tablets and then inject them allow showers of insoluble tablet fillers like talc and cornstarch to enter their circulation. These patients usually develop pulmonary granulomata.[26] Eventually, they develop pulmonary hypertension with pulmonary arteriovenous fistulae, providing a path for insoluble tablet fillers to enter the cerebral circulation. Patients have been reported with retinal lesions[42] and cerebral infarcts[43] following apparent paradoxical embolism of tablet fillers, and one Ts and Blues addict was believed to have developed his frontal hematoma from such a mechanism.[26]

Individual Drugs

Cocaine

Cocaine is a sympathomimetic, a central nervous system stimulant and a local anesthetic. It prevents norepinephrine and serotonin reuptake, producing hypertension and vasoconstriction. There are two forms: cocaine hydrochloride (HCl) has an average purity of 58% and cannot be smoked. The alkaloidal forms, "crack" and "freebase," became available around 1983. They are purer, cheaper, can be smoked, and are quite popular. The two forms of cocaine seem to differ in the types of strokes they typically cause.[44] The hydrochloride salt (powder) of cocaine is more commonly associated with hemorrhagic stroke (ICH or subarachnoid hemorrhage) and an underlying cerebrovascular malformation than alkaloidal cocaine.[44] Cocaine hydrochloride-associated stroke is hemorrhagic about 4 of 5 times, compared to about half of the time with alkaloidal cocaine.

Cocaine abuse in the United States has reached alarming proportions. In a survey of U.S. households in 1972, 9.1% of people aged 18 to 25 years admitted to using cocaine. In 1985, this figure rose to 25.2%. In 1985, 7.6% of those aged 18 to 25 years admitted to using cocaine in the past month. Figures were lower for those outside this age range, but they were still alarming.[45] In two recent studies of recreational drug-associated strokes, cocaine was the most common drug implicated. Cocaine use occurred in 57% of drug-related strokes admitted between 1979 and 1988,[1] and in 45% of 11 patients with stroke historically associated with drug abuse between 1988 and 1989.[5]

Most cocaine-related strokes occur in close temporal relationship to drug use. A history of cocaine use immediately before symptom onset was obtained in 6 of 9 patients with intracranial hemorrhages. All nine patients had cocaine metabolites in their urine.[46] In a series of 28 patients with "crack"-associated stroke, patients were only included if their stroke occurred within 72 hours of drug administration, and 18 of these patients (64%), had neurologic symptoms either immediately or within 1 hour of using cocaine.[47] Hemorrhagic strokes have been described after intranasal use ("snorting"), smoking of the alkaloidal forms, or intravenous use. In utero exposure to cocaine can result in ICH, cerebral infarcts, and other abnormalities in infants.[48]

It is difficult to blame adulterants for cocaine-related ICH. Of common cocaine adulterants, only phenylpropanolamine (PPA) can cause stroke, but PPA was not identified in any of 16 patients with cocaine-associated stroke who had toxicology testing.[44,47] Concomitant use of alcohol and heroin might conceivably cause stroke, but in one large series, 39% of patients with cocaine-associated stroke were discovered to have used only cocaine. Alcohol is associated with hemorrhagic stroke, but the evidence is strongest for chronic habitual drinking rather than acute recent binge drinking.[49] The importance of concomitant alcohol use is its ability to depress the degradation of cocaine. As will be mentioned below, heroin rarely causes ICH unless it has caused endocarditis, liver disease, or nephropathy.

Of 105 cocaine-related strokes, 34 were ICHs.[44] Of these, 27 had an angiogram or an autopsy, 6 had arteriovenous malformations, 4 had aneurysms, 1 had a venous angioma, and 15 had normal vasculature. Cocaine-related ICHs have usually been lobar or in the basal ganglia. One patient who smoked "crack" and consumed large quantities of alcohol developed simultaneous multiple, bilateral, deep and superficial intracerebral hematomas.[50]

Amphetamines

Amphetamines are sympathomimetics and central nervous system stimulants that act by stimulating the release of biogenic amines from axon terminals. They produce acute hypertension and vasoconstriction, and may result in vasculitides of different types.

Most amphetamine-related strokes have been hemorrhagic strokes. Brust[33] reviewed the literature and found 32 patients with amphetamine-related hemorrhagic stroke. Patients were 16 to 60 years of age. Eighteen had taken the drug orally, 9 intravenously, 2 orally and intravenously, 1 nasally and intravenously, and 2 by uncertain route. Most were chronic users, but in 5 patients stroke followed a first exposure. The dose in one case was quite low. Severe headache usually occurred within minutes of drug administration. Blood pressure was elevated in many in whom it was taken early enough. Eight patients died. Angiography revealed beading in 12 patients, and vasculitis was found at autopsy in 3 patients, including 1 whose angiogram did not show features of vasculitis. Only 1 patient had an underlying cerebral vascular malformation.

Phenylpropanolamine

Phenylpropanolamine, sometimes with ephedrine or other drugs, is contained in many over-the-counter diet pills and decongestant medications. It can also be sold illicitly as an amphetamine-like stimulant, as it is structurally and pharmacologically similar to amphetamines. Compared to amphetamines, phenylpropanolamine is more potent in its peripheral sympathomimetic effects such as hypertension and vasoconstriction, and less potent as a central nervous system stimulant. In healthy volunteers, acute severe hypertension can occur after ingesting even recommended over-the-counter doses of phenylpropanolamine.

Kase et al[28] reported two patients with ICHs secondary to phenylpropanolamine and reviewed the literature on the subject. Most patients with phenylpropanolamine-related ICHs have been young, predominantly women, without a prior history of hypertension. Most ICH occurred within hours of first time ingestion. Some patients were taking only phenylpropanolamine, while others were taking tablets that contained other drugs. The amounts of phenylpropanolamine taken were, in nearly half of the cases, within the recommended dose of 75 mg/day for appetite control. One patient had multiple simultaneous ICHs, a rare presentation for nontraumatic ICH.[51] Several of the patients reviewed by Kase et al had beading on their angiogram, while other patients had normal angiograms. Only one patient has had histologically documented vasculitis secondary to phenylpropanolamine.[18] She was taking a diet pill that contained phenylpropanolamine, stopped using it for several months while she was pregnant, then ingested one pill 3 weeks postpartum and developed ICH 90 minutes later.

Other Amphetamine-Like Over-the-Counter Sympathomimetics

Ephedrine has been used for many years as a bronchodilator and nasal decongestant and is generally safe when used in recommended doses. In recent years it has been used illicitly as a stimulant. One man[23] developed a subarachnoid hemorrhage within 1 hour of taking what he thought was amphetamines. Urinary drug screening using highly-specific techniques revealed only ephedrine. Angiography on the day of admission was normal. However, 1 week later repeat angiography revealed beading. A biopsy of normal skin revealed evidence for immune complex deposition. Wooten et al[23] believe this man had vasculitis secondary to ephedrine, but others[24] believe the evidence was not conclusive.

Pseudoephedrine is a very weak sympathomimetic. It is not a drug of addiction or abuse. A 17-year-old girl attempted suicide by ingesting 20 pseudoephedrine tablets, and 24 hours later developed a frontal ICH. Seven days after hemorrhage, angiography revealed beading of the intracranial arteries.[25]

Heroin

Most heroin-associated strokes are ischemic.[52] Hemorrhagic strokes in heroin addicts may be secondary to infective endocarditis or to liver disease. Heroin commonly causes nephropathy, and one heroin addict has been reported[51] with massive ICH, likely secondary to severe hypertension and azotemia. There is only one reported case of ICH related to heroin not due to endocarditis or renal or liver disease.[53]

Phencyclidine

Phencyclidine (PCP) is a dissociative anesthetic used in veterinary medicine. In recent years its abuse has been increasing. The mechanism of action is not well understood and may involve interference with association pathways linking the cerebral cortex with deeper structures in the brain. PCP is also thought to be a strong central and weak peripheral anticholinergic agent. Other investigators stress the adrenergic effects of PCP, which may be taken orally, smoked, or injected intravenously. It is sometimes smoked inadvertently by persons who think it is marijuana. PCP can cause vasoconstriction and hypertension. In one study[54] of 1,000 cases of PCP intoxication, 570 (57%) had hypertension which occasionally was severe, but none of these patients had stroke. There are three case reports of hemorrhagic stroke secondary to PCP.[55–57] One patient had an ICH,[56] one a subarachnoid hemorrhage,[57] and one a subarachnoid and intraventricular hemorrhage.[55] None of them was over 20 years old. One was found to have a perforation in the ventral surface of his basilar artery,[57] the particular site where the embryologic development and regression of the trigeminal artery occurs. No vasculitis was found histologically. Rupture presumably occurred due to the combination of acute severe hypertension and congenital structural weakness at this site.

Treatment mainly involves supportive care. There is no specific antidote, but excretion from the body can be enhanced by acidification of urine and gastric lavage. Psychosis is a serious problem, and there is a risk of suicide and violence to others. Phenothiazines should not be used in these patients because they may potentiate PCP's anticholinergic effects. Haloperidol (5-mg intramuscularly, hourly as needed) may be used.

Pentazocine and Tripelennamine

Pentazocine and tripelennamine ("Ts and Blues") abuse began in Chicago in the late 1970s. Pentazocine has both opioid agonist and antagonist effects. Its cerebral effects are similar to those of the opioids. Tripelennamine is an antihistamine which is said to prolong and heighten the euphoria attributed to pentazocine. Both compounds are produced only as oral forms, but addicts dissolve them in water and inject them.

Caplan et al[26] reported 13 patients with neurologic complications of "Ts and Blues." Two of these patients had ICH. One had infective endocarditis and a ruptured mycotic aneurysm. The other patient had a frontal hematoma.

Angiography revealed occlusions in some branches of the middle cerebral artery, with several areas of extravasated contrast and irregular beading of small arteries. Possible mechanisms included vascular damage by foreign material or by immunologic mechanisms.

Toxicology Screens

Issues involved in toxicology screening have been well reviewed by Mullen and Bracha.[58] Ideally, the following should be sent to the laboratory:

1. The suspected agents, the time of ingestion, and the time of sampling.
2. A 50-ml sample of urine.
3. Two 3-ml samples of blood, one containing whole blood (anticoagulated with oxalate and preserved with fluoride) and one containing blood clots from which serum can be obtained. Some assays are traditionally performed on whole blood, while others are performed on serum. Phencyclidine is usually searched for only in the urine, and the only agents screened for in blood and not urine are the alcohols and propranolol. However, without blood screening the potential exists for missing an ingested substance because it has not yet been excreted in the urine, either because of long half-life or very recent ingestion.
4. Gastric fluid (obtained by emesis or lavage) may be a useful adjunct.
5. Pills and contraband.

Many different tests are available to screen for drugs, including immunoassay (radioimmunoassay, enzyme-multiplied immunoassay, fluorescent polarized immunoassay), ultraviolet spectroscopy, thin-layer chromatography, gas chromatography coupled with mass spectrometry, and high-pressure liquid chromatography.

All these tests are highly sensitive. Rare false-negatives occur when:

1. The wrong patient's sample is sent.
2. The urine sample is taken too early (very soon after ingestion) or too late. Duration of excretion is discussed later in this section.
3. Patients may try to avoid detection by using someone else's urine, or adulterating their urine with various substances such as salt, vinegar, soap, or blood. Whenever possible, urine samples should be collected under direct observation.

Gas chromatography coupled with mass spectrometry and thin-layer chromatography are highly specific. False-positive results are almost impossible. Large laboratories often only report a positive result after it has been tested by three different procedures, so false-positive results are even less likely. The more specific tests tend to be expensive and require skillful technicians, while other tests are easily performed and inexpensive but less specific. For example, the enzyme-multiplied immunoassay for amphetamines cross-reacts with phenylpropanolamine and ephedrine, the opiate test may be positive if poppy seeds have been ingested, and the marijuana enzyme-multiplied immunoassay can react with ibuprofen. Generally, problems are avoided where the simpler techniques are complemented by more specific tests available on a regional basis.

The duration of urinary detectability varies for different drugs and under different circumstances. For example, the duration of detectability may be lengthened by significant kidney, liver, or heart disease; by alkalinizing or acidifying the urine; or with chronic abuse as opposed to first time use. Cocaine is very rapidly eliminated, but cocaine metabolites such as benzoylecgonine can be detected in the urine for 2 to 3 days in first time users and for 10 to 22 days in chronic users of large doses.[59] The duration of detectability is generally about four urine half-lives. The urine half-life of amphetamine ranges from 7 to 34 hours. When the urine is acidified, the half-life is at the shorter end of the range, and when the urine is alkaline, it reaches the longer end. Thus, under alkalinization amphetamine is detectable for about a week. PCP's urine half-life ranges from 7 to 16 hours. In severe poisoning, a half-life up to 4 days has been recorded, perhaps due to renal dysfunction. The urine half-life of ephedrine is 5 to 7.5 hours, for morphine 1.3 to 6.7 hours, and for pentazocine 2.1 to 3.5 hours.

Summary and Recommendations

Any patient with ICH, particularly if the patient is young, needs a systematic inquiry into the use of recreational drugs, diet pills, or sympathomimetic decongestants (Table 4). Urine, blood, and possibly also gastric fluid and the drugs themselves should be sent for toxicology screening. The duration of detectability of most drugs is over 24 hours in the urine, and chronic abusers of cocaine may have cocaine metabolites detectable in their urine for many days. Toxicology screens are highly sensitive, and the more expensive techniques are highly specific. Cocaine is the commonest drug to be associated with ICH.

Consideration should also be given to the mechanism of ICH. Endocarditis needs to be diligently ruled out because, while uncommon, it must be treated with antibiotics. HIV infection should also be considered, and thrombocyto-

---

Table 4
Intracerebral Hemorrhage and Drug Use

1. Any user is at risk, including first time users.
2. Any route is dangerous.
3. Any dose can lead to ICH.
4. Regardless of long-term prognosis for recurrence, ICH mortality is high.

---

penia should be ruled out. Thrombocytopenia in a young patient with ICH should prompt a search for HIV and cocaine and heroin use.

Four-vessel conventional cerebral angiography is indicated in patients with drug-related ICH. This may reveal a vascular anomaly, beading, or no abnormalities. Regardless of the presence of beading, the diagnosis of vasculitis requires histologic examination of involved brain along with a sample of leptomeninges. The natural history of drug-related vasculitis and its treatment are not known. No specific treatment can be recommended because an impression exists that, if the patient can abstain from drug use, recurrent stroke is unlikely. Others have empirically used high doses of corticosteroids plus cyclophosphamide. If the patient abstains from drugs, vascular anomalies are repaired, endocarditis or thrombocytopenia are treated, and prognosis from the point of view of recurrent stroke is excellent. However, mortality and morbidity from the presenting ICH is still unacceptably high.

References

1. Kaku DA, Lowenstein DH: Emergence of recreational drug abuse as a major risk factor for stroke in young adults. *Ann Intern Med* 1990;113:821.
2. Jick H, Aselton P, Hunter JR: Phenylpropanolamine and cerebral hemorrhage (letter). *Lancet* 1984;1:1017.
3. Jacobs IG, Roszler MH, Kelly JK, et al: Cocaine abuse: neurovascular complications. *Radiology* 1989;170:223.
4. Sloan MA, Kittner SJ, Rigamonti D, et al: Occurrence of stroke associated with use/abuse of drugs. *Neurology* 1991;41:1358.
5. Toffol GJ, Biller J, Adams HP: Nontraumatic intracranial hemorrhage in young adults. *Arch Neurol* 1987;44:483.
6. Lacey JR, Fillely CM, Earnest MP: Brain infarction and hemorrhage in young and middle-aged adults. *West J Med* 1984;141:329.
7. Caplan L: Intracerebral hemorrhage revisited. *Neurology* 1988;38:624.
8. Hart RG, Foster JW, Luther MF, et al: Stroke in infective endocarditis. *Stroke* 1990;21:695.
9. Hart RG, Kagan-Hallet K, Joerns SE: Mechanisms of intracranial hemorrhage in infective endocarditis. *Stroke* 1987;18:1048.
10. Masuda J, Yutani C, Waki R, et al: Histopathological analysis of the mechanisms of intracranial hemorrhage complicating infective endocarditis. *Stroke* 1992;23:843.
11. Brust JCM, Dickinson PCT, Hughes JEO, et al: The diagnosis and treatment of cerebral mycotic aneurysms. *Ann Neurol* 1990;27:238.
12. Frazee JG, Cahan LD, Winter J: Bacterial intracranial aneurysms. *J Neurosurg* 1980;53:633.
13. Citron BP, Halpern M, McCarron M, et al: Necrotizing angiitis associated with drug abuse. *N Engl J Med* 1970;283:1003.
14. Kessler JT, Jortner BS, Adapon BD: Cerebral vasculitis in a drug abuser. *J Clin Psychiatry* 1978;39:559.

15. Bostwick DG: Amphetamine induced vasculitis. *Hum Pathol* 1981;12:1031.
16. Rumbaugh CL, Fang HCH, Higgins RE, et al: Cerebral microvascular injury in experimental drug abuse. *Investig Radiol* 1976;11:282.
17. Rumbaugh CL, Bergeron RT, Scanlan RL, et al: Cerebral vascular changes secondary to amphetamine abuse in the experimental animal. *Radiology* 1971;101:345.
18. Glick R, Hoying J, Cerullo L, et al: Phenylpropanolamine: an over-the-counter drug causing central nervous system vasculitis and intracerebral hemorrhage. Case report and review. *Neurosurgery* 1987;20:969.
19. Judice DJ, LeBlanc HJ, McGarry PA: Spinal cord vasculitis presenting as a spinal cord tumor in a heroin addict. Case report. *J Neurosurg* 1987;48:131.
20. Krendel DA, Ditter SM, Frankel MR, et al: Biopsy-proven cerebral vasculitis associated with cocaine abuse. *Neurology* 1990;40:1092.
21. Fredericks RK, Lefkowitz DS, Challa VR, et al: Cerebral vasculitis associated with cocaine abuse. *Stroke* 1991;22:1437.
22. Trugman JM: Cerebral arteritis and oral methylphenidate (letter). *Lancet* 1988;1:584.
23. Wooten MR, Khangure MS, Murphy MJ: Intracerebral hemorrhage and vasculitis related to ephedrine abuse. *Ann Neurol* 1983;13:337.
24. Nadeau SE: Intracerebral hemorrhage and vasculitis related to ephedrine abuse (letter). *Ann Neurol* 1984;15:114.
25. Loizou LA, Hamilton JG, Tsementzis SA: Intracerebral hemorrhage in association with pseudoephedrine overdose (letter). *J Neurol Neurosurg Psychiatry* 1982;45:471.
26. Caplan LR, Thomas C, Banks G: Central nervous system complications of addiction to "T's and Blues." *Neurology* 1982;32:623.
27. Forman HP, Levin S, Steward B, et al: Cerebral vasculitis and hemorrhage in an adolescent taking diet pills containing phenylpropanolamine: case-report and review of literature. *Pediatrics* 1989;33:737.
28. Kase CS, Foster TE, Reed JE, et al: Intracerebral hemorrhage and phenylpropanolamine use. *Neurology* 1987;37:399.
29. Stafford CR, Bogdanoff BM, Green L, et al: Mononeuropathy multiplex as a complication of amphetamine angiitis. *Neurology* 1975;25:570.
30. Matick H, Anderson D, Brumlik J: Cerebral vasculitis associated with oral amphetamine overdose. *Arch Neurol* 1983;40:253.
31. Margolis MT, Newton TH: Methamphetamine ("speed") arteritis. *Neuroradiology* 1971;2:179.
32. Salanova V, Taubner R: Intracerebral hemorrhage and vasculitis secondary to amphetamine use. *Postgrad Med J* 1984;60:429.
33. Brust JCM: Stroke and substance abuse. In: Barnett HJM, Mohr JP, Stein BM, et al., eds: *Stroke: Pathophysiology, Diagnosis and Management.* New York: Churchill-Livingston Inc., 1986:903.
34. Engstrom JW, Lowenstein DH, Bredesen DE: Cerebral infarctions and transient neurological deficits associated with acquired immunodeficiency syndrome. *Am J Med* 1989;86:528.

35. Mizusawa H, Hirano A, Llene JF, et al: Cerebrovascular lesions in acquired immune deficiency syndrome (AIDS). *Acta Neuropathol* 1988;76:451.

36. Walsh C, Krigel R, Lennette E, et al: Thrombocytopenia in homosexual patients, prognosis, response to therapy, and prevalence of antibody to the retrovirus associated with the acquired immunodeficiency syndrome. *Ann Intern Med* 1985;103:542.

37. Schwartzman RJ, Hill JB: Neurologic complications of disseminated intravascular coagulation. *Neurology* 1992;32:791.

38. Adams WH, Rufo RA, Talarico L, et al: Thrombocytopenia and intravenous heroin use. *Ann Intern Med* 1978;89:207.

39. Karpatkin S: Immunologic thrombocytopenic purpura in HIV-seropositive homosexuals, narcotic addicts and hemophiliacs. *Semin Hematol* 1988;25: 219.

40. Leissinger CA: Severe thrombocytopenia associated with cocaine use. *Ann Intern Med* 1990;112:708.

41. Togna G, Tempesta E, Togna AR, et al: Platelet responsiveness and biosynthesis of thromboxane and prostacyclin in response to in vitro cocaine treatment. *Hemostasis* 1985;15:100.

42. Tse DT, Ober RR: Talc retinopathy. *Am J Ophthal* 1980;90:624.

43. Mizutani T, Lewis RA, Gonatas NK: Medial medullary syndrome in a drug abuser. *Arch Neurol* 1980;37:425.

44. Levine SR, Brust JCM, Futrell N, et al: A comparative study of the cerebrovascular complications of cocaine: alkaloidal versus hydrochloride — a review. *Neurology* 1991;41:1173.

45. Rouse BA: Trends in cocaine use in the general population. In: Schober S, Schede C, eds: *The Epidemiology of Cocaine Use and Abuse.* National Institute on Drug Abuse Research Monograph 110, Alcohol, Drug Abuse and Mental Health Administration, U.S. Public Health Services, Department of Health and Human Services. 1991:5.

46. Mangiardi JR, Daras M, Geller ME, et al: Cocaine related intracerebral hemorrhage. Report of nine cases and review. *Acta Neurol Scand* 1988;77: 177.

47. Levine SL, Brust JCM, Futrell N, et al: Cerebrovascular complications of the use of the "crack" form of alkaloidal cocaine. *N Engl J Med* 1990;323: 699.

48. Dominguez R, Vila-Coro AA, Slopis JM, et al: Brain and ocular abnormalities in infants with in utero exposure to cocaine and other street drugs. *Am J Dis Child* 1991;145:688.

49. Camargo CA: Moderate alcohol consumption and stroke, the epidemiologic evidence. *Stroke* 1989;20:1611.

50. Green RM, Kelly KM, Gabrielsen T, et al: Multiple intracerebral hemorrhages after smoking "crack" cocaine. *Stroke* 1990;21:957.

51. Weisberg L: Multiple spontaneous intracerebral hematomas: clinical and computed tomographic correlations. *Neurology* 1981;31:897.

52. Brust JCM, Richter RW: Stroke associated with addiction to heroin. *J Neurol Neurosurg Psychiatry* 1976;39:194.

53. Knoblauch AL, Buchholz M, Koller MG, et al: Hemiplegie nach injektion von heroin. *Schweiz Med Wochenschr* 1983;113:402.
54. McCarron MM, Schulze BW, Thompson GA, et al: Acute phencyclidine intoxication: incidence of clinical findings in 1,000 cases. *Ann Emerg Med* 1981;10:237.
55. Bessen HA: Intracranial hemorrhage associated with phencyclidine abuse. *JAMA* 1982;248:585.
56. Eastman JW, Cohen SN: Hypertensive crisis and death associated with phencyclidine poisoning. *JAMA* 1975;231:1270.
57. Boyko OB, Burger PC, Heinz R: Pathological and radiological correlation of subarachnoid hemorrhage in phencyclidine abuse. Case report. *J Neurosurg* 1987;67:446.
58. Mullen J, Bracha HS: Toxicology screening, how to assure accurate results. *Postgrad Med* 1988;84:141.
59. Weiss RD, Gawin FH: Protracted elimination of cocaine metabolites in long-term, high dose cocaine abusers. *Am J Med* 1988;85:879.

Chapter 5

Anticoagulation

Conrado J. Estol, MD

During the last two decades, there has been dramatic progress in stroke diagnosis. However, these advances have not been paralleled by therapeutic developments. Public awareness regarding cerebrovascular diseases is very low, considering that stroke is the third most common cause of death after cardiovascular disease and cancer.[1] Anticoagulation (ATC) is one of the few modalities presently accepted in the treatment of stroke, but the lack of scientific data supporting its efficacy results in more debate than agreement.

Some of the unanswered questions on this issue include: Which patients benefit from ATC? When and for how long should ATC be used? What agent should be selected? What is the optimal therapeutic range of oral ATC? The answers to these questions may have an impact on the incidence of ATC-related hemorrhages.

Unlike other treatments in the daily management of stroke, with ATC the physician confronts the risk of an intracranial hemorrhage as a potential complication. This fear is especially high in physicians without expertise in stroke treatment. For patients who receive ATC, strict monitoring of the anticoagulant status according to standardized tests is the most effective mechanism available against ATC-related hemorrhages.

This chapter focuses on the importance of standardized laboratory determinations of the prothrombin time (PT); the relation of specific risk factors to the occurrence of ATC-related hemorrhage; the incidence of hemorrhage in different studies; the clinical findings; the probable mechanisms of bleeding, treatment, and analysis of hemorrhagic infarctions; and a review of special situations, such as patients with prosthetic heart valves and bacterial endocarditis.

Indications for Anticoagulation

After a presumptive stroke mechanism has been identified, ATC should be considered in appropriate patients after a thorough discussion of benefits

From Feldmann E (ed). *Intracerebral Hemorrhage*. Armonk, NY: Futura Publishing Company, Inc., © 1994.

versus risks with patient and family. Obviously, if the patient cannot be followed carefully or the PT cannot be measured reliably, ATC carries a risk which will outweigh its potential benefit.

Anticoagulation is used empirically in certain patients with stroke. A recent review of 25 patients with angiographically-documented large artery disease of the carotid and vertebrobasilar circulation addressed the issue of ATC in atherothrombotic stroke.[2] All patients presented with symptoms appropriate to their large artery disease and were followed on warfarin for 5 months to 8 years. Eighteen patients were treated for 2 years or more. During follow-up, 17 patients had no further ischemic events, 4 had only single, minor transient ischemic attacks (TIAs), and 4 had recurrence of their original ischemic events. A hemorrhagic complication was observed in one patient who recovered fully on conservative therapy. The authors' recommendations for ATC therapy included: acute occlusion of a large extracranial or intracranial artery with only a mild to moderate deficit, symptomatic stenosis of a large intracranial artery such as the middle cerebral artery or basilar artery, and symptomatic extracranial internal carotid artery disease in patients with contraindications for endarterectomy.

More conclusive evidence that ATC is effective in primary and secondary stroke prevention is available for patients with atrial fibrillation and cardiogenic cerebral embolism.[3-5] The role of ATC for hypercoagulable states, such as the antiphospholipid antibody syndrome, is under study.[6,7]

Some studies have analyzed the efficacy of heparin separately from oral anticoagulants. Miller and Hart[8] found support to use heparin in progressing stroke, acute, partial stroke, recent TIA, and cardioembolic stroke, although they discourage the use of heparin in completed thrombotic stroke. On the other hand, reviews by Phillips[9] and Scheinberg[10] strongly argue against the use of heparin.

These contradictory opinions arise from shortcomings in the literature such as the lack of blinded, randomized, controlled trials, small numbers of patients, inclusion of multiple stroke subtypes, no information on past cerebrovascular symptoms, larger number of male patients, and overlapping of heparin and warfarin use.[11] The data available do not provide proof of ATC efficacy in atherothrombotic stroke, but rather suggest that it is safe to use ATC in a few, well-defined, cerebrovascular scenarios.[2]

Therapeutic Anticoagulation: What Do We Mean?

The term "therapeutic" depends heavily on the origin of the literature analyzed. Important differences arise, with serious clinical implications, when comparing the hematologic and neurologic British and U.S. literature on ATC.[12-14] This problem derives from the use of different reagents in the determination of the PT. The PT in patients treated with ATC measures the activity of oral anticoagulants in neutralizing vitamin K dependent factors X, IX, VII, and II from the clotting cascade. To perform the test, thromboplastin is added to a sample of citrated blood and the time that it takes to form a clot is measured. The PT in patients not receiving ATC (control) is 10 to 12 seconds. This value will be prolonged proportional to the dose of oral anticoagulants received by the patient.

Different thromboplastins used for this test have different sensitivities. Some thromboplastins are more sensitive for deficiency in vitamin K dependent factors, thus better reflecting the actual anticoagulant status of the patient. If a less sensitive thromboplastin is used, the PT obtained will underestimate the actual degree of ATC for that patient.

The thromboplastin used in the United Kingdom and in some countries of South America is derived from human brain and is very sensitive. In the U.S., however, the thromboplastin is derived from rabbit brain, which is less sensitive. In the U.S., a in PT ratio of 2 (patient time/control time) represents a PT ratio of 4 for assays employing human brain thromboplastin. This results in excessively prolonged PTs, which correlate with an increase in the risk of hemorrhage. To reach a 2- to 2.5-fold increase of the PT ratio (for human brain thromboplastin), the PT employing rabbit thromboplastin should be increased to only 1.3 to 1.5 times the normal control.

In 1977 and 1982, in an attempt to standardize results, the World Health Organization established a preparation of human brain thromboplastin to be used as reference for calibration of other thromboplastins. Following these guidelines, the International Society of Hematology proposed that the PT should be reported as an International Normalized Ratio (INR).[13,15] The INR is obtained by plotting the logarithm of the PT value using the reference thromboplastin against the logarithm of the PT value corresponding to the plasma sample to be calibrated. The slope of the line obtained represents the International Sensitivity Index (ISI). The conversion of the PT *ratio* obtained from an anticoagulated plasma to the INR is performed by applying the ISI as the power of the ratio: $INR = ratio^{ISI}$. The INR is the PT ratio that would be obtained if the reference thromboplastin were used for the test. To perform these calculations, one must know the ISI, which is available for most thromboplastins in use. Conversion tables are available.

When a laboratory in the U.S. (using rabbit brain thromboplastin) reports a PT value that is 1.5 times control, the INR using the reference human thromboplastin is approximately 2.1. The INR is the ATC value that should be considered when deciding on the degree of ATC necessary for each patient.

Until a few years ago, these corrections were not taken into consideration when treating patients. It was common to have patients with PT ratios of 2 to 2.5 times control in the U.S., equivalent to an INR of 4.5 to 7.[16] These PT values were excessively prolonged and might account for some of the hemorrhages occurring during anticoagulant treatment.[17-26] Another confounding factor is the variable method of reporting PT: as a percent of a control plasma sample, as time (seconds), or as a ratio (patient time/control time).

A questionnaire performed at six medical centers involving 52 house officers and 30 attending neurologists assessed the actual ATC parameters used, measured as the PT ratio.[27] The average PT ratio was 1.82 for attending neurologists and 1.69 for house officers. Prothrombin time ratios of 2 or greater were used by 40% of attending neurologists and 18% of house officers. The authors concluded that many physicians, especially those whose training had taken place 15 or more years earlier, were using oral ATC parameters above the presently recommended values; therefore increasing the risk of hemorrhagic complications. Various studies have shown that a PT of 1.3 to 1.4 times the control (INR = 2–3), using the less sensitive rabbit brain thromboplastin is effective for treatment of venous thrombosis, high-risk surgical patients, and prevention of stroke related to myocardial infarction or cardioversion of atrial fibrillation.[28–31]

Based on empiric data, a PT increase to 1.3 to 1.5 the control (INR = 2-3) has been used for treatment of symptomatic atherostenotic cerebrovascular lesions.[1,2] However, cerebrovascular diseases have underlying mechanisms different from venous thrombosis and other disorders. The PT ratio effective of other conditions might not be effective for stroke. Levine and Hirsh reviewed 15 studies of patients treated with ATC for TIA and minor stroke to determine the safety and efficacy of this treatment.[12] The authors concluded that since the risk of major bleeding was greater than 2% per year and the reduction for stroke and death was approximately 20% to 30% overall, the use of anticoagulant therapy in minor stroke was not justified. These conclusions are strongly influenced by the shortcomings inherent in the studies analyzed, most of which were designed and completed several decades ago.

Well-designed studies to assess the efficacy of anticoagulant therapy in cerebrovascular disease are lacking, but recently have been initiated. Keith and colleagues estimated that approximately 1,200 patients would be necessary to determine, with statistical power, a 30% to 50% reduction in stroke risk within a month of a TIA.[32]

Epidemiology and Risk Factors for Anticoagulation-Related Hemorrhages

Anticoagulation-related bleeding is clinically similar for warfarin and heparin and is responsible for 10% to 20% of all ICH in different series.[33–36] Of patients treated with ATC, the incidence of ICH can approach 7%,[37,38] but the data vary greatly from study to study. Forfar followed 501 anticoagulated patients for 7 years and found an 8.2% incidence of hemorrhage, with 0.4% of them intracranial.[39] In another study of 3,862 patients, there were 263 (6.8%) episodes of bleeding, but only 5 (0.1%) were intracranial.[37] Whisnant et al.[40] studied patients with TIAs and noted an eightfold increased risk of intracerebral hemorrhage (ICH) in patients receiving ATC. Furlan et al[41] observed a sixfold increased risk of ATC-related ICH among 20 patients. Anticoagulation-related hemorrhage is believed to be especially prevalent in older[18–20,42] or hypertensive[12,18,20–22,37,43] patients. In one retrospective study of patients with ICH secondary to oral ATC, the relative risk of ICH was increased to 7.7 in patients older than 50 years of age.[44]

The role of hypertension in ATC-related ICH is controversial. Caplan posited that ICH could occur in patients with chronic hypertension as a result of sudden increase in blood pressure from, for example, withdrawal of antihypertensive medications, trigeminal nerve stimulation, or use of sympathomimetic drugs.[45] In older patients, the effects of long-standing hypertension may be more severe than in the younger population, and compliance with medication may be worse. Thus, a sudden increase in blood pressure is more likely.

Other authors, however, have not found a relationship between ATC-related ICH and hypertension.[18,40,41,46] The findings of the Sixty-Plus study,[46] a double-blind, randomized placebo controlled study of ATC treatment in elderly patients after myocardial infarction, reported eight cerebral hemorrhages and nine deaths in the treated group, and one hemorrhagic cerebral infarct and 12 deaths in the placebo group. The prevalence of hypertension was similar in both groups.

Many hemorrhages occurring during ATC therapy are related to abnormally prolonged PTs.[18–26] However, other studies have not shown a clear correlation between excessive ATC and hemorrhagic complications. Hemorrhagic complications may occur in the presence of a PT within "therapeutic" range.[22,44,47–50] One study showed that the most severe hemorrhages were related to a prolonged PT, whereas minor hemorrhages occurred even in the presence of a therapeutic PT.[39] Hemorrhages in patients with a therapeutic PT could be secondary to the combination of ATC and incidental or minor brain injuries or from alteration of coagulation factors that are not commonly measured.[47] Further study is necessary to determine the relationship between different PT values, the occurrence of hemorrhage, and its mechanisms.

Location of ATC-Related ICH

Hemorrhage can occur in any location in the central and peripheral nervous system in patients treated with ATC. Patients receiving ATC for recent cerebral infarction deserve special attention, since hemorrhage may occur at the site of infarction. Hemorrhage unrelated to the infarction most commonly manifests as subdural hematoma (SDH), although subarachnoid and remote ICH also occur.[47] According to different series, ATC-related SDHs comprise between 12% and 38% of all SDHs.[22,49,51–53] Other areas of the nervous system affected include the spinal cord, in the form of epidural hematomas, or the peripheral nervous system.[49,54,55] The femoral nerve is most frequently affected, as a result of compression from hematoma in the iliacus muscle.

While some physicians believe that ATC-related hemorrhage often occurs at multiple simultaneous sites, in one study there were no cases of multifocal involvement in any of the patients with parenchymatous hemorrhage.[23] In the same survey, the location of intracerebral bleeding in 16 patients reproduced the sites affected in hypertensive hemorrhages except for an unusually high incidence (37.5%) of cerebellar involvement.

Clinical Features

Kase and colleagues reviewed 24 patients with ICH during anticoagulant treatment.[23] In contrast to the sudden onset of symptoms described in other types of ICH, the course of symptoms was progressive over several hours or days in 58% of patients. This progression may be due to prolonged bleeding or blood transudation from small arteries or capillaries directly damaged by anticoagulants.[56] The majority of episodes occurred during the first year of anticoagulant therapy, with most occurring in the first 6 months. As in other types of ICH, headache is also a frequent finding, but in ATC patients it can precede the onset of focal signs by many hours. One retrospective study[57] analyzed the clinical characteristics of 79 patients with ICH secondary to ATC with warfarin. The average time that patients received ATC before the hemorrhage was 4.3 years. There was no correlation between the degree of ATC and hemorrhage size. The PT was an average of 1.7 times the control value.

Other important features noted in the patients reported by Kase et al. included a very low incidence of trauma preceding the ICH, the lack of associated systemic bleeding in all but one of the patients, and the occurrence of only one instance of ICH in a previously infarcted area in the nine patients who received ATC for a cerebral infarction.[23] This series highlights the dramatic *lack* of "classic" signs of ATC-related ICH: rapid and dramatic onset, history of trauma, multiple bleeding sites on computed tomography (CT), associated systemic bleeding, and involvement of infarcted areas are uncommon.

ATC-related ICH may not have a higher mortality than ICH from other causes.[36,57,58] Higher mortality might be expected with blood accumulating for periods up to 72 hours.[23] Askey reported 30 ICHs in 1,626 patients on long-term anticoagulant therapy. Two thirds of the affected patients died.[43] As expected, in Kase's et al. report mortality predominated in patients with the largest hemorrhages, and reached 62.5%.[23] At least one other study, however, has shown no difference in the degree of recovery between ATC-related and spontaneous ICH.[20]

A number of factors determine outcome from ICH. Large hemorrhages carry a worse prognosis, especially those with a volume greater than 60 mm³.[59] Small hemorrhages may mimic lacunar syndromes and have a much better prognosis. Hemorrhages in the cerebellum or diencephalic region fare worse than those located in the hemispheres. One study suggested a predilection for the cerebellum in anticoagulant-related hemorrhages.[23] The volume of ventricular blood, the number of ventricles involved, and the presence of associated hydrocephalus all have a negative effect on outcome.[60] The initial neurologic deficit was identified as a useful predictor for outcome in one study.[60] Patients presenting with severe clinical deficits had a higher mortality.

Treatment

The management of ATC-related ICH follows guidelines appropriate for other types of ICH. Large cerebellar and accessible hemorrhages in the nondominant hemisphere, refractory to medical therapy, are often evacuated surgically after reversing the ATC effects. SDHs thicker than 1 cm are usually treated surgically. To avoid missing an SDH, it should be remembered that SDHs become isodense on CT 2 weeks after bleeding.

Although hemorrhages may abate and reabsorb spontaneously,[61,62] when they are the result of excessive ATC appropriate medical treatment to stop a potentially continuous source of bleeding must be employed. Discontinuation of anticoagulants, administration of fresh frozen plasma (FFP) and vitamin K in patients treated with warfarin, and protamine sulfate in those treated with heparin, can be sufficient to stop bleeding. In warfarin treated patients, FFP is used when rapid correction is necessary. Otherwise, vitamin K (AquaMephyton) 10 mg i.m. reverses the effects of warfarin in 6 hours.

ATC and Hemorrhagic Infarction

Hemorrhagic infarctions (HI) deserve a special focus, as most physicians stop ATC when HI is found on a patient's CT scan. Interestingly, these CTs are usually obtained as a follow-up of the initial ischemic lesion, not because clinical worsening has occurred. HI is thus often an incidental finding rather than the cause of clinical worsening in a patient. However, HI must be differentiated from parenchymatous hemorrhage (PH), a greater degree of bleeding complicating a cerebral infarction and usually associated with clinical worsening.

A history of embolic infarction is usually considered a significant risk factor for hemorrhagic transformation in patients who receive ATC.[21,63,64] However, only one of the patients reported by Kase et al.[23] had an ICH in the previously infarcted territory, and no episodes of bleeding were noted among 85 patients from different studies who were treated with ATC following an embolic stroke.[65-68] Other studies have documented the occurrence of ICH related to the initiation of heparin[43,47,69,70] or warfarin[26,47,64,65,70] therapy in patients with cerebral infarction.

Autopsy Data

In a post mortem study, Fisher and Adams[71] noted an incidence of 66 (18%) HIs in 373 brains with arterial occlusions. Sixty-three of the cases with HI occurred in patients with cerebral embolism. In other autopsy series, the frequency of HI in cerebral embolism varies between 50% and 70%.[72-74]

Imaging Studies

HI appears radiographically as a heterogeneous, serpiginous, finger-like hyperdensity on CT, frequently following the gyral pattern, lying within the area of infarction without mass effect and, as mentioned above, usually not associated with clinical deterioration. Parenchymatous hemorrhage, on the other hand, is a dense, homogeneous, hyperdense area which exceeds the area of infarction, often produces mass effect with ventricular shift, and is usually associated with clinical deterioration. The frequency of 50% to 70% for HI observed in autopsy series decreases 5% to 43% with CT data.[75-79] Autopsies obviously are biased towards more severely affected cases, reporting a higher incidence of HI. CT studies are likely to miss small hemorrhages, resulting in falsely lower values. Parenchymatous hemorrhage is an uncommon complication of ischemic infarction in untreated patients. Two studies showed an incidence of 2%. No cases of PH were found in The Cerebral Embolism Study Group.[80]

Mechanism

Fisher and Adams[71] proposed that HI results from embolus migration, with reperfusion and subsequent bleeding within an area of ischemic infarction. Injured capillaries and small venules are the sources of hemorrhage.

Tempo

The timing of these hemorrhages has been analyzed with serial CT studies, which have shown that they usually occur between 2 days and 2 weeks after stroke onset.[81-84] Futrell et al[85] analyzed the incidence of HI in small cerebral infarcts in a rat model. No evidence of HI was found on day 1, and a small number (5.5%) of infarcts became hemorrhagic between days 2 and 7.[85] Other studies have shown that HI can occasionally be detected within the first day after embolic arterial occlusion. However, no study has proven hemorrhagic conversion of an infarct in the first 6 hours following the onset of ischemia. These first 6 hours following a stroke constitute an important therapeutic window for administration of thrombolytic drugs which carry a potential hemorrhagic effect.

Role of ATC

Spontaneous hemorrhagic conversion of *untreated* ischemic infarction is common, especially in embolic stroke. However, the evidence suggests that HIs are rarely the cause of clinical worsening. Because of the risk of reembolization in stroke patients with a known embolic source, many neurologists favor continuation of anticoagulant therapy even in the presence of hemorrhagic transformation of an infarct in patients with no hemorrhage-related deterioration. One study followed all patients in whom anticoagulants were continued after HI was observed on CT.[86] A total of 10 patients between 33 and 77 years of age were identified, all being treated with warfarin or heparin at full anticoagulant dosage when an HI developed. A cardiac source for emboli was identified in all patients. Infarction had occurred in the middle cerebral artery territory in nine patients and in the posterior cerebral artery territory in one. All infarcts were of moderate to large size. Anticoagulation was continued at therapeutic levels after HI was detected. The clinical status remained unchanged or improved in all patients, and CT evidence of hemorrhagic conversion disappeared in the serial CTs obtained (Figure 1).

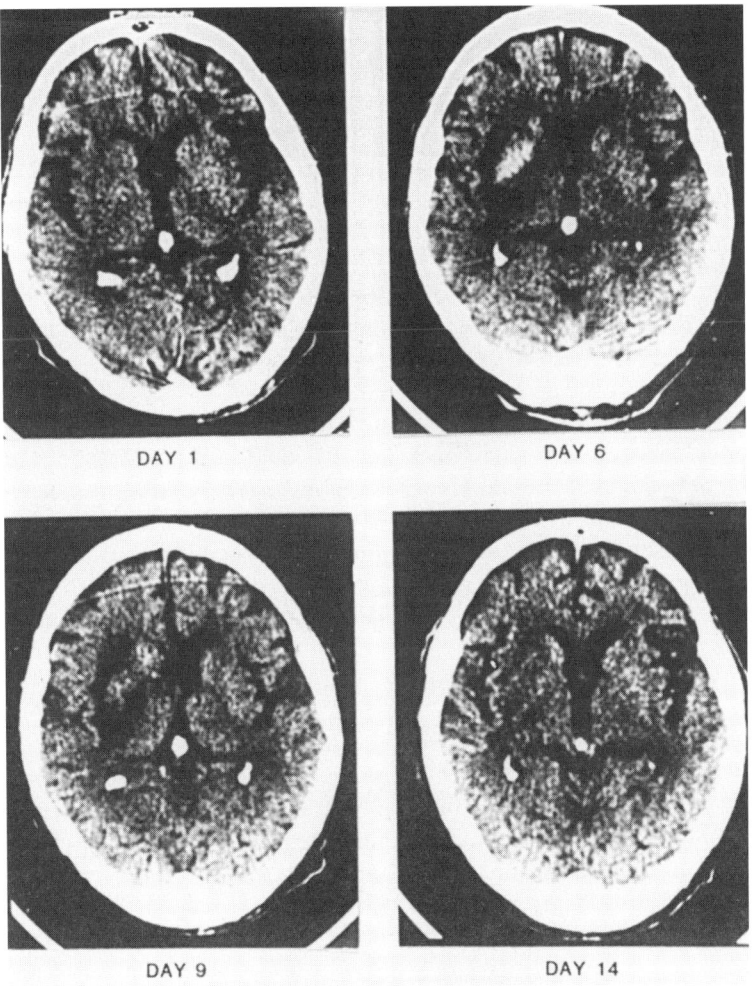

Figure 1: Serial CT scans in a patient with a hemorrhagic infarction occurring in the right basal ganglia during ATC. There is almost complete resolution of the hemorrhage.

ATC-Related ICH and Prosthetic Heart Valves: When To Restart ATC?

This question has been addressed only in anecdotal reports. Gomez et al reported a 63-year-old woman with a Bjork-Shiley valve who developed a left thalamic hemorrhage while receiving warfarin therapy.[87] On day 10 after bleeding, the patient became unresponsive, with worsening of motor deficit. After CT failed to show new areas of bleeding, she was started on heparin, with improvement of her symptoms. The authors suggested restarting anticoagulant therapy after the first 10 days following an ICH.

Babikian et al reviewed their experience with the timing for resumption of ATC in eight instances of ICH in six patients with prosthetic valves.[88] Warfarin therapy was resumed after a mean interval of 19 days. No episodes of thromboembolism off warfarin, or rebleeding after warfarin was resumed, were noted. The number of patients in this report was small, and the resumption of ATC varied from 5 to 42 days after bleeding. The choice of a probable safe time to restart warfarin was arbitrary. Also, the cause of intracranial hemorrhage in these patients may not be representative of other patients with prosthetic valves treated with ATC, because all but two of the patients had excessively prolonged PTs.

Another variable that may influence the resumption of ATC is the location and size of the hemorrhage. A shorter time off ATC will be indicated for a patient with a small, parencymal ICH, while a longer time may be appropriate for a patient with a large subdural hematoma and associated mass effect.

Prosthetic heart valve recipients have an increased risk of thromboembolic events, which are reduced with the use of anticoagulant therapy.[89,90] The reports presented here suggest that ATC can be resumed safely, in some cases, between 5 and 42 days after ICH. Unless a larger number of cases is analyzed, a specific number of days off ATC cannot be recommended. The best approach is to individualize the decision.

Embolism from Bacterial Endocarditis: To Treat or Not To Treat?

Many neurologists will not consider anticoagulating patients with infective embolic lesions secondary to bacterial endocarditis (BE).[11,91,92] This decision results from human and animal studies showing an increased incidence of ICH with the use of anticoagulants in infective endocarditis.[21,93] In the Massachusetts General Hospital series of 218 patients with BE, 23% of the intracranial hemorrhages occurred in the 3% of patients who were treated with ATC.[94] Hart and Davenport and colleagues indirectly supported this position by reporting a low incidence of reembolization in patients not receiving anticoagulants when infection was controlled.[95,96] The authors also found that in cases of recurrence, emboli were small. In another study of 175 patients with BE, ATC was given to 20 patients.[97] Six ischemic strokes and one ICH occurred. Treatment was discontinued in 3 of the patients and the remaining 17 had an uneventful course of ATC. The authors concluded that hemorrhagic transformation in patients with BE treated with ATC was lower than previously reported. However, they also suggested that due to the low risk of recurrent cerebral embolism they observed, it was advisable to withhold ATC in patients who had suffered a single septic embolic event.

The high incidence of neurologic complications in BE, and the associated increase in mortality, justify an aggressive approach to the evaluation and treatment of this disease.[98] The decision to use ATC to prevent recurrent embolism hinges on the likelihood of recurrence on one side, and the potentially devastating consequences of a hemorrhage on the other. Anticoagulation should not be used routinely. A group of patients at high risk for embolization should be identified and treated. This group is represented mostly by patients with prosthetic valves. Those who have large vegetations and mitral valve involvement are probably at higher risk. Wilson et al showed probable beneficial effects in patients with prosthetic heart valves and BE who were anticoagulated.[99] The authors proposed a delay of 2 weeks before starting ATC therapy in patients who had suffered a recent embolic infarct. It is also prudent to obtain an angiogram in patients who have suffered a cerebral embolic event to exclude the presence of a mycotic aneurysm. If a decision is made to anticoagulate the patient, this should be performed with extreme caution and strict control of PT values to avoid excessive ATC.

Conclusions

If possible, a nurse with special training should follow all patients receiving chronic outpatient ATC, and readjust their anticoagulant dose depending on the values obtained with each PT. Optimally, a brochure with details of the reasons for treatment and related risks should be given to each patient. In the case of significant changes of the PT value in a patient who had previously been under control, a reassessment is justified. In patients with a family or personal history suspicious for hematologic disease, or in those in whom it is difficult to achieve a good PT value de novo, it is reasonable to obtain a detailed battery measuring coagulation factors not evaluated in routine examinations.

Although ICHs can occur even with strictly controlled ATC treatment, the frequency of this complication is low. Fear that is not based on scientific analysis should not preclude the use of anticoagulants in patients who can benefit from treatment.

References

1. Estol CJ, Caplan LR: Therapy of acute stroke. *Clin Neuropharmacol* 1989; 13:91.

2. Estol CJ, Pessin MS: Anticoagulation: is there still a role in atherothrombotic stroke? *Stroke* 1990;21:820.

3. Petersen P, Boysen G, Godtfredsen J, et al: Placebo-controlled, randomized trial of warfarin and aspirin for prevention of thromboembolic complications in chronic atrial fibrillation: the Copenhagen AFASAK study. *Lancet* 1989;1:175.

4. Stroke prevention in atrial fibrillation study group investigators: preliminary report of the stroke prevention atrial fibrillation study. *N Engl J Med* 1990;322:863.

5. The Boston area anticoagulation trial for atrial fibrillation investigators: the effect of low-dose warfarin on the risk of stroke in patients with non-rheumatic atrial fibrillation. *N Engl J Med* 1990;323:1505.

6. Estol CJ, Pessin MS, DeWitt LD, et al: Stroke and increased Factor VIII activity. *Neurology* 1989;39(suppl. 1):159.

7. The Antiphospholipid Antibodies and Stroke Study Group. Recurrent thromboembolic and stroke risk in patients with neurological events and antiphospholipid antibodies. *Ann Neurol* 1990;28:226.

8. Miller VT, Hart RG: Heparin anticoagulation in acute brain ischemia. *Stroke* 1988;19:403.

9. Phillips SJ: An alternative view of heparin anticoagulation in acute focal brain ischemia. *Stroke* 1989;20:295.

10. Scheinberg P: Heparin anticoagulation. *Stroke* 1989;20:173.

11. Caplan LR: Anticoagulation for cerebral ischemia. *Clin Neuropharmacol* 1986;9:399.

12. Levine M, Hirsh J: Hemorrhagic complications of long-term anticoagulant therapy for ischemic cerebral vascular disease. *Stroke* 1986;17:111.

13. Loeliger EA: The optimal therapeutic range in oral anticoagulation: history and proposal. *Thromb Haemost* 1979;42:1141.

14. Poller L, Taberner DA: Dosage and control of oral anticoagulants: an international collaborative survey. *Br J Haematol* 1982;51:479.

15. Ingram GIC, Schmidt RM, Filers RJ, et al: Report of the expert panel on oral anticoagulant control. *Thromb Haemost* 1979;42:1073.

16. Wright IS, Beck DF, Marple CD: Myocardial infarction and its treatment with anticoagulants. *Lancet* 1954;1:92.

17. Hirsh J, Levine M: Therapeutic range for the control of oral anticoagulant therapy. *Arch Neurol* 1986;43:1162.

18. Husted S, Andreasen F: Problems encountered in long-term treatment with anticoagulants. *Acta Med Scand* 1976;200:379.

19. Ruff RL, Dougherty JH: Evaluation of acute cerebral ischemia for anticoagulant therapy: computed tomography or lumbar puncture. *Neurology (NY)* 1981;31:736.

20. Wintzen AR, de Jonge H, Loeliger EA, et al: The risk of intracerebral hemorrhage during oral anticoagulant treatment: a population study. *Ann Neurol* 1984;16:553.

21. Barron KD, Fergusson G: Intracranial hemorrhage as a complication of anticoagulant therapy. *Neurology (Minneap)* 1959;9:447.

22. Wells CE, Urrea D: Cerebrovascular accidents in patients receiving anticoagulant drugs. *Arch Neurol* 1960;3:553.

23. Kase CS, Robinson RK, Stein RW, et al: Anticoagulant-related intracerebral hemorrhage. *Neurology* 1985;35:943.

24. Iizuka J: Intracranial and intraspinal hematomas associated with anticoagulant therapy. *Neurochirurgia (Stuttg)* 1972;1:15.

25. Lieberman A, Hass WK, Pinto R, et al: Intracranial hemorrhage and infarction in anticoagulated patients with prosthetic heart valves. *Stroke* 1978; 9:18.

26. Kanoff RB, Ruberg RL: Bilateral spontaneous intracerebral hematomas following anticoagulation therapy: report of case with recovery following surgery. *J Am Osteopath Assoc* 1979;79:174.

27. Alberts MJ, Wayne Massey E, Dawson D: A multicenter study of anticoagulation parameters when using heparin and warfarin. *Arch Neurol* 1987; 44:1229.

28. Clagett GP, Salzman EW: Prevention of venous thromboembolism. *Prog Cardiovasc Dis* 1975;17:345.

29. Hull R, Delmore T, Carter C, et al: Adjusted subcutaneous heparin versus warfarin sodium in the long-term treatment of venous thrombosis. *N Engl J Med* 1982;306:189.

30. Drapkin A, Merskey C: Anticoagulant therapy after acute myocardial infarction: relation of therapeutic benefit to patient's age, sex and severity of infarction. *JAMA* 1972;222:541.

31. Bjerkelund CJ, Orning OM: The efficacy of anticoagulant therapy in preventing embolism related to DC electrical conversion of atrial fibrillation. *Am J Cardiol* 1969;23:208.

32. Keith DS, Phillips SJ, Whisnant JP, et al: Heparin therapy for recent transient focal cerebral ischemia. *Mayo Clin Proc* 1987;62:1101.

33. Mohr J, Caplan L, Melski J, et al: The Harvard Cooperative Stroke Registry: a prospective registry. *Neurology* 1978;28:754.

34. Yarnell P, Earnest M: Primary non-traumatic intracranial hemorrhage. A municipal emergency hospital viewpoint. *Stroke* 1976;7:608.

35. Kase CS: Intracerebral hemorrhage: non hypertensive causes. *Stroke* 1986; 17:590.

36. Feldmann E: Intracerebral hemorrhage. *Stroke* 1991;22:684.

37. Coon WW, Willis PW: Hemorrhagic complications of anticoagulant therapy. *Arch Intern Med* 1974;133:386.

38. Ramirez-Lasepas M, Quinones MR: Heparin therapy for stroke. Hemorrhagic complications and risk factors for intracerebral hemorrhage. *Neurology* 1984;34:114.

39. Forfar JC: A 7-year analysis of hemorrhage in patients on long-term anticoagulant treatment. *Br Heart J* 1979;42:128.

40. Whisnant JP, Cartlidge NEF, Elveback LR: Carotid and vertebral-basilar transient ischemic attacks: effects of anticoagulants, hypertension and cardiac disorders on survival and stroke occurrence — a population study. *Ann Neurol* 1978;3:107.

41. Furlan AJ, Whisnant JP, Elveback LR: The decreasing incidence of primary intracerebral hemorrhage: a population study. *Ann Neurol* 1979;5:367.
42. Muller HR, Radu EW: Intracerebral hematoma. In: Harrison MJG, Dyken ML, eds: *Cerebral Vascular Disease*. London: Butterworths, 1983:320.
43. Askey JM: Hemorrhage during long-term anticoagulant drug therapy. Intracranial hemorrhage. *Calif Med* 1966;104:6.
44. Vastola EF, Frugh A: Anticoagulants for occlusive cerebrovascular lesions. *Neurology (Minneap)* 1959;9:143.
45. Caplan LR: Intracerebral hemorrhage revisited. *Neurology* 1988;38:624.
46. Sixty-Plus reinfarction study research group. Risks of long-term oral anticoagulant therapy in elderly patients after myocardial infarction. *Lancet* 1982;1:64.
47. Silverstein A: Neurological complications of anticoagulant therapy. *Arch Intern Med* 1979;139:217.
48. Riddick FA: Long-term anticoagulation therapy in an outpatient department: techniques and complications. *J Chronic Dis* 1960;12:622.
49. Wiener LN, Nathanson M: The relationship of subdural hematoma to anticoagulant therapy. *Arch Neurol* 1962;2:282.
50. Dooley DM, Perlmutter I: Spontaneous intracranial hematomas in patients receiving anticoagulation therapy. *JAMA* 1964;187:396.
51. Sreerama V, Ivan LP, Dennery JM, et al: Neurosurgical complications of anticoagulant therapy. *Can Med Assoc J* 1973;108:305.
52. Nathanson M, Cravioto H, Cohen B: Subdural hematoma related to anticoagulation therapy. *Ann Intern Med* 1958;49:1368.
53. Snyder M, Renaudin J: Intracranial hemorrhage associated with anticoagulation therapy. *Surg Neurol* 1977;7:31.
54. Spurney OM, Rubin S, Wolf JW, et al: Spinal epidural hematoma during anticoagulant therapy. *Arch Intern Med* 1964;114:103.
55. Parkes JD, Kidner PH: Peripheral nerve and root lesions developing as a result of hematoma formation during anticoagulant therapy. *Postgrad Med* 1970;46:146.
56. McCarter JC, Bingham JB, Meyer OO: Studies on the hemorrhagic agent 3,3'-methylenebis (4-hydroxicoumarin) IV. The pathologic findings after the administration of Dicumarol. *Am J Pathol* 1944;20:651.
57. Franke CL, de Jonge J, van Swieten JC, et al: Intracerebral hematomas during anticoagulant treatment. *Stroke* 1990;21:726.
58. Fieschi C, Carolei A, Fiorelli M, et al: Changing prognosis of primary intracerebral hemorrhage: results of a clinical and computed tomographic follow up study of 104 patients. *Stroke* 1988;19:192.
59. Kase CS, Mohr JP: General features of intracerebral hemorrhage. In: Barnett HJM, Mohr JP, Stein BM, et al., eds: *Stroke*. New York: Churchill Livingstone, 1986:497.
60. Young WB, Lee KP, Pessin MS, et al: Prognostic significance of ventricular blood in supratentorial hemorrhage: a volumetric study. *Neurology* 1990;40:616.

61. Ojemann RG, Heros RC: Spontaneous brain hemorrhage. *Stroke* 1983;14: 468.
62. Helweg-Larsen S, Sommer W, Strange P, et al: Prognosis for patients treated conservatively for spontaneous intracerebral hematomas. *Stroke* 1984;15:1045.
63. Shields RW, Laureno R, Lachman R, et al: Anticoagulant related hemorrhage in acute cerebral embolism. *Stroke* 1984;15:426.
64. Drake ME, Shin C: Conversion of ischemic to hemorrhagic infarction by anticoagulant administration: report of two cases with evidence from serial computed tomographic brain scans. *Arch Neurol* 1983;40:44.
65. Furlan AJ, Cavalier SJ, Hobbs RE, et al: Hemorrhage and anticoagulation after nonseptic embolic brain infarction. *Neurology (NY)* 1982;32:280.
66. Koller RL: Recurrent embolic cerebral infarction and anticoagulation. *Neurology (NY)* 1982;32:283.
67. Lodder J, van der Lugt PJM: Evaluation of the risk of immediate anticoagulant treatment in patients with embolic stroke of cardiac origin. *Stroke* 1983;14:42.
68. Hakim AM, Furlan AJ, Hart RG, et al: Immediate anticoagulation of embolic stroke: a randomized trial. *Stroke* 1983;14:668.
69. Hart RG, Lockwood KI, Hakim AM, et al: Immediate anticoagulation of embolic stroke: brain hemorrhage and management options. *Stroke* 1984; 15:779.
70. Hart RG, Coull BM, Miller VT: Anticoagulation and embolic infarction (letter). *Neurology (NY)* 1983;33:252.
71. Fisher CM, Adams RD: Observations on brain embolism with special reference to the mechanism of hemorrhagic infarction. *J Neuropath Exp Neurol* 1951;10:92.
72. Fisher CM, Adams RD: Observations on brain embolism with special reference to hemorrhagic infarction. In: Furlan AJ, ed: *The Heart and Stroke.* New York: Springer-Verlag, 1987:17.
73. Jorgensen L, Torvik A: Ischemic cerebrovascular diseases in an autopsy series Part 2. Prevalence, location, pathogenesis, and clinical course of cerebral infarcts. *J Neurol Sci* 1969;9:285.
74. Lodder J, Krijne-Kubat B, Broekman J: Cerebral hemorrhagic infarction at autopsy: cardiac embolic cause and the relationship to the cause of death. *Stroke* 1986;17:626.
75. Hornig CR, Dorndorf W, Agnoli AL: Hemorrhagic cerebral infarction—a prospective study. *Stroke* 1986;17:179.
76. Lodder J: CT-detected hemorrhagic infarction: relation with the size of the infarct, and the presence of midline shift. *Acta Neurol Scand* 1984;70:329.
77. Fisher CM, Zito JL, Silva A, et al: Hemorrhagic infarction: a clinical and CT study. *Stroke* 1984;15:192.
78. Okada Y, Yamaguchi T, Minematsu K, et al: Hemorrhagic transformation in cerebral embolism. *Stroke* 1989;20:598.
79. Weisberg LA: Nonseptic cardiogenic cerebral embolic stroke: clinical-CT correlations. *Neurology* 1985;35:896.

80. Cerebral Embolism Study Group: Immediate anticoagulation of embolic stroke: brain hemorrhage and management options. *Stroke* 1984;15:779.

81. Hornig CR, Dorndorf W, Agnoli AL: Hemorrhagic cerebral infarction—a prospective study. *Stroke* 1986;17:179.

82. Ott BR, Zamani A, Kleefield J, et al: The clinical spectrum of hemorrhagic infarction. *Stroke* 1986;17:630.

83. Hart RG, for Cerebral Embolism Study Group: Timing of hemorrhagic transformation of cardioembolic stroke. In: Stober T, ed: *Central Nervous System Control of the Heart.* Boston: Martinus Nijhoff Publishing, 1986: 229.

84. Okada Y, Yamaguchi T, Minematsu K, et al: Hemorrhagic transformation in cerebral embolism. *Stroke* 1989;20:598.

85. Futrell N, Garcia JH, Millikan C: Hemorrhagic transformation of small cerebral infarcts in the rat. *Ann Neurol* 1990;28:227.

86. Pessin MS, Estol CJ, Lafranchise F, et al: Safety of anticoagulation in hemorrhagic infarctions. *Neurology* 1991;41(suppl.):346.

87. Gomez CR, Sandhu J, Mehta P: Resumption of anticoagulation during hypertensive cerebral hemorrhage with prosthetic heart valve. *Stroke* 1988; 19:407.

88. Babikian VL, Kase CS, Pessin MS, et al: Resumption of anticoagulation after intracranial bleeding in patients with prosthetic heart valves. *Stroke* 1988;19:407.

89. Edmunds LH: Thromboembolic complications of current cardiac valvular prostheses. *Ann Thorac Surg* 1982;34:96.

90. Larsen GL, Alexander JA, Stanford W: Thrombo-embolic phenomena in patients with prosthetic aortic valves who did not receive anticoagulants. *Ann Thorac Surg* 1977;23:323.

91. Cohen SM: Massive cerebral hemorrhage following heparin therapy in subacute bacterial endocarditis. *J Mt Sinai Hosp NY* 1949;16:214.

92. Kanis HA: The use of anticoagulants in bacterial endocarditis. *Postgrad Med* 1974;50:312.

93. Foote RA, Reagan TV, Sandok BA: Effects of anticoagulants in an animal model of septic cerebral embolization. *Stroke* 1978;9:573.

94. Pruitt AA, Rubin RH, Karchner AW, et al: Neurologic complications of bacterial endocarditis. *Medicine* 1978;57:329.

95. Hart RG, Foster JW, Luther MF, et al: Stroke and infective endocarditis. *Stroke* 1990;21:695.

96. Davenport J, Hart RG: Prosthetic valve endocarditis 1976–1982: antibiotics, anticoagulation and stroke. *Stroke* 1990;21:993.

97. Salgado AV, Furlan AJ, Keys TF, et al: Neurologic complications of endocarditis: a 12 year experience. *Neurology* 1989;39:173.

98. Greenlee JE, Mandell GL: Neurological manifestations of infective endocarditis: a review. *Stroke* 1973;4:958.

99. Wilson WR, Geraci JE, Danielson GK, et al: Anticoagulant therapy and central nervous system complications in patients with prosthetic valve endocarditis. *Circulation* 1978;57:1004.

Chapter 6

Thrombolysis and Intracranial Hemorrhage

Michael A. Sloan, MD

Intracranial hemorrhage is the most dreaded complication of thrombolytic therapy. Early studies of thrombolysis in presumed ischemic stroke patients reported an unacceptably high incidence of cerebral hemorrhage.[1-6] These investigations were subject to several limitations.[7-9] Patients were enrolled with a worsening clinical deficit and clear spinal fluid, but computed tomographic (CT) scans were not available to exclude hematomas before enrollment in clinical trials. In some cases, significant hypertension was present before or during neurologic worsening.[1,2,5,6] Combined anticoagulant and thrombolytic therapy was common, with the latter often accompanied by induction of a systemic fibrinolytic state in some studies.[1,2,5,6] Nonetheless, these experiences delayed further investigation of therapeutic thrombolysis.

In the 1970s, 1980s, and 1990s, there has been a resurgence of interest in the use of thrombolytic therapy for treatment of a wide variety of thromboembolic disorders, including myocardial infarction (MI),[10-85] pulmonary embolism,[86,87] deep vein thrombosis,[7] peripheral arterial occlusive disease,[7,88] and ischemic stroke.[89-152] The results of therapy with various thrombolytic agents have been most dramatic for MI[10,11,13-19] and are promising for acute ischemic stroke.[111,113,114,127-131,145-152] In the last 11 years, there has also been an interest in using thrombolytic agents as an adjunctive measure in patients with aneurysmal subarachnoid hemorrhage (SAH),[153-168] intracranial hematoma,[169-183] and cerebral venous sinus thrombosis.[184-187]

Even though therapeutic thrombolysis is valuable for selected disorders and shows promise in others, intracranial hemorrhage remains the most important adverse effect. Proper use of thrombolytic therapy requires careful patient selection, knowledge of risk factors for intracranial hemorrhage, recognition of symptoms and signs of intracranial hemorrhage, determination of the type of intracranial hemorrhage, and aggressive management to optimize patient outcomes.

From Feldmann E (ed). *Intracerebral Hemorrhage.* Armonk, NY: Futura Publishing Company, Inc., © 1994.

This review has three parts. First, the types of, risks for, and causes of intracranial hemorrhage following thrombolytic therapy will be evaluated, specifically in the MI setting. Second, an analysis of current knowledge of the types of and potential risk factors for intracranial hemorrhage following thrombolytic therapy for acute ischemic stroke will be presented. Finally, the rationale for and preliminary results from open studies of thrombolytic therapy in hemorrhagic cerebrovascular disease will be discussed.

Types of Intracranial Hemorrhage Following Thrombolysis

Intracranial hemorrhage has been reported to complicate thrombolytic therapy for each thromboembolic disorder. The clinical and radiologic features of these hemorrhages have been best studied in the acute MI setting.[10–84] The occurrence of parenchymatous intracerebral hemorrhage (PIH),[10–84] cerebral infarction with hemorrhagic transformation or hemorrhagic infarction (HI),[15,24, 25,31,37,38,51,56,73] subdural hemorrhage (SDH),[20,24,26,31,78] SAH,[24,25,42,44,45,78] intraventricular hemorrhage (IVH),[25,57,78] and epidural hematoma (EPH)[60] has been reported. In some cases, multiple types of intracranial hemorrhage may coexist.[26,78] It is therefore essential to define the characteristics of these different types of hemorrhagic complications in order to identify risk factors and causes for intracranial hemorrhage and to facilitate optimal patient care.

Parenchymatous intracerebral hemorrhage (PIH) refers to primary bleeding within brain parenchyma. Primary hemorrhages are thought to be nonterritorial, compact, or confluent collections of blood that have, on CT scans, a homogeneous density and sharp edge, often with a surrounding mass effect occurring after several days.[188,189] In one study,[31] PIH was classified on the basis of focal neurologic deficits associated with focal collections of blood in brain parenchyma seen on CT scan with neither a normal brain image at the time of onset of neurologic symptoms nor evidence for preceding ischemic cerebral infarction. In patients with ischemic cerebral infarction treated with thrombolytic agents, the definition of PIH requires that it be located in a region remote from the presumed ischemic cerebral infarct site.

Hemorrhagic transformation or conversion of an ischemic cerebral infarction (HI) refers to secondary bleeding believed to occur either with early reperfusion into a damaged vascular bed with impaired autoregulation[190–192] or because of development of collateral circulation into the same vascular bed.[190,193,194] HIs are strictly territorial, and CT scans show mixed areas of hypodensity and hyperdensity, with an indistinct edge and no significant mass effect at an early stage.[188,189] Recent work suggests that confluent HI can occur early after onset of ischemic stroke.[195,196] Thus, it may be extremely difficult to distinguish confluent HI from PIH on a CT scan.[31,82,83,190,195] In the setting of thrombolytic therapy, HI or confluent HI may be diagnosed if blood appears within an area of cerebral infarction on the first CT scan or there is no abnormality on the first

CT scan but hemorrhage is seen in the infarct location on a subsequent CT scan.[31]

Extraparenchymal hemorrhage may also occur. SDH may be diagnosed if a high- or mixed-density fluid collection is seen in the subdural space. There may be sulcal effacement and mass effect on CT scan.[31,83] EPH may be diagnosed if a high-density fluid collection is seen in the epidural space.[60] SAH may be diagnosed if a high-density fluid collection is seen in the subarachnoid space. It may be primary or secondary to PIH extension.[26] Intraventricular hemorrhage may be diagnosed if a high-density fluid collection is seen in the ventricular system on CT scan. It may be primary, secondary to PIH extension, or associated with SAH.

Intracranial Hemorrhage Following Thrombolytic Therapy for Acute MI

General Aspects

In the thrombolytic era, the reported occurrence rate of stroke complicating acute MI in several large placebo-controlled,[10-20] comparative,[21,22,24-26,30,31,34] and many smaller trials[35-79] has decreased compared with studies reported in the prethrombolytic era (1.7% to 3.2%).[83] This has been observed in trials using streptokinase (SK),[10-15,21,22,26,35-46,63,72] anisoylated plasminogen-streptokinase activator complex (APSAC),[16,17,25,67] recombinant tissue-type plasminogen activator (rt-PA),[18-22,24-26,29,31,47-59,64,70-72] recombinant single chain urokinase plasminogen activator (rscu-PA),[30,46] and various combination[61-63] or front-loaded[69-71] thrombolytic therapy regimens. The incidence of stroke in treated groups is 0.5% to 2.5% (mean 1.13%) and in control groups it is 0% to 1.0% (mean 0.81%) (Tables 1, 2). This apparent reduction in stroke risk in the thrombolytic era may result from improved treatment of acute MI patients in general and high-risk patients in particular. It may also be due to exclusion of patients at high risk of stroke.[12,18,21,22,31,82-85] The wide variation in stroke rates across studies could be due to chance, different effects of the various thrombolytic agents, or different intensity of the evaluation and reporting of stroke complications.[12,15,16,18,21-25,31,33,82-84] Intracranial hemorrhage reportedly occurred in 0.36% of treated patients (Table 2). In large thrombolytic therapy trials, the mean reported intracranial hemorrhage occurrence rates after treatment with SK, rt-PA, APSAC, and rscu-PA were 0.22%, 0.51%, 0.40%, and 0.78%, respectively.

Clinical Presentation

Intracranial hemorrhage has frequently been reported to occur during[18,31,33,48,53,54] and usually 24 hours or less after infusion[11,12,14,15,18,24,25,31,33] of the

Table 1
Incidence of Stroke in Placebo Controlled Trials of Coronary Thrombolysis

Study (Agent)*	Ref	Treatment		Control	
		No.	%	No.	%
1. GISSI (SK)	10–12	63/5860	1.1	54/5852	0.9
2. ISAM (SK)	13,14	5/859	0.6	0/882	0.0
3. ISIS-2 (SK)	15	61/8592	0.7	67/8595	0.8
Subtotal		129/15311	0.84	121/15329	0.79
1. ASSET (rt-PA)	18,19	28/2516	1.1	25/2495	1.0
2. ECSG (rt-PA)	20	8/722	1.1	2/366	0.5
Subtotal		36/3238	1.11	27/2861	0.94
1. AIMS (APSAC)	16,17	8/624	1.3	4/634	0.63
TOTAL		173/19173	0.90	152/18824	0.81

* SK = streptokinase; APSAC = anisoylated plasminogen-streptokinase activator complex; rt-PA = recombinant tissue plasminogen activator. Used with permission.[83]

fibrinolytic agent. In one study,[31,33] 65% of cases occurred within 12 hours and 83% of cases within 24 hours of study entry. Limited data suggest that as many as 70% of these hemorrhages are lobar, occurring in the cortex and subcortical white matter.[26,29,33,57] They are frequently (15% to 33%) multiple.[26,29] This pattern of intracranial hemorrhage location is typical of coagulopathy-induced and other nonhypertensive causes of PIH.[189,197] Patients typically develop a change in level of consciousness, unifocal or multifocal neurologic symptoms and signs, nausea, vomiting, headache, and seizures.[27] In many cases, the mode of onset is catastrophic and rapidly fatal.[14,15,18,31,74,75,79] Thus, changes in neurologic function during this time period should be regarded as highly suspicious of intracranial hemorrhage. Emergent CT scanning is necessary to distinguish intracranial hemorrhage from the effects of ischemic cerebral infarction, severe cardiac dysfunction, or concomitant MI therapy (lidocaine, morphine, etc.), or both.[82,83]

Precision of Diagnosis

In several large trials,[12,21,24,25,31,33,34] there was an excess of early strokes, particularly hemorrhages, in patients treated with thrombolytic therapy. Inspection of Table 2 indicates that the delineation of stroke subtypes in large comparative studies was uncertain or not specified in 35% of stroke cases. In GISSI-1,[12] GISSI-2,[21,23] ISG,[22] and ISIS-3,[25] CT scans were obtained within 14 or 15[23] days of stroke onset, or autopsies were performed in fatal cases, and the exact number of CT-documented hemorrhages was not stated. Analysis of GISSI-2[23] was also limited by the lack of adequate definitions for hemorrhagic stroke, use of combined analysis of cases reviewed and cases not reviewed by

Table 2
Cerebrovascular Complications in Large Comparative Coronary Thrombolysis Trials

		Stroke Incidence			Stroke Subtypes		
Study	Ref	N	%	ICH (n/%)	CI (n/%)	NS (n/%)	SDH (n/%)
A. Streptokinase (SK)							
GISSI-1	[10–12]	49/5860	0.8	8(16)	9(19)	32(65)	—
ISIS-2	[15]	61/8592	0.7	7(11)	—	54(89)	—
GISSI-2	[21]	54/6199	0.9	15(28)	24(44)	15(28)	—
ISG	[22]	44/4197	1.0	15(34)	22(50)	7(16)	—
(1)Netherlands	[24]	24/2469	1.0	24(100)	—	—	—
(2)ISIS-3	[25]	141/13607	1.0	25(18)	66(47)	50(35)	—
Subtotal		373/40924	0.91	94(25)	121(32)	158(43)	—
% of all patients				(0.22)	(0.30)	(0.39)	(0.0)
B. Recombinant Tissue Plasminogen Activator (rt-PA)							
ASSET	[18,19]	28/2516	1.1	7(25)	11(39)	10(36)	—
(3)TAMI	[26–28]	13/1696	0.8	11(85)	—	—	6(45)
Burroughs-Wellcome	[29]	9/1900	0.5	9(100)	—	—	—
TIMI-2	[31–33]						
150mg		23/908	2.5	12(52)	9(39)	—	2(9)
100mg		33/3016	1.1	11(33)	20(61)	—	2(6)
GISSI-2	[21]	70/6182	1.1	19(28)	28(40)	23(32)	—
ISG	[22]	68/4190	1.6	25(37)	26(38)	17(25)	—
(2)ISIS-3	[25]	188/13569	1.4	76(40)	55(29)	57(31)	—
Subtotal		359/27865	1.29	143(40)	129(36)	83(23)	10(2.5)
% of all patients				(0.51)	(0.46)	(0.30)	(0.03)
C. Anisoylated Plasminogen-Streptokinase Activator Complex (APSAC)							
(2)ISIS-3	[25]	172/13599	1.26	54(31)	45(26)	73(43)	—
% of all patients				(0.40)	(0.33)	(0.53)	—
D. Recombinant Single Chain Urokinase Plasminogen Activator (rscu-PA)							
	[30]	15/1032	1.45	8(53)	7(47)	—	—
% of all patients				(0.78)	(0.68)	—	—
TOTAL		919/83420	1.10	299(33)	302(33)	314(34)	10(1.1)
% of all patients				(0.36)	(0.36)	(0.38)	(0.01)

GISSI-1 = Gruppo Italiano per lo studio della Streptochinasi nell'Infarto Miocardico; ISIS-2 = Second International Study of Infarct Survival; GISSI-2 = Gruppo Italiano per lo studio della Sopravvivenza nell'Infarto Miocardico; ISG = International Study Group; Netherlands = Netherlands Cooperative Registry, Thoraxcenter, University Hospital of Erasmus University; ISIS-3 = Third International Study of Infarct Survival; ASSET = Anglo-Scandinavian Study of Early Thrombolysis; TIMI-2 = Thrombolysis in Myocardial Infarction, Phase II; and TAMI = Thrombolysis and Angioplasty in Myocardial Infarction I–III. N = number of stroke patients in entire study population; n = number of patients with specific stroke subtypes in each study; ICH = definite intracerebral hemorrhage; CI = definite ischemic cerebral infarction; NS = stroke subtype unspecified or "probable" ischemic infarction or "probable" intracranial hemorrhage; and SDH = subdural hematoma. In the "subtotal" and "total" lines, the numbers in parentheses refer to the percentage of strokes in each subgroup. In the line, "% of all patients," the numbers in parentheses refer to the reported occurrence rate of each stroke subtype in the entire population treated with each agent or all agents in the cited studies.
(1) For the Netherlands study, 1791 of 2469 (72.5%) patients were treated with streptokinase. In this study, no attempt was made to distinguish parenchymatous ICH from hemorrhagic transformation of ischemic infarction.
(2) In ISIS-3, only definite stroke subtype diagnoses were categorized as ICH or CI, while probable diagnoses were assigned to the NS category. In addition, "definite" ICH included patients with PIH, SAH, and HI.
(3) In the TAMI study, 6 of 13 (46.2%) stroke patients had been treated with rt-PA, 4 of 13 (30.8%) stroke patients had been treated with SK, 2 of 13 (15.4%) stroke patients had been treated with UK, and 1 of 13 (7.7%) stroke patients had been treated with rt-PA and UK. Since the number of individuals treated with each thrombolytic regimen in this study (N = 1,696) was not stated, all intracranial hemorrhages were assigned to the rt-PA group to facilitate analysis. In TAMI, multiple lesion types were described in 4 cases.

the Study Committee (ie, noncomparative groups), bias inherent in a large stroke group of unknown type, and weak statistical associations. In the Netherlands multicenter trial,[24] no attempt was made to differentiate between PIH and HI. In ISIS-3,[25] "definite hemorrhagic stroke" included cases of PIH, HI, and SAH based on evidence from CT, autopsy, or lumbar puncture with limited data collection and analysis. In several studies, the reported central nervous system hemorrhagic complication was most likely to be hemorrhagic transformation of single[14,31,37,38,50,51,71] or multiple[86] cerebral infarctions. The frequency of this phenomenon is unknown, but it may be more common than suspected since in many studies,[10–13,15,16,21–25] knowledge of the nature of all cerebrovascular complications is incomplete. Of the 56 cerebrovascular complications in TIMI-2,[31,32] 8 of 29 (28%) ischemic cerebral infarcts were proven to have HI. If these 8 are added to the 23 PIH,[31,33] then up to 25% of "intracranial hemorrhage" in other studies might be due to HI. The contribution of thrombolytic therapy to the occurrence of HI is not well defined.[81] It is thus probable that misclassification of HI as intracranial hemorrhage has occurred in large comparative studies, with resultant overestimation of the occurrence rate of PIH.[83,84]

Risk Factors

On the basis of currently available data, putative risk factors for intracranial hemorrhage in the setting of thrombolytic therapy have been identified. These determinations rely upon stroke rates which should be considered as estimates of the true rates. The actual strength of the association between these factors and the occurrence of intracranial hemorrhage, particularly PIH, therefore, remains to be determined. Attention to the following markers for intracranial hemorrhage may nonetheless permit more careful patient selection for thrombolytic therapy (Table 3).

Age

The mortality rate in elderly patients with acute MI, even if treated with SK[45,66] or rt-PA,[25,66,198] increases dramatically from less than 65 years to greater

---

Table 3
Risk Factors for Intracranial Hemorrhage After
Thrombolytic Therapy

1. Age
2. Hypertension
3. Type and dosage of thrombolytic agent
4. Anticoagulant therapy at study entry
5. Prior neurologic disease
6. Weight <70 kg
7. Female sex
8. ? Cardiopulmonary resuscitation

than 75 years.[199,200] Since the elderly constitute an ever increasing proportion of the population at risk, and only 18% of eligible patients with acute MI receive thrombolytic therapy, a number of investigators are seeking to extend treatment to this age group.[85,201–206] A recent meta-analysis[201] of five large trials[11,12, 14–16,18] suggests that thrombolytic therapy may significantly reduce mortality in the elderly (17.9%) when compared with control subjects (22.1%). However, elderly patients may be more likely to have bleeding complications.[66,198,207] Some investigators have expressed the concern that elderly patients may have more defects in cerebrovascular integrity,[28,53] particularly since older age is associated with silent vascular disease. In small studies,[28,55,66] older age was not clearly found to be a risk factor for intracranial hemorrhage in patients treated with rt-PA. In recent large trials,[21–23] both SK and rt-PA were associated with an excess of strokes in older patients (greater than 70 years: 2.7% rt-PA, 1.6% SK; less than 70 years: 0.9% rt-PA, 0.8% SK). In another large study,[31] older patients had a significantly increased frequency of PIH when age was treated as a continuous variable.

Some investigators have recommended that a randomized, placebo-controlled trial is necessary to determine safety and efficacy of thrombolytic therapy in patients who are greater than 75 years old,[45,198] although such efforts may be difficult in practice.[208] A recent cost-effectiveness analysis[205] suggests that thrombolytic therapy with SK in elderly patients may be beneficial. In the aggregate, while thrombolytic therapy for elderly patients with acute MI may be associated with more strokes, the overall reduction in mortality suggests that the benefits of careful thrombolysis may outweigh the risks.[83]

Hypertension

Hypertension may produce intracranial hemorrhage by one of three mechanisms: 1) damage to cerebral arteries which eventually rupture (as in chronic hypertension); 2) acute hypertension of sufficient degree to overcome cerebral autoregulation and lead to "breakthrough perfusion"; or 3) reperfusion of ischemic brain tissue.[209,210] For many years, patients with blood pressure greater than 180 systolic or greater than 110 diastolic ("uncontrolled hypertension") were excluded from receiving thrombolytic therapy based on recommendations from the National Institutes of Health.[211]

More recent work has examined the relation between a history of hypertension or acute hypertension and the occurrence of intracranial hemorrhage after thrombolytic therapy. In ISIS-2,[15] although persistent severe hypertension was a relative contraindication, the mortality rate with systolic blood pressure greater than 175 mm Hg was 5.7% in patients treated with SK versus 8.7% in controls. In another trial, O'Connor and colleagues[28] found lower blood pressure in four patients with intracranial hemorrhage than in nine patients with ischemic stroke. Anderson and colleagues[66] reported that transient systolic blood pressure greater than 150 mm Hg was associated with intracranial hemorrhage, although the study had small numbers of patients and was retrospective. Althouse and colleagues[55,212] reported that 2 of 9 (22%) patients with transient systolic blood pressure greater than 180 mm Hg before treatment with rt-PA versus 1 of 147 (0.7%) patients without this level of blood pressure before treatment with rt-PA had intracranial hemorrhage. In TIMI-2,[31] PIH was more frequent among patients with chronic hypertension than among patients without such a history (0.9% versus 0.4%), although this difference was not statistically significant. However, PIH occurred in 2 of 22 (9.1%) patients with systolic blood pressure greater than 180 mm Hg or diastolic blood pressure greater than 110 mm Hg before study entry compared with 9 of 647 (1.4%) patients without elevated blood pressure. One patient, who initially had severe hypertension which was then controlled at the time of study entry, subsequently had recurring severe hypertension despite treatment and suffered a PIH. Gorelick and colleagues[75] reported a patient with poorly controlled hypertension who had a fatal cerebellar PIH after intracoronary SK. Finally, in GISSI-2,[23] diastolic blood pressure greater than 110 mm Hg was associated with intracranial hemorrhage. Although a significant incremental elevation in blood pressure may contribute to occurrence of intracranial hemorrhage in some cases, it is still possible that severe hypertension at the time of recognition of a change in neurologic function may reflect a systemic response to an acute cerebrovascular insult and not be its cause.

Type and Dosage of Thrombolytic Agent

The occurrence of intracranial hemorrhage in large thrombolytic therapy trials ranges from 0.22% (SK)[10–12,15,21–23,25] to 0.78% (rscu-PA).[30] In TIMI-2,[31,33] 12 of 908 (1.3%) patients treated with 150 mg alteplase rt-PA and intravenous heparin and 11 of 3016 (0.4%) patients treated with 100 mg alteplase rt-PA and intravenous heparin developed PIH. This apparent dose-response relationship is confounded by the effect of more restrictive entry criteria in the 100 mg group, such as exclusion of patients with any blood pressure greater than 180/110 mm Hg or history of acute cerebrovascular disease.[213,214] In other large trials using 100 mg alteplase rt-PA or 1.5×10^6 units SK with or without heparin,[19,21,22] intracranial hemorrhage occurred in 0.4% to 0.6% of patients.

The type of agent used may be as important as its dosage. In ISIS-3,[25] "definite or probable intracranial hemorrhage" occurred in 0.24% of SK patients, 0.66% of duteplase rt-PA patients, and 0.55% of APSAC patients, respectively. It has recently been stated that the 30 U dose of APSAC contains approximately 1.2 million units of SK, somewhat less than the 1.5 million units of SK used in clinical practice. Thus, the higher intracranial hemorrhage rate for APSAC is difficult to explain on the basis of dosage.[215,216] Whether the even higher reported frequency of intracranial hemorrhage in patients treated with rt-PA reflects the varying definitions for intracranial hemorrhage in different studies,[10–12,15,19,21–23,25,30,31,33] varying intensity of diagnostic or pathologic investigation,[10–12,15,21–25,31–33] differences in thrombolytic activity between rt-PA preparations (alteplase = single chain rt-PA, duteplase = double chain rt-PA),[215,216] other systematic differences or some combination is unknown. It has recently been argued that the dose of duteplase rt-PA (0.6 million IU/kg), given its lower plasminogen activating activity (as determined in the standard clot lysis assay), actually corresponds to a dose with higher kinetic activity than the standard 100 mg of alteplase rt-PA.[215,216] At the present time, the conclusion that the risk of hemorrhagic stroke is higher in patients treated with the standard dose of rt-PA than in patients treated with SK[21-23,25] or APSAC[25] is poorly supported by the available data.

Patients with body weight less than 70 kg,[24] particularly women,[28,53] have higher rt-PA concentrations during the infusion and, with more fibrinogenolysis, may have a greater risk of bleeding complications. However, in one study,[23] body mass index was not associated with risk of any stroke or hemorrhagic stroke, although data collection was limited. The effect of weight-adjusted thrombolytic regimens on intracranial hemorrhage occurrence remains to be determined.[59]

Recently, there has been interest in altering the timing of delivery or combining various thrombolytic agents in order to maximize thrombolytic efficacy. Several studies have employed various accelerated or "front-loaded" rt-PA regimens.[69-71,73,217,218] In four studies,[69-71,73] 3 of 721 (0.42%) patients had intracranial hemorrhage. In eight small studies (total of 760 patients) using combination thrombolytic therapy (rt-PA plus SK or rt-PA plus UK), the reported intracranial hemorrhage occurrence rate is 0.7% for rt-PA plus UK and 0.5% for rt-PA plus SK.[62] As more experience with these regimens is gained, estimation of the actual risk of intracranial hemorrhage with various modified thrombolytic regimens will be possible.

Concomitant Medications

It is possible that use of other medications in conjunction with thrombolytic therapy places patients at risk for intracranial bleeding. One recent study[24] found that patients taking oral anticoagulants at study entry had an increased risk of intracranial hemorrhage. A number of drugs, such as nonsteroidal anti-inflammatory agents, nitrates, and propranolol may affect platelet function and contribute to bleeding.[219-221] Calcium antagonists have been shown to inhibit platelet aggregation[222] and arachidonic acid metabolism.[223] In TIMI-2,[31] use of calcium antagonists at study entry was associated with an increased frequency of PIH (1.5%) compared with patients not taking these drugs (0.045%) and was not the result of any one agent's effect. Whether or not this association is due to chance, pre-existing cerebrovascular disease, or an effect of calcium antagonists is unknown.

Prior Neurologic Disease

In coronary thrombolysis trials, potential study patients with histories of acute ischemic cerebrovascular disease within 3 months of entry have generally been excluded.[82,85,211] In the TIMI-2 pilot and early clinical trial,[31] patients with acute cerebrovascular disease within the 6 months before acute MI presentation were excluded. In the initial phase of the study, prior to the use of more stringent exclusion criteria, 3 of 30 (10%) patients with a history of stroke, intermittent cerebral ischemic attack, or other neurologic disease had PIH compared with 8 of 639 (1.2%) without such histories. At this point, the protocol was changed to make patients with histories of stroke or intermittent cerebral ischemic attacks ineligible. Since the observed excess risk of PIH is based on the observation of only three patients who had PIH in the high-risk group, the estimated increased risk is not precise (95% confidence interval about the odds ratio, 1.94 to 22.81). Unfortunately, no data from other large trials is available.[10–12,15,21–25] At the present time, a major international trial, Global Utilization of Streptokinase and t-PA for Occluded Coronary Arteries (GUSTO), excludes patients with any history of neurologic disease.[62]

Cardiopulmonary Resuscitation

It has recently been suggested that brief (less than 10 minutes) cardiopulmonary resuscitation (CPR) should not be a contraindication to thrombolytic therapy.[202] Califf and colleagues[224] found no difference in transfusion requirements or in the incidence of pneumothorax and pneumopericardium in 62 patients receiving brief CPR when compared to 646 patients not requiring CPR. Scholz and colleagues[225] found that prolonged CPR (mean duration 36 ± 32 minutes, range 4 to 120 minutes) was not associated with an increased risk of bleeding complications. However, prolonged CPR may lead to global hypoxic-ischemic encephalopathy, parenchymal and vascular tissue disruption, and increased risk of intracranial hemorrhage.[202] At the present time, there has been no formal examination of this issue from the standpoint of intracranial bleeding.

Causes

A number of conditions and pre-existing lesions may contribute to the occurrence of intracranial hemorrhage in specific individuals. These factors are summarized in Table 4.

Combined Thrombolytic, Anticoagulant, and Antiplatelet Therapy

Basic aspects of the control of fibrinolysis and mechanisms of action of the various thrombolytic agents have recently been reviewed.[7–9,219,221,226,227] Briefly, SK binds to plasminogen, induces a conformational change, and forms plasminogen activator. Spontaneous deacylation of APSAC regenerates the active site of plasmin. Urokinase directly activates plasminogen. These plasminogen activators can produce severe hypofibrinogenemia with a resulting bleeding dia-

Table 4

Causes of Intracranial Hemorrhage After Thrombolytic Therapy

1. Acute hypertension
2. Combined thrombolytic/anticoagulant/antiplatelet therapy
3. Cerebrovascular pathology
   a. Arteriovenous malformations
   b. Congophilic amyloid angiopathy
   c. Microaneurysms/other microvascular lesions
   d. Berry aneurysms
4. Head injury before treatment
5. Hemorrhagic transformation of ischemic cerebral infarction
6. Following invasive cardiovascular procedures
7. Brain tumors

thesis. On the other hand, rt-PA forms a complex with plasminogen and fibrin that allows for plasmin generation on the fibrin surface. And rscu-PA may act via fibrin-dependent neutralization of a competitive inhibitor.[8,219,227] Both rt-PA and rscu-PA are endowed with fibrin selectivity, but at clinically effective doses significant hypofibrinogenemia can still occur. In some studies using rt-PA, a dose-response relationship for induction of a systemic fibrinolytic state has been shown.[31,53,59,228,229] Plasmin may also cleave factors V and VIII, which are essential for thrombin generation. As a result, marked prolongation of the prothrombin time (PT) and activated partial thromboplastin time (PTT) is common, particularly with the exogenous agents, SK and UK.

Plasma fibrinogen degradation products (FDP) are higher in patients treated with SK than patients treated with rt-PA.[219,230] In patients treated with rt-PA, there are modest, direct correlations between rt-PA levels at 50 minutes and FDP at 5 hours, and modest inverse correlations between rt-PA levels at 50 minutes and fibrinogen and plasminogen levels at 5 hours.[229] However, several other studies have shown a poor correlation between residual plasma rt-PA level and residual functional fibrinogen level,[230,231] as well as between the extent of the fibrinolytic state and bleeding complications.[44,53,219,230] Although the levels of fibrinogen[53,229] and FDP[230,231] appear to correlate with the frequency of bleeding within treatment groups,[230] the occurrence of systemic bleeding appears to relate more to the lysis of hemostatic plugs at sites of vascular invasion[219,226,229,230] and concomitant anticoagulation.[230] While pathologic[232,233] and therapeutic fibrinolysis clearly lead to bleeding, use of the "standard" measurements of coagulation and fibrinolysis as well as special markers (D-dimer, B-b15-42, B-b1-42) do not have sufficient sensitivity and specificity to predict the risk of bleeding in individual patients.[234,235]

The effect of fibrinolytic therapy on platelet function may contribute to bleeding complications. Both SK[236] and rt-PA[237] may prevent platelet aggregation, and rt-PA may promote dispersion of platelet aggregates.[238] Several other studies suggest that SK[239–241] and rt-PA[242] may promote platelet aggregation. Discrepant results may be due to the fact that these in vitro observations reflect use of different SK preparations,[238,240] patient populations, and experimental conditions. The in vivo effects are difficult to predict on the basis of in vitro studies and will depend upon the nature of the insult, involved vascular bed, type and dose of agent, local conditions, and other factors.[243]

Adjunctive anticoagulant and antiplatelet therapies may contribute to the occurrence of bleeding.[230,244] One recent study[24] found that patients taking oral anticoagulants before admission had an increased risk of intracranial hemorrhage. Increased bleeding may in part relate to the use of intravenous[15,229,230] or subcutaneous[15,21–23,25] heparin. In ISIS-2,[15] there was a small excess (0.3%) of major bleeding requiring transfusion whether or not aspirin was used, but it was dependent upon planned use of intravenous and subcutaneous heparin. Preliminary data suggest that use of aspirin may enhance the effects of rt-PA on platelet disaggregation in vitro.[238] In one recent study,[220] prolongation of the bleeding time to greater than 9 minutes (Ivy method) at 90 minutes after treatment initiation correlated with spontaneous bleeding, and bleeding was more frequent in patients taking aspirin. Moreover, the use of activated plasminogen activator inhibitor (PAI-1) may correct the prolonged bleeding time and arrest bleeding.[245]

The role of the various hemostatic perturbations in the production of intracranial hemorrhage is not clear. In nine published cases,[29,53,54,57,75,77] intracranial hemorrhage occurred in association with severe hypofibrinogenemia. On occasion, marked elevation of fibrin(ogen) degradation products have also been observed.[53,54] In the majority of case reports, the PTT has been markedly prolonged.[29,44,53,54,57,74,75,77–79] In two recent small studies,[67,72] use of intravenous heparin was associated with increased bleeding complications in patients treated with APSAC,[67] but not SK[72] or rt-PA.[72] In TIMI-2,[31] limited data suggest that there were no important differences in fibrinogen, FDP, rt-PA antigen, or plasminogen levels between patients with PIH, cerebral infarction, or between these groups and the other patients without cerebrovascular complications who had plasma specimens analyzed. In addition, the proportion of patients with or without PIH or cerebral infarction who had at least 1 PTT greater than 90 seconds were not different. The occurrence rate of intracranial hemorrhage was similar in patients who received 100 mg alteplase rt-PA alone,[19,21,22,31] 100 mg alteplase rt-PA and intravenous heparin,[29,31] and 100 mg alteplase rt-PA and subcutaneous heparin,[21,22,25] though the latter is not likely to be therapeutic in the first 24 hours of use.[246] Taken together, these data confirm the observations of others[20,44,53,218] that there is a poor correlation between the existence of a systemic fibrinolytic state and the occurrence of intracranial hemorrhage.

The role of concomitant aspirin therapy in these patients is also controversial. Recent work suggests that the use of aspirin may be associated with an increased risk of hemorrhagic stroke in U.S. physicians.[247] This concern has prompted several investigators to hypothesize that aspirin use may contribute to the occurrence of intracranial hemorrhage after thrombolytic therapy,[28] and to therefore delay use of aspirin until one day after treatment.[31] Prolongation of the bleeding time by combined rt-PA and aspirin therapy appears to be maximal within the first 4 hours after initiation of rt-PA administration.[220] However, intracranial hemorrhage did not occur in that small study, and intracranial hemorrhage often occurs greater than 4 hours after initiation of thrombolytic therapy.[21,26,29,31,57] In GISSI-2,[23] use of aspirin was associated with a lower incidence of hemorrhagic stroke. In ISIS-3,[25] a small but significant excess of strokes attributed to "definite or probable" cerebral hemorrhage occurred among patients treated with aspirin plus heparin (0.56%) versus heparin alone (0.40%). The relevance of this latter finding is unclear. Finally, tests of platelet aggregation in patients with intracranial hemorrhage are impractical, and it would be difficult to interpret an abnormal test result in patients with bleeding who did not have such testing done before thrombolytic therapy.[219]

Cerebrovascular Pathology

Even though diverse hemostatic derangements following thrombolytic therapy may contribute to intracranial hemorrhage, its occurrence, particularly in elderly patients, may well reflect unmasking of pre-existing cerebrovascular lesions. While autopsy investigations have been performed in a number of studies,[12,15,23,25,26,57,78,79] specific results have rarely been reported[26,57,78,79] and may be unrevealing.[26,27] A number of cerebrovascular lesions have been described which may be the underlying cause of bleeding in patients treated with thrombolytic agents.

Arteriovenous malformations (AVMs) are vascular anomalies composed of tangles of abnormally fragile arteries and veins that are prone to parenchymatous, subarachnoid, and intraventricular bleeding. Pathologic and magnetic resonance studies have demonstrated that the natural history of AVMs may be complicated by subclinical episodes of thrombosis or bleeding.[248] It is possible that blood clots formed either spontaneously or to limit the extent of bleeding episodes may be inadvertently lysed by thrombolytic agents. Two cases of PIH due to AVM rupture after thrombolytic therapy have been reported.[31,76] Proner and colleagues,[76] described a patient who developed a right frontotemporal PIH 10 hours after initiation of therapy with 100 mg alteplase rt-PA. At surgery, an AVM with gross signs of recent bleeding was removed. In TIMI-2,[31] one patient who received 100 mg alteplase rt-PA developed PIH on day 2. Computed tomography scan showed an AVM adjacent to the hemorrhage.

Cerebral amyloid angiopathy (CAA) is recognized as an important cause of intracranial hemorrhage in elderly people.[197,249] Cerebral amyloid angiopathy is characterized by an acellular thickening in the walls of arterioles and small-to medium-sized arteries and veins. Both media and adventitia are infiltrated by amyloid. Such changes are found in vessels in the superficial cerebral cortex.[249] In rare cases, CAA may be found in the brainstem and cerebellum.[249,250] Ultrastructural studies of patients with multiple hemorrhages[250–252] or infarcts[250] associated with CAA have demonstrated segmental fibrinoid degeneration of small vessels,[252,253] petechiae in cortical and subcortical locations,[252] and occasional microaneurysms.[252,253] The microaneurysms have sometimes been present in the basal ganglia.[250] Many serum proteins are present in vessel walls affected by CAA, implying "leakiness" of the vessels.[253] Blood vessels infiltrated by amyloid are believed to be brittle, unable to withstand trauma or blood pressure changes.[249] Cerebral amyloid angiopathy-related intracranial hemorrhage typically occurs in elderly patients who are frequently demented, and many cases have also been reported in the sixth and seventh decades.[250] The hemorrhages are single, multiple, or sequential. They are located in the lobar and subcortical or cortical regions.

Limited pathologic data are available to explore the relationship between CAA and intracranial hemorrhage after thrombolytic therapy for acute MI. Ramsay and colleagues[78] reported a 56-year-old man with an inferior wall MI who developed fatal multiple left temporoparietal hemorrhages and a left subdural hemorrhage after receiving 1.5 million units SK. Histologic sections were positive for amyloid. Kase and colleagues[57] reported a 67-year-old hypertensive woman with an inferior wall MI who developed three hemorrhages after receiving 100 mg alteplase rt-PA. Evacuation of one hemorrhage was performed and histologic sections revealed no evidence of amyloid. Pendlebury and colleagues[79] reported a 60-year-old woman with an inferior wall MI who developed fatal right frontal and left temporal lobar hemorrhages after receiving 100 mg alteplase rt-PA. On microscopic examination, blood vessels in intact and hemorrhagic areas stained positive for amyloid. Only one other case of CAA-associated intracranial hemorrhage following thrombolytic therapy has been reported.[61] The suspicion that CAA may be a potential cause of intracranial hemorrhage in patients treated with thrombolytic agents may be based on the lobar location, multiplicity, and the increasing frequency in older patients.[82–84]

Various microscopic lesions have been described in patients with spontaneous PIH. These include Charcot-Bouchard microaneurysms,[254–259] miliary aneurysms with lipohyalinosis,[259] fibrin globes ("bleeding globes"),[259,260] and pseudoaneurysm.[261] Microaneurysms are saccular or fusiform dilations of small arteries, 250 to 400 μm in diameter, with degenerative changes in the adventitia. Ross Russell[256] and Cole and Yates[258] found that these lesions could occur in any part of the brain, particularly in elderly hypertensive patients. Aneurysms were commonly found on lateral branches of striate arteries in the basal ganglia or on penetrating vessels supplying cerebral cortex. In the study of Cole and Yates,[258] 30% were found at the gray-white junction, 15% in the pons, and 4% in the cerebellum. In some aneurysms, large quantities of fibrin were present or near the luminal surface, with thrombus in the cavity. On occasion, several small hemorrhages (usually six to seven) were found in the subcortical white matter, basal ganglia, and internal capsule.[259] In rare instances, microaneurysms coexist with CAA.[250] Cole and Yates[261] also described pseudoaneurysms consisting of laminated extravascular blood coagulum, fibrin in the walls of the hemorrhage cavity, and perivascular collections of blood. Fisher[259,260] described fibrin ("bleeding") globes, which he believed to represent secondary distortion of small arteries resulting in an "avalanche" effect to produce hematoma enlargement.

Some investigators[262–264] have suggested that other lesions in hypertensive patients may be important in the production of spontaneous PIH. In two studies, Takebayashi and colleagues[262,263] obtained ruptured lenticulostriate arteries from patients who had emergency surgery for PIH and found evidence of severe arteriosclerosis and degeneration of smooth muscle cells in the media at or near bifurcations. When examined by electron microscopy, these changes were most prominent in the distal portions of the vessels.[263] Ruptured miliary aneurysms were seen in only two cases.[262] Fibrinoid necrosis, present in more peripheral arterioles, has been described by several investigators.[263,264] Fibrinoid necrosis has also been demonstrated in normotensive patients, at times in association with miliary aneurysms in small arteries on the cerebral surface.[264]

Since these lesions exist, particularly in elderly hypertensive patients, it is tempting to speculate that they may be responsible for the occurrence of some cases of PIH after thrombolytic therapy for MI. For example, their location, multiplicity, fragility, and microscopic evidence of hemorrhage suggest that some instances of single or multiple PIH could be explained on this basis. However, in spontaneous PIH cases it has often been difficult to demonstrate the presence of these lesions in surgical specimens.[262,265] At the present time, no direct evidence exists to prove that these lesions could be unmasked by thrombolytic therapy to produce PIH. Furthermore, these lesions are generally associated with chronic hypertension and the association of chronic hypertension with PIH in patients treated with thrombolytic agents is not strong.[31]

Only a handful of cases of SAH occurring after thrombolysis for MI have been documented in the literature.[25,26,42,44,45] Clinical details have been provided in only two cases.[26,44] The paucity of reported cases may reflect incomplete evaluation of stroke cases, or lack of susceptibility of congenital aneurysms to rupture after thrombolytic therapy.

Head Injury Before Treatment

Subdural hematomas are a rare (0.01%) complication of thrombolytic therapy for acute MI.[20,26,31] Acute and chronic SDHs are believed to grow by direct rebleeding.[266,267] Experimental[267] and clinical[268–271] studies suggest that the fibrinolytic system is activated in chronic SDH. Once an SDH is formed, red blood cells accumulate in the hematoma at a daily rate of 5% to 10% of total volume.[269] The outer wall of the subdural neomembrane surface contains plasminogen and plasminogen activator,[270] whereas the subdural fluids have low plasminogen values, the latter presumably due to consumption. Fibrinogen degradation products are present in high concentrations[269–271] and are incorporated into newly formed fibrin strands. Such clots are defective and can not provide effective local hemostasis. Any minor trauma can produce rebleeding or plasmatic effusion. Moreover, these events can lead to a self-perpetuating growth cycle and clinical symptoms.[267]

Thrombolytic agents may enhance fibrinolytic activity within an SDH, promote bleeding, and produce symptoms. In TIMI-2,[31] one patient who developed a symptomatic SDH had a history of head injury 8 years previously. Another patient had syncope and a trivial head injury following an acute inferior wall MI and developed an acute SDH during the rt-PA infusion.[82] In another study,[20] one patient developed a cerebellar hematoma after unrecognized syncope and head trauma. Finally, a recent study[26] indicates that SDH may be single or multiple and accompany other forms of intracranial hemorrhage in patients treated with thrombolytic agents. While it is true that SDH may result from trivial head trauma preceding thrombolytic therapy, it is not known how often head injury precedes thrombolytic treatment in patients who did not develop the complication.

Following Invasive Cardiovascular Procedures

Both ischemic[14,272,273] and hemorrhagic[31,47,58,59,274] stroke have been reported to occur after coronary artery bypass graft surgery[14,31,47,59,272–274] and percutaneous transluminal coronary angioplasty.[58] Abnormal bleeding after cardiopulmonary bypass is well known and is believed to be due to an acquired defect in formation of the platelet plug. Platelets are activated by passage through the oxygenation apparatus, causing secondary release and partial depletion of α granules. Severity of the defect relates to duration of cardiopulmonary bypass and use of platelet-active drugs. This defect is, in general, rapidly reversible[273,275] and can be prevented.[276] Hemostatic effects of rt-PA may contribute to systemic bleeding if cardiac surgery is performed soon after thrombolytic treatment.[276]

Despite the risk, the role played by concomitant invasive cardiovascular procedures remains unclear. Intracranial hemorrhage following invasive cardiovascular procedures has been reported to occur between less than 24 hours and 4 weeks after thrombolytic treatment.[14,31,47,58,59,272,274] Important parameters such as clinical features, profile of illness, and presence or absence of anticoagulant therapy have not been reported. In only one instance has the site of hemorrhage (posterior fossa) been specified.[47] In TIMI-2,[31] there was no increase in PIH occurrence in patients who received immediate or delayed coronary angiography and percutaneous transluminal coronary angioplasty. On the basis of published data,[14,47,58,59,272,274] it is not possible to distinguish between PIH and HI in these cases. In addition, it may not be possible to differentiate between the catheter procedure itself, the thrombolytic therapy, concomitant anticoagulant therapy, or the underlying cardiac or cerebrovascular disease as the cause of the stroke.[83]

Brain Tumors

Both primary and metastatic brain tumors may occasionally be complicated by intratumoral hemorrhage.[197] Anecdotal experience suggests that the rate of intracranial hemorrhage in brain tumors following thrombolytic therapy for acute MI has been excessively high.[207]

Management of Intracranial Hemorrhage Following Thrombolytic Therapy for Acute MI

Any change in neurologic function, particularly during the first 24 hours after treatment, should be regarded as strongly indicative of intracranial hemorrhage until proven otherwise. Emergent CT scanning and application of the aforementioned definitions will aid in identification of the type of intracranial hemorrhage. Early involvement of neurologists, hematologists, and neurosurgeons will optimize management decisions.[82]

It is reasonable to discontinue thrombolytic, anticoagulant, or combined therapies as soon as symptoms and signs are recognized. Since intracranial hemorrhage is a serious complication, it is useful to document the severity of the coagulopathy to the extent possible. For fibrinogen determinations, the sulfite precipitation test provides higher and more accurate levels than the Clauss chronometric method, although the Clauss method is believed to provide the best indication of functional fibrinogen levels. The presence of a lytic state is best documented by the reptilase time. Assays for coagulation factors V and VIII have not been routinely performed in coronary thrombolysis trials since they are repleted during cryoprecipitate and fresh frozen plasma therapy.[219] However, knowledge of coagulation factor levels at or near the time of symptom onset may be important, from academic and clinical perspectives. The bleeding time has been shown to correlate with spontaneous bleeding after rt-PA therapy[220] and should be measured. However, more work is necessary to delineate the effect of SK, UK, APSAC, rt-PA, or rscu-PA on the bleeding time and its importance.[221]

Once PIH, SAH, or SDH is documented, the patient should be given 10 U of cryoprecipitate, which will increase the fibrinogen level about 0.70 gm/L and the factor VIII level by about 30% in a 70 kg adult. Fresh frozen plasma may be used as a source of factors V and VIII and as a volume expander in carefully selected cases. In patients who are receiving heparin therapy, 1 mg protamine for every 100 units of heparin given in the preceding 4 hours may be administered. If the bleeding time is abnormal, infusion of 6 to 8 units of platelets is indicated. In rare cases, antifibrinolytic agents, such as epsilon aminocaproic acid (Amicar®) may be necessary. It should be recognized that these replacement therapies may theoretically be complicated by coronary reocclusion.[219] Blood pressure should be managed judiciously, with a careful balance between competing cardiologic and neurologic concerns. Angiography may be necessary when an arteriovenous malformation or berry aneurysm is suspected. Neurosurgical intervention, such as craniotomy with clot removal, lesion obliteration, stereotactic procedures, or ventriculostomy should be based on joint consideration of the patient's clinical and hematologic status.[82,84]

If an HI is present, then anticoagulant therapy may be withheld and restarted 7 to 10 days later, unless clinical circumstances dictate otherwise. Since patients with confluent HI potentially have a more serious hemorrhagic transformation, it may be prudent to withhold anticoagulant therapy for at least 7 to 10 days. If the hematoma is accompanied by mass effect, therapy similar to that for PIH should be considered. The utility of angiography in this setting is unclear. However, in the patient with a carotid territory stroke, evidence of surgically important carotid disease (greater than 70% stenosis) should be sought. Long-term antithrombic or surgical therapy for secondary stroke prevention may be planned by consideration of the site of acute MI, cardiologic and neurologic status, documented vascular lesions, and other factors.[84]

Prognosis of Intracranial Hemorrhage Following Thrombolytic Therapy for Acute MI

The overall mortality for PIH following thrombolytic therapy may be as high as 70%.[11–14,16,18,29–33,53,54,57] Recent studies suggest that the acute mortality has been reduced to between 44%[29] and 52%.[31] With 100 mg alteplase rt-PA, the mortality rate may be as low as 36%. Recovery with little residual deficit may occur in 54%.[31] The reduction in mortality and more favorable outcome may reflect more careful patient selection, better control of the dosage of the fibrinolytic agent and concomitant therapies, timely diagnosis, and, in some instances, aggressive medical or surgical management. In trials of anticoagulation therapy for acute cardioembolic stroke, patients who have HI often deteriorate, and a 55% mortality rate has been reported.[277] In TIMI-2,[31] 1 of 8 (12.5%) patients who had HI died, implying a more favorable outcome after thrombolytic therapy for acute MI. The occurrence of SDH appears to have a high mortality rate[20,26,31] but complete recovery is possible.[31]

Intracranial Hemorrhage Following Thrombolytic Therapy for Acute Ischemic Cerebral Infarction

In cases of thrombolytic therapy for acute ischemic stroke, one must be concerned about bleeding into both normal brain and ischemic brain. It is therefore necessary to review current concepts and existing data pertaining to hemorrhagic transformation of ischemic infarcts. This will provide the background for comparison with the occurrence of intracranial hemorrhage following thrombolysis for experimental and clinical stroke.

Hemorrhagic Infarction

It is well known that transformation of a "bland" cerebral infarction to an HI[190,278–306] or parenchymatous hemorrhage (confluent HI[16,190,194,195,285–287]) may occur. In clinical studies, the causes, incidence, risk factors, and suspected pathogenesis are difficult to evaluate, as many studies describe both nonanticoagulated and anticoagulated patients.[277,283–285,289–292,294,295,298,299] Hemorrhagic infarction describes multifocal secondary bleeding into brain infarcts via diapedesis through damaged capillary and venular walls, forming petechiae of varying sizes. When large areas of petechiae merge to form confluent purpura or parenchymatous hematoma, a CT scan detectable intracerebral hemorrhage may occur.[190]

Early investigators[2,296,305,306] believed that HI in a variety of settings resulted from restoration of blood flow into a recently ischemic area that contained abnormal blood vessels lacking autoregulatory capacity,[307,308] and was perhaps potentiated by hypertension.[306,307] Restoration of blood flow may occur either by reopening the occluded vessel or by establishment of collateral circulation.[190,296] Experimental studies in rats,[309] cats,[310,311] and monkeys[312] have shown that when ischemia is followed by reperfusion, permeability changes in the blood-brain barrier occur at some time between 2 and 6 hours after the onset of ischemia. Brain capillaries may expand and rupture in areas of ischemia and reperfusion.[312] The extent of disruption of endothelial junctions and capillary rupture are related to the duration and degree of ischemia. Thus, mild (petechial) to moderate HIs are believed to result from diapedesis through ischemic endothelium, usually without vessel rupture. When vessel walls necrose, hemorrhage may be focal and severe. However, it remains unsettled whether parenchymatous hematoma in this setting represents a severe form of multicentric bleeding from reperfusion of injured capillaries as in HI or is due to rupture of one or more arterioles.[304] Four experimental studies[306,313–315] using norepinephrine infusion,[314] hypercarbia,[314] or aortic obstruction[306,313,315] and one clinical report of patients with permanently occluded MCAs[193] have shown that induction of significant acute hypertension may produce HI. It is believed that restoration and accentuation of blood flow through leptomeningeal collaterals via retrograde flow into damaged cerebral vessels is the mechanism of HI in this situation.[315]

In autopsy series, cardioembolic strokes appear to have a higher propensity for hemorrhagic transformation (51% to 76% prevalence[278,290,296,298,299]) than nonembolic strokes (2% to 21% prevalence[191,284–297]). The reported difference may reflect ascertainment bias, because lethal infarcts are more often large with mass effect, brain herniation, or hemorrhagic transformation.[290] However, HI has also been documented in patients with small- to moderate-sized infarctions.[295,316] Clinical CT studies of nonanticoagulated patients indicate that HI occurs in 5% to 43% of cases.[194,287,289,316] Autopsy[298] and clinical CT[289,291,292,295] studies suggest that the majority of HIs occur within 3 to 4 days after stroke onset. Some HIs may occur as early as several hours after onset[195] or as late as the end of the second week post-stroke.[289,295] Parenchymatous hematomas (confluent HIs) occur in 2% to 8.6% of cases.[194,285–287]

It is estimated that as many as 95% of HIs in nonanticoagulated patients are asymptomatic,[289,291,292] while parenchymatous hematomas are generally associated with clinical worsening, except for the smallest ones.[302] One experimental study[317] suggests that anticoagulation does not increase the likelihood of HI, but may accentuate the degree of hemorrhage on CT. Several studies report that the estimated incidence of clinical deterioration is 5% to 20%.[283,285,291,294,305] The period of active bleeding is transient, and anticoagulation therapy administered after the appearance of HI on CT does not usually result in clinical or roentgenographic worsening.[281,284]

Thrombolysis — Experimental Studies

A number of workers have developed various experimental models and protocols to test the hypothesis that timely administration of thrombolytic therapy will be effective in recanalizing occluded cerebral blood vessels and reducing cerebral infarct size.[121,318-351] The results, limitations, and relevance of experimental stroke models in general[352-356] and in the setting of thrombolytic therapy in particular[9,81,357-359] have recently been reviewed. Experimental studies in baboons,[320,330,342] mongrel dogs,[324,325,329,338,346] rabbits,[318,319,321,328,331-334,337,341,343-345,349,350] and rats[121,322,326,327,351] have utilized SK,[318,320,321,329,338,341,343,347] UK,[324,325,344] prourokinase,[325,346] rt-PA,[121,319-323,326-328,330-334,337,341-345,348-350] and rt-PA analogues[336,347] by employing a wide variety of methods of ischemic injury to investigate issues of timing, dosage, and duration of therapy. The duration of ischemia has ranged from 5 minutes to 24 hours. These studies have shown that thrombolytic therapy induces angiographically demonstrable recanalization,[320,322-326,328,331-333,337,339,340,347,351] improved neurologic outcome,[319,320,323,326,334,338,351] smaller infarct volume,[320,323,328,344,345,349,350] and improved regional cerebral blood flow[326,345,351] and metabolism.[121,329,338]

The occurrence of HI is common in animals subjected to experimental focal cerebral ischemia followed by thrombolysis. In six studies designed to assess changes in coagulation status,[325,326,339,340,342,346] systemic fibrinolysis was marked in one[346] and briefly observed (30 minutes) in another.[326] In animals treated with SK[329,333,338,341,343,347] or UK,[324] infarct-associated hemorrhages have been noted but were severe only in animals treated with high doses of SK 24 hours after vascular occlusion with severe ischemia.[321] In animals treated with rt-PA, petechial hemorrhages have been observed with similar frequency in control[321,329-333,336,337,339,341,342] and experimental[321,329-334,337,339,341,342] groups. In one study,[349,350] coadministration of heparin to prolong the PTT to greater than 300 seconds did not lead to macroscopic or microscopic HI. In some studies,[318,336,339] a small amount of SAH or IVH was seen microscopically.

Parenchymatous hemorrhage (confluent HI or macroscopic hemorrhages) has been observed in animals treated at 60 minutes,[341] 3 hours,[347] 3 1/2 hours,[342] 6 hours,[341] 8 hours,[337] and 24 hours[321,337] after occlusion. In rare instances, a parenchymatous hemorrhage may occur in placebo-treated animals.[342] In one small study,[342] no neurologic deterioration was observed in animals with HI. In two studies,[342,343] there was no relation between rt-PA dose and the occurrence of HI. In addition, one study[342] showed that there was no relation between volume of infarction and volume of HI. Preliminary evidence suggests that administration of SK,[321,341,343] particularly when delayed for 6 to 24 hours, may be associated with a greater frequency of hemorrhagic complications.[321,341] If treatment is delayed for 8 hours, animals with severe or fatal stroke are more likely to have microscopic hemorrhage at post mortem examination.[337]

These findings have several implications for therapeutic thrombolysis in acute ischemic stroke. Early thrombolytic therapy may accelerate the natural history of the ischemia-spontaneous recanalization process by promoting reperfusion into a damaged vascular bed after varying durations and degrees of ischemia.[302,304,309,311,357] There appears to be a therapeutic window after which clinically significant hemorrhagic phenomena may be encountered. The risk of hemorrhage at various times between 90 minutes and 6 hours of ischemia remains to be demonstrated. Extrapolation from animal studies to the clinical setting involving human stroke victims should be made with caution. Such patients are usually elderly, are frequently hypertensive, have a variety of macro- and microvascular lesions, and may be more likely to suffer adverse consequences from hemorrhagic complications.[81,357,358]

Thrombolysis—Clinical Studies

For recent studies of thrombolytic therapy in acute ischemic stroke,[95-152] the rationale, data on safety and efficacy, and ongoing analyses have recently been reviewed.[7,9,81,112,299-301,360,361] These reports have been designed as either angiographically controlled[1,2,89-93,102,103,111-114,116,120,127,129-133,139,144,148,149,152] or clinical outcome[5,90,91,98,99,106,107,109,111-114,124,145-147,149,152] evaluations of intravenous[1,2,4,5,89-91,98,99,106,107,109,115,124,128-132,138,144-147,152] or intra-arterial[91-93,102,103,110-114,116,117,120,127,133,134] therapy with SK,[102,111,113,116,134] UK,[4,5,99,102,106,107,111,113-116,120,124,127,133,134,142] rt-PA,[109,110,112,115,117,124,128-132,139,144-149,152] prourokinase,[142] and ancrod.[119] Patients with carotid,[2,4,89-93,103,109,111,112,114,116,127-133,142,144,146,147,149,152] vertebrobasilar,[4,90,102,110,113,117,120,129-134,139,142] or any[1,106,107,115,145,148] territory stroke have been treated by a variety of protocols initiated at various times after symptoms onset. Recanalization in the carotid[4,89,91-93,103,111,112,114,116,127-133,142,144,152] and vertebrobasilar[102,110,113,117,120,129-132,134,139,142,145] territories has been reported in 41.8% (range 8% to 100%) and 59.4% (range 40% to 100%) of cases, respectively. Clinical improvement was documented in 61 of 245 (24.9%) of patients treated in older studies[1-6,89-93,95-97] and 218 of 447 (48.8%) of patients treated in more recent studies.[102,103,110-117,122,129-135,138-142,145-149,152]

Intracranial hemorrhages have been reported in numerous studies from the pre-CT scan[1,2,5,6] and CT scan[98,99,106,107,111-117,119-124,127-133,135,137-139,141-149,152] eras (Table 5). Using the definitions outlined before, the types of hemorrhage include HI,[1,5,106,107,111-115,120-122,124,127-133,135,137,139,142,144-146,148,149,152] confluent HI,[1,5,112-114,116,118,120,129-131,133,135,137,144-146,149,152] PIH,[123,129-131,144-146] intracranial hemorrhage of unspecified type,[5,98,99,117,128] extension to the subarachnoid or intraventricular space,[5,114,120,127,135,146] or SDH.[129-131] Hemorrhages have occurred in patients treated with SK,[111,113,116] UK,[5,98,99,106,107,111,113-116,121,122,124,133,142] alteplase rt-PA,[112,117,122-124,129-132,137,139,145,146,148,149] duteplase rt-PA,[118,128,144,152] and prourokinase[142] by intravenous[1,5,98,99,106,107,115,121,123,124,128-132,137,142,144-146,148,149,152] and intra-arterial[111,112,114,116-118,120,122,127,133,135,139,149] routes. Of the 2,173 reported patients treated with thrombolytic agents, the proportions of HI, confluent HI, PIH, and intracranial hemorrhage of unspecified type are 136 of 2,173 (6.3%), 46 of 2,173 (2.1%), 6 of 2,173 (0.3%) and 6 of 2,173 (0.3%), respectively. If one only considers the major recent trials (total n = 905),[111,113,114,120,121,127-133,135,137,144-147,149,152] the proportions of HI, confluent HI, PIH, and other intracranial hemorrhage are 99 of 905 (10.9%, range 2.3% to 42.1%), 37 of 905 (4.1%, range 5% to 25%), 4 of 905 (0.4%, range 0% to 5%) and 2 of 905 (0.2%, range 0% to 10.5%). In recent studies, the proportions of HI, confluent HI, PIH, and intracranial hemorrhage of unspecified type in the carotid distribution trials[111,114,116,122,123,127-131,133,137,142,144-146,149,152] are 75 of 394 (19%,

Table 5

Published Studies Describing Central Nervous System Hemorrhage (ICH) Following Thrombolytic Therapy for Acute Ischemic Stroke

Author	Ref	Agent	Route	Δt_{t-o}	Vascular Territory	N	HI (n/%)	CHI (n/%)	PIH (n/%)	ICH-NS (n/%)
A. Intravenous Studies
Meyer	1	SK	IV	< 72h	Carotid	37	1(2.7)	3(8.1)	—	—
Fletcher	5	u-PA	IV	< 36h	—	31	1(3.2)	1(3.2)	—	2(6.5)
Abe	98,99	u-PA	IV	< 720h	—	216	—	—	—	1(0.5)
Atarashi	106	u-PA	IV	< 120h	—	191	2(1)	—	—	—
Otomo	107	u-PA	IV	< 120h	—	176	2(1.1)	—	—	—
Otomo	115	u-PA	IV	< 120h	—	184	3(1.6)	—	—	—
Otomo	115	rt-PA	IV	< 120h	—	171	2(1.2)	—	—	—
Terashi	121	rt-PA	IV	< 72h	—	171	8(4.7)	—	—	—
Terashi	121	u-PA	IV	< 72h	—	171	8(4.7)	—	—	—
Hennerici	123	rt-PA	IV	2–18h	MCA/BA	12	—		1(8.3)	—
Abe	124	rt-PA	IV	< 72h	—	14	3(2.1)	—	—	—
Abe	124	u-PA	IV	< 72h	—	77	6(4.1)	—	—	—
Mori	128	drt-PA	IV	< 6h	Carotid	19	8(42.1)	—	—	2(10.5)
von Kummer	129–131	rt-PA	IV	< 6h	ICA/MCA	32	9(28.1)	3(9.4)	1(3.1)	—
Yamaguchi	132	rt-PA	IV	< 6h	—	58	12(21)	—	—	—
Pilz	137	rt-PA	IV	< 8h	BA	17	1(5.9)	3(17.7)	—	—
Pilz	137	rt-PA	IV	< 6h	MCA	5	1(20)	—	—	—
Hamann	142	u-PA + rscu-PA	IV	< 6h	MCA	3	1(33.3)	—	—	—
Brott	145	rt-PA	IV	< 1.5h	ICA/MCA/ACA	74	3(4.1)	2(2.7)	1(1.4)	—
Haley	146	rt-PA	IV	1.5–3.0h	ICA/MCA	20	4(20.0)	1(5)	1(5)	—
Sperling	148	rt-PA	IV	< 6h	—	12	1(8.3)	—	—	—
Brucker	149	rt-PA + u-PA	IV/IA	< 6h	ICA/MCA = 19; BA =9	28	8(28.6)	2(7.1)	—	—
Okada	152	rt-PA	IV	< 6h	ICA/MCA	10	4(40)	1(10)	—	—
del Zoppo	144	drt-PA	IV	< 8h	ICA/MCA	104	21(20.2)	11(10.6)	2(1.9)	—
B. Intraarterial Studies
del Zoppo	111	SK/u-PA	IA	< 8h	Carotid	20	4(20)	—	—	—
del Zoppo	112	rt-PA	IA	< 1h	MCA	3	1(33.1)	1(33.3)	—	—
Hacke	113	SK/u-PA	IA	< 24h	VBA	43	1(2.3)	3(7.0)	—	—
Mori	114,127	u-PA	IA	< 12h	ICA = 8; MCA = 31; BA = 5	44	4(9.1)	6(13.6)	—	—
Theron	116	SK/u-PA	IA	< 1h	ICA/MCA	12	—	3(25)	—	—
Buteux	117	rt-PA	IA	—	PCA	1	—	—	—	1(100)
Brückmann	118	drt-PA	IA	< 6h	MCA	1	—	1(100)	—	—
Pfeiffer	120,135	SK/u-PA	IA	< 8h	VBA	20	3(15)	1(5)	—	—
Ikeda	122	u-PA	IA	< 3h	ICA/MCA	13	3(23.1)	—	—	—
Matsumoto	133	u-PA	IA	< 24h	ICA/MCA	39	9(23.1)	4(10.3)	—	—
Matsumoto	133	u-PA	IA	< 24h	BA/PCA	11	1(9.1)	—	—	—
Herderscheé	139	rt-PA	IA	< 6h	BA	2	1(50)	—	—	—
TOTAL						2173	136(6.3)	46(2.1)	6(0.3)	6(0.3)

N = total number of patients in study population
n = total number of patients with specified type of hemorrhagic complication
HI = hemorrhagic infection
CHI = Confluent hemorrhagic infection
PIH = parenchymatous intracerebral hematoma
ICH = intracranial hemorrhage
ICH-NS = intracranial hemorrhage of unspecified type
Δt_{t-o} = time interval from onset of symptoms to initiation of thrombolytic therapy

SK = streptokinase
u-PA = urokinase
rt-PA = alteplase recombinant tissue plasminogen activator
drt-PA = duteplase recombinant tissue plasminogen activator
ICA = internal carotid artery
MCA = middle cerebral artery
ACA = anterior cerebral artery
PCA = posterior cerebral artery
BA = basilar artery
VBA = vertebral and basilar arteries

range 0% to 42.1%), 31 of 394 (7.9%, range 0% to 25%), 5 of 394 (1.3%, range 0% to 20%) and 2 of 394 (0.5%, range 0% to 10.5%), respectively. Similarly, the proportions of HI, confluent HI, PIH and intracranial hemorrhage of unspecified type reported in the vertebrobasilar distribution trials[113,120,127,133,135,137,139] are 5 of 98 (5.1%, range 0% to 50%), 8 of 98 (8.2%, range 0% to 20%), 0%, and 0%, respectively. In some trials,[121,122,132] the exact nature of the hemorrhagic complication could only be inferred. In one study,[147] confluent HI occurred in one patient in the placebo group.

Limited data are available on the hematologic aspects of thrombolytic therapy for acute ischemic stroke. In several studies, concomitant heparin[111,113,129–131,142,149] and a hemorheologic agent[111,113] were administered. In one study,[128] there was a dose-response relationship between rt-PA dose and changes in fibrinolytic parameters. In another study,[113] changes in hemostasis were not different between patients who did and did not have hemorrhage. In two studies,[145,146] cerebellar PIH occurred in association with sustained, severe hypofibrinogenemia. However, in another study,[151] the 3 hour post-treatment fibrinogen level was not related to the combined occurrence of confluent HI and PIH.

A number of clinical aspects may be important in the genesis of intracranial hemorrhage in this setting. Evidence of a relation between blood pressure and intracranial hemorrhage is conflicting. In one study,[144] there was no relation between blood pressure and the occurrence of intracranial hemorrhage, but in two other studies[145,146,151] diastolic blood pressure (104 ± 10 versus 86 ± 14 mm Hg) and mean blood pressure (127 ± 18 versus 108 ± 17 mm Hg) were higher in patients with intracranial hemorrhage versus patients without intracranial hemorrhage.

Evidence for a relation between rt-PA dose and occurrence of intracranial hemorrhage is also conflicting. In two studies using alteplase rt-PA,[145,146,151] an apparent dose-response relationship with combined HI, confluent HI, and PIH was observed (0.97 mg/kg with hemorrhage versus 0.74 mg/kg without hemorrhage), although it was not seen in terms of dose/meter^2 or actual dose administered. In a study using duteplase rt-PA,[144] no dose-response relationship was apparent between rt-PA dose and combined HI, confluent HI, and PIH. The reasons for these conflicting data may include small numbers of patients, differences in thrombolytic activity between agents, differences in rt-PA dosages, and other factors. In two studies,[145,146,151] there was a trend for patient weight to be inversely correlated with combined HI, confluent HI and PIH, with hemorrhage patients weighing 65.1 ± 11.9 kg and nonhemorrhagic patients weighing 78.5 ± 17.5 kg. In three studies,[144–146,151] there was no relationship between intracranial hemorrhage and patient age, gender, history of hypertension, history of diabetes, subsequent heparin use, pretreatment glucose level,[145,146] tobacco use,[144] cardiac arrhythmias, prior aspirin use or subsequent heparin use. In one study,[129–131] the three patients with confluent HI or PIH had PTTs greater than 120 seconds. However, since few patients have been treated with concomitant heparin therapy, the actual effect of heparin in producing intracranial hemorrhage is not yet clear.

Many patients have moderate to severe deficits before treatment is given. While one study[114,127] suggests that intracranial hemorrhage may be more common in unconscious patients, two other studies[145,146,151] suggest no relationship between intracranial hemorrhage and initial summed NIH Stroke Scale Score. In three studies,[114,127,132,144] patients treated later, particularly greater than 6 hours after symptom onset, were more likely to suffer intracranial hemorrhage. Patients with HI,[111,114,117,118,127,137,142,144,149] confluent HI,[114,120,127,135,137,144-146] and PIH[123,145,146] may be clinically stable[111,114,117,118,127,144-146,148] or deteriorate[113,120,123,129-131,133,135,137,142,144-146,149] following the hemorrhagic complication. In many cases, patients with intracranial hemorrhage die,[113,114,122,123,127,129-131,133,137,142,146] either as a result of the severity of the ischemic stroke or the hemorrhage.

Limited data are available on the radiologic aspects pertaining to thrombolytic therapy for acute ischemic stroke. Intracranial hemorrhage (including HI, confluent HI, and PIH) may occur in patients who do[111,113,114,116,117,127,133,137,144,152] or do not[113,114,127-131,133,137,144,152] recanalize after thrombolytic therapy. In three studies,[128-131,144] there was no relationship between recanalization or degree of collateral circulation[129-131] and the occurrence of HI, confluent HI, and PIH.

The relation between the ischemic lesion appearance on CT scan, brain hemorrhage, and prognosis is not clear. Three recent studies[152,316,362] have shown that CT scans obtained within 2 hours,[316] 3 hours,[152] and 12 hours[362] of stroke onset may demonstrate evidence of ischemic cerebral injury. One study[362] suggests that early demonstration of a lesion on CT may not correlate with patient outcome, as defined by Glasgow Outcome Scale Score and the attending physician's assessment of the patient at hospital discharge. In one study[152] of 10 patients with anterior circulation stroke who received CT scan within 3 hours of stroke onset and intravenous rt-PA therapy within 6 hours of stroke onset, four patients with early CT abnormalities did not experience recanalization and one developed a symptomatic confluent HI. In another study,[144] patients with confluent HI were more likely to deteriorate than patients with HI (6 of 11 versus 4 of 21). In that study,[144] there was no relationship between intracranial hemorrhage and the presence of infarction on the first CT scan or in the ultimate infarct size.

These results are encouraging, in that the overall occurrence of intracranial hemorrhage in treated patients does not appear to be increased compared with studies in untreated patients.[194,287,289,291] Limited data also appear to indicate that bleeding into normal brain is infrequent, as in patients treated with thrombolytic therapy for acute myocardial infarction. In view of the relatively small numbers of patients treated by a variety of thrombolytic therapy regimens in individual reports, many questions remain regarding the role of the various clinical, laboratory, and radiologic factors which may relate to brain hemorrhage in this setting. Future investigations in large, controlled trials should consider prospective analysis of the role of age, sex, blood pressure (at entry, during treatment, after treatment but before hemorrhage), weight, presence of cardiac disease, type of thrombolytic agent, dose of thrombolytic agent, time to treatment, vascular territory, stroke severity (as determined by various Stroke Scale scores or other means), CT scan features (hypodensity on first scan, infarct volume, infarct location) reperfusion, collateral patterns, use of concomitant antithrombotic drugs, and use of other drugs (Table 6).

Table 6
Potential Risk Factors for Intracranial
Hemorrhage Following Thrombolytic Therapy
for Acute Ischemic Stroke

I. Demographics
   A. Age
   B. Sex
   C. Blood pressure
   D. Weight
   E. Cardiac disease
II. Thrombolytic Agents
   A. Type
   B. Dose
   C. Presence of fibrinolytic state
III. Clinical Factors
   A. Time to treatment
   B. Stroke severity
   C. Vascular territory
   D. CT scan
   E. Reperfusion
IV. Concomitant Therapy
   A. Antiplatelet
   B. Anticoagulant
   C. Other

Thrombolytic Therapy for PIH Intracerebral or IVH

In recent years, the management of spontaneous parenchymatous hematoma has been evolving, including the indications for surgery, timing of surgical intervention, and methods of hematoma evacuation. There are several reasons to consider surgical evacuation of PIH. Parenchymal hemorrhage leads to primary tissue destruction and mass effect with compression. Early removal of the mass might relieve compression of the microcirculation, reduce edema formation, reduce intracranial pressure, remove toxic and vasoactive blood by-products, and perhaps improve outcome.[182]

Using stereotactic techniques,[169–174,178–180,182] the hematoma coordinates are determined. Through a burr hole, a catheter is passed into the hematoma. Aspiration of the liquid or solid part of the hematoma is attempted. Bleeding vessels are occluded or coagulated. If a significant amount of clot persists, then a silicone catheter is inserted into the hematoma bed and 5,000 to 6,000 units of UK may be infused at 6 to 8 hour intervals for up to several days. Similarly, thrombolytic agents may be infused via a ventricular catheter to facilitate removal of the ventricular clot in selected cases. Several CT scans are obtained to document the response to therapy. Experimental studies in macaques,[169] rabbits,[170,172] rats,[169] dogs,[175–177] and in vitro[173] using UK[169,172,175–177] and rt-PA[178] demonstrate that thrombolytic agents promote clot lysis,[169,172] clot absorption,[175,178] and clot aspiration.[176] In one study,[172] clot lysis at 3 hours occurred in 9 of 10 (90%) of UK treated animals and 1 of 7 (14%) controls, while clot lysis at 24 hours occurred in 10 of 12 (83%) UK treated animals and 2 of 6 (33%) controls. In another study,[169] serial CT scans demonstrated more rapid resolution of the mass associated with partial motor recovery.

Stereotactic aspiration with the assistance of UK[170,171,174,179,181,182] or rt-PA[173] has been carried out in preliminary open studies in patients with putaminal,[171,173] basal ganglion,[170] subcortical lobar,[170] thalamic,[170] cerebellar,[170,179] and intraventricular[181,183] hematomas. Use of thrombolytic agents has increased the amount of clot removed.[170,171,179,181] In one study of 241 patients with putaminal hemorrhage treated more than 6 hours after onset of bleeding, 81% were able to return to useful lives.[173] However, 76% were alert to somnolent on admission and might have done well even without surgery. In another study,[170] there was no significant difference in mortality between craniotomy and stereotactic aspiration with UK in cases treated within the first 3 days or later after onset. In another study of putaminal hemorrhage,[174] clot lysis was optimized by treatment within 24 hours of onset and was associated with rapid improvement in many patients. In another study of putaminal hemorrhage,[171] a double track aspiration technique was applied between 6 and 24 hours after onset with similar results. In one study of 14 patients with hypertensive cerebellar hemorrhage,[179] 13 (91%) had a good to very good quality of life 6 months later. Finally, in one study of six patients with severe IVH,[181] five (83%) showed excellent or good outcome. One recent patient with severe IVH and hydrocephalus after rupture of an anterior cerebral artery aneurysm made a substantial recovery after intraventricular rt-PA therapy.[183] In these preliminary studies, bleeding complications occurred in 0%[171,179,181] to 4%[170,173,174] of patients. These findings support the experimental data[172,178] and suggest that this promising approach may be safe in properly selected patients.

Thrombolytic Therapy for Aneurysmal SAH

Use of CT scans has convincingly shown that the extent and location of thick subarachnoid clot can accurately predict the site and severity of vasospasm after SAH and resultant delayed ischemic neurologic deficits.[363,364] Two recent reviews[365,366] summarize the literature on the role and mechanisms by which subarachnoid blood induces cerebral vasospasm. Analysis of diverse experimental and clinical investigations indicate that early rather than later removal of subarachnoid blood offers the best chance to prevent vasospasm.[365,366] However, aggressive surgical intervention to remove extensive clot or tightly adherent blood from vessels may be associated with damage to brain or perforating vessels.[160,365,366] Under normal circumstances, cerebrospinal fluid (CSF) lacks intrinsic fibrinolytic (t-PA) activity.[153,158] Irritation of the endothelium of small meningeal vessels, such as by hemorrhage or trauma, induces release of t-PA into the CSF, but in concentrations too small to affect rapid or efficient pharmacologic clot removal. The rationale for intrathecal thrombolytic therapy following aneurysm clipping is to augment the limited fibrinolytic activity of the CSF, promote rapid clot lysis, and thereby promote clearance of entrapped erythrocytes prior to hemolysis and release of spasmogens near vessels in the subarachnoid space.[158,183]

Experimental studies with small numbers of pigs,[155,156] cynomolgus monkeys,[157-159,161] dogs,[160] and cats,[162] using plasmin[155,156] or various doses of rt-PA[157-162] have demonstrated several potentially valuable effects of intrathecal thrombolytic therapy after SAH. In general, early (30 minutes[162] to 54 hours[160] after first induced SAH) application of single[160,162] or multiple[157] bolus injections through an Ommaya reservoir[157] or use of sustained-release gel rt-PA[158,159,161] has resulted in near complete disappearance of subarachnoid clot in treated animals. Angiographic studies[157-159,161] have shown significant reduction in the occurrence of vasospasm, especially severe vasospasm, in treated animals compared with controls. Cerebral infarction occurred only in an occasional placebo treated animal.[157,159] In pathologic studies,[155,156,160] intimal proliferation[155,156] and proliferative vasculopathy (luminal narrowing, corrugation of the elastic lumina, and subendothelial thickening and proliferation)[160] were significantly less likely to be seen in treated animals. In one study,[162] intrathecal application of rt-PA abolished the elevation in CSF outflow resistance by permitting near normal CSF absorption, thus facilitating rapid clearance of the breakdown products of subarachnoid blood. In these studies, no histologic evidence of brain inflammation was seen.[157,160,161] In one study,[157] no significant change in coagulation status occurred in treatment or placebo groups. In two studies,[157,159] incisional bleeding occurred in four animals, presumably due to epidural leakage. In one study,[159] petechial hemorrhages occurred in one animal in each group. No intracerebral, intraventricular, epidural, or subdural hematomas occurred in these studies.[157-162]

In the last 2 years, five preliminary open clinical studies using single[165,167,168] or multiple[164,166] injections of various doses of rt-PA have been reported. Many patients have been classified as Hunt and Hess grade III or IV[166] or at high risk of developing vasospasm (Fisher grade III[363-366]). Unilateral[165-168] or bilateral[164] craniotomies and continuous ventricular drainage[164-166] were performed within 48[164-166] to 72[167,168] hours of symptom onset. In most patients, partial to total blood clot removal was demonstrated by serial postoperative CT scans over several days.[164,165,167,168] Of the 85 treated patients,[164-168] only two patients developed fatal symptomatic vasospasm.[165,168] In four studies,[165-168] mild to moderate vasospasm has been demonstrated by angiography[165,166] and transcranial Doppler (TCD).[168] In one study,[167] the severity of angiographic vasospasm was significantly less when the highest rt-PA dose (13 mg) was used. In another study,[168] serial TCD studies revealed flow velocity elevation of a mild to moderate degree in 16 of 20 (80%) patients. Fatal symptomatic vasospasm was present in one patient. In one study,[164] there were no regions of low perfusion on single photon emission CT scans. Despite these results, one study[167] demonstrated no significant difference in 3 month outcome between 3 mg, 10 mg, and 13 mg treatment groups, although the incidence of hypodense areas on CT scan was reduced when the rt-PA dose was increased.

Thrombolytic therapy did not result in systemic fibrinogenolysis in three studies.[164-166] However, bleeding complications have been reported. In three studies,[165-167] bleeding complications were frequent and included subgaleal bleeding,[167] oozing from the incision site, oozing from the ventriculostomy site,[166] and facial bruising.[167] In one study,[165] 1 of 15 patients received 15 mg of rt-PA after clipping of a large right PCoA aneurysm. Postoperatively, he did not awaken and CT scan showed a large right SDH which was evacuated. However, the next day, residual right SDH and a right temporal hematoma were removed. A second patient in that study[165] had a thin asymptomatic EPH which was partially aspirated the day following surgery. In another study,[166] 1 of 10 patients developed a small EPH that required delayed burr hole drainage. In another study,[167] 2 of 30 patients developed intracranial hemorrhage. One had development of PIH after operation from which a good recovery was made with conservative therapy. The second patient required evacuation of an EPH from which a good recovery was made.

REFERENCES

1. Meyer JS, Gilroy J, Barnhart ME, et al: Anticoagulants plus streptokinase therapy in progressive stroke. *JAMA* 1963;189:373.
2. Meyer JS, Gilroy J, Barnhart ME, et al: Therapeutic thrombolysis in cerebral thromboembolism: randomized evaluation of intravenous streptokinase. In: Millikan CH, Siekert W, Whisnant JP, eds: *Cerebral Vascular Diseases*. New York: Grune & Stratton, 1964:200.
3. Hass WK, Clauss RM, Goldberg AF: Special problems associated with surgical and thrombolytic treatment of strokes. *Arch Surg* 1966;92:27.
4. Araki G, Minakami K, Mihara H: Therapeutic effects of urokinase in cerebral infarction. *Rinsho to Kenkyu* 1973;50:3317.
5. Fletcher AP, Alkjaersig N, Lewis M: A pilot study of urokinase therapy in cerebral infarction. *Stroke* 1976;7:135.
6. Hanaway J, Torack R, Fletcher AP, et al: Intracranial bleeding associated with urokinase therapy for acute ischemic hemispheral stroke. *Stroke* 1976;7:143.
7. del Zoppo GJ, Zeumer H, Harker LA: Thrombolytic therapy in stroke: possibilities and hazards. *Stroke* 1986;17:595.
8. Verstraete M, Collen D: Thrombolytic therapy in the 80s. *Blood* 1986;67:1529.
9. Sloan MA: Thrombolysis and stroke: past and future. *Arch Neurol* 1987;44:748.
10. Gruppo Italiano per lo Studio della Streptochinasi nell'Infarto Miocardico

(GISSI): Effectiveness of intravenous thrombolytic treatment in acute myocardial infarction. *Lancet* 1986;i:397.

11. Rovelli F, Devita C, Feruglio GA, et al: GISSI trial: early results and late follow-up. *J Am Coll Cardiol* 1987;10(suppl):33B.

12. Maggioni AP, Franzosi MG, Farnia ML, et al: Cerebrovascular events after myocardial infarction. *Br Med J* 1991;302:1428.

13. The ISAM Study Group: A prospective trial of intravenous streptokinase in acute myocardial infarction (ISAM). *N Engl J Med* 1986;314:1465.

14. Schroder R, Neuhaus KL, Leizorovicz A, et al: A prospective placebo-controlled double-blind multicenter trial of intravenous streptokinase (ISAM): Long-term mortality and morbidity in acute myocardial infarction. *J Am Coll Cardiol* 1987;9:197.

15. ISIS-2 (Second International Study of Infarct Survival): Randomized trial of intravenous streptokinase, oral aspirin, both or neither among 17,187 cases of suspected acute myocardial infarction: ISIS-2. *Lancet* 1988;ii:349.

16. AIMS Trial Study Group: Effect of intravenous APSAC on mortality after acute myocardial infarction: preliminary report of a placebo-controlled clinical trial. *Lancet* 1988;i:545.

17. AIMS Trial Study Group: Long-term effects of intravenous anistreplase in acute myocardial infarction: final report of the AIMS study. *Lancet* 1990;335:427.

18. Wilcox RG, Olsson CG, Skene AM, et al: Trial of tissue plasminogen activator for mortality reduction in acute myocardial infarction: Anglo-Scandinavian Study of Early Thrombolysis (ASSET). *Lancet* 1988;ii:525.

19. Wilcox RG, von der Lippe G, Olsson CG, et al: Effects of alteplase on acute myocardial infarction: 6-month results from the ASSET Study. *Lancet* 1990;335:1175.

20. Van de Werf F, Arnold AER, for the European Cooperative Study Group: Intravenous tissue plasminogen activator and size of infarct, left ventricular function, and survival in acute myocardial infarction. *Br Med J* 1988; 297:1371.

21. Gruppo Italiano per lo Studio della Sopravvivenza nell'Infarto Miocardico: GISSI-2: a factorial randomized trial of alteplase versus streptokinase and heparin versus no heparin among 12,490 patients with acute myocardial infarction. *Lancet* 1990;336:65.

22. International Study Group: In-hospital mortality and clinical course of 20,891 patients with suspected acute myocardial infarction randomized between alteplase and streptokinase with or without heparin. *Lancet* 1990;336:71.

23. Maggioni AP, Franzosi MG, Santoro E, et al: The Gruppo Italiano per lo Studio della Sopravvivenza nell'Infarto Miocardico II (GISSI-II), and the International Study Group: the risk of stroke in patients with acute myocardial infarction after thrombolytic and antithrombotic treatment. *N Engl J Med* 1992;327:1.

24. de Jaegere PP, Arnold AP, Balk AH, et al: Intracranial hemorrhage in

association with thrombolytic therapy: incidence and clinical predictive factors. *J Amer Coll Cardiol* 1992;20:289.

25. ISIS-3: A randomised comparison of streptokinase vs. tissue plasminogen activator vs. anistreplase and of aspirin plus heparin vs. aspirin alone among 41,299 cases of suspected acute myocardial infarction. ISIS-3 (Third International Study of Infarct Survival) Collaborative Group. *Lancet* 1992;339:753.

26. Uglietta JP, O'Connor CM, Boyko OB, et al: CT patterns of intracranial hemorrhage complicating thrombolytic therapy for acute myocardial infarction. *Radiology* 1991;181:555.

27. O'Connor CM, Aldrich H, Massey EW, et al: Intracranial hemorrhage after thrombolytic therapy for acute myocardial infarction: clinical characteristics and in hospital outcome (abstract). *J Am Coll Cardiol* 1990; 15(suppl):213A.

28. O'Connor CM, Califf RM, Massey EW, et al: Stroke and acute myocardial infarction in the thrombolytic era: clinical correlates and long-term prognosis. *J Am Coll Cardiol* 1990;16:533.

29. Kase CS, Pessin MS, Zivin JA, et al: Intracranial hemorrhage after coronary thrombolysis with tissue plasminogen activator. *Am J Med* 1992; 92:384.

30. Vermeer F, Massberg I, Meyer J, et al: Saruplase, a new fibrin specific thrombolytic agent: efficacy and safety in the first 1000 patients (abstract). *J Am Coll Cardiol* 1991;17(suppl):152A.

31. Gore JM, Sloan M, Price TR, et al: Intracerebral hemorrhage, cerebral infarction, and subdural hematoma after acute myocardial infarction and thrombolytic therapy in the thrombolysis in myocardial infarction study. Thrombolysis in Myocardial Infarction, Phase II, Pilot and Clinical Trial. *Circulation* 1991;83:448.

32. Sloan MA, Price TR, Terrin ML, et al: Ischemic cerebral infarction after rt-PA and heparin therapy for acute myocardial infarction: the TIMI-II pilot and randomized trial combined experience. *Ann Neurol* 1992;32:238.

33. Sloan MA, Price TR, Randall AM, et al: Intracerebral hemorrhage after rt-PA and heparin for acute myocardial infarction: the TIMI II pilot and randomized trial combined experience. *Stroke* 1990;21(suppl):182.

34. Longstreth WT, Litwin PE, Weaver WD, for the MITI Project Group: Myocardial infarction, thrombolytic therapy, and stroke. *Stroke* 1993;24: 587.

35. Amery A, Roeber G, Vermeulen HJ, Verstraete M: Single blind randomized multicenter trial comparing heparin and streptokinase treatment in recent myocardial infarction. *Acta Med Scand (Suppl)* 1969;505:5.

36. European Working Party: Streptokinase in recent myocardial infarction: a controlled multicenter trial. *Br Med J* 1971;3:325.

37. Bett JHN, Castaldi PA, Hale GS, et al: Australian multicenter trial of streptokinase in acute myocardial infarction. *Lancet* 1973;i:57.

38. Ness PM, Simon TL, Cole C, et al: A pilot study of streptokinase therapy

in acute myocardial infarction: observations on complications in relation to trial design. *Am Heart J* 1974;88:705.

39. European Cooperative Study Group: Streptokinase in acute myocardial infarction. *N Engl J Med* 1979;301:794.

40. Rutsch W, Schartl M, Mathey D, et al: Percutaneous transluminal coronary recanalization. Procedure, results, and acute complications. *Am Heart J* 1981;102:1178.

41. Weinstein J: Treatment of myocardial infarction with intracoronary streptokinase: efficacy and safety data from 209 United States cases in the Hoechst-Roussel Registry. *Am Heart J* 1982;104:894.

42. Gans W, Gelt I, Shaw PK, et al: Intravenous streptokinase in evolving acute myocardial infarction. *Am J Cardiol* 1984;53:1209.

43. Urban PL, Cowley M, Goldberg S, et al: Intracoronary thrombolysis in acute myocardial infarction: clinical course following successful myocardial reperfusion. *Am Heart J* 1984;108:873.

44. Aldrich MS, Sherman SA, Greenberg HS: Cerebrovascular complications of streptokinase infusion. *JAMA* 1985;253:1777.

45. Lew AS, Hod H, Cercek B, et al: Mortality and morbidity rates of patients older and younger than 75 years with acute myocardial infarction treated with intravenous streptokinase. *Am J Cardiol* 1987;59:1.

46. PRIMI Study Group: Randomized double blind trial of recombinant pro-urokinase against streptokinase in acute myocardial infarction. *Lancet* 1989;i:863.

47. Topol EJ, Morris DC, Smalling RD, et al: A multicenter, randomized, placebo-controlled trial of a new form of intravenous recombinant tissue-type plasminogen activator (Activase) in acute myocardial infarction. *J Am Coll Cardiol* 1987;9:1205.

48. Topol EJ, Califf RM, George BS, et al: A randomized trial of immediate versus delayed elective angioplasty after intravenous tissue-plasminogen activator in acute myocardial infarction. *N Engl J Med* 1987;317:581.

49. de Bono DP: Thrombolysis with intravenous human recombinant tissue-type plasminogen activator in acute myocardial infarction: the European experience. *J Am Coll Cardiol* 1987;10(suppl):75B.

50. Passamani E, Hodges M, Herman M, et al: The Thrombolysis in Myocardial Infarction (TIMI) Phase II Pilot Study: tissue plasminogen activator followed by percutaneous transluminal coronary angioplasty. *J Am Coll Cardiol* 1987;10(Suppl):51B.

51. National Heart Foundation of Australia Coronary Thrombolysis Group: Coronary thrombolysis and myocardial salvage by tissue plasminogen activator given up to four hours after onset of a myocardial infarction. *Lancet* 1988;i:203.

52. Neuhaus K-L, Tebbe U, Gottwik M, et al: Intravenous recombinant tissue plasminogen activator (rt-PA) and urokinase in acute myocardial infarction. Results of the German Activator Urokinase Study (GAUS). *J Am Coll Cardiol* 1988;12:581.

53. Califf RM, Topol EJ, George BS, et al: Hemorrhagic complications associ-

ated with the use of intravenous tissue plasminogen activator in treatment of acute myocardial infarction. *Am J Med* 1988;85:353.

54. Carlson S, Aldrich MS, Greenberg HS, et al: Intracerebral hemorrhage complicating intravenous tissue plasminogen activator treatment. *Arch Neurol* 1988;45:1070.

55. Althouse R, Maynard C, Olsufka M, et al: Risk factors for hemorrhagic and ischemic stroke in myocardial infarct patients treated with tissue plasminogen activator. *J Am Coll Cardiol* 1989;13(suppl):153A.

56. Tebbe U, Tanswell P, Seifried E, et al: Single bolus injection of recombinant tissue-type plasminogen activator in acute myocardial infarction. *Am J Cardiol* 1989;64:448.

57. Kase CS, O'Neal AN, Fisher M, et al: Intracranial hemorrhage after use of tissue plasminogen activator for coronary thrombolysis. *Ann Intern Med* 1990;112:17.

58. Hsia J, Hamilton WP, Kleiman N, et al: A comparison between heparin and low dose aspirin as adjunctive therapy with tissue plasminogen activator for acute myocardial infarction. *N Engl J Med* 1990;323:1433.

59. Smalling RW, Schumacher R, Morris D, et al: Improved infarct-related arterial patency after high dose, weight adjusted, rapid infusion of tissue-type plasminogen activator in myocardial infarction: results of a multicenter randomized trial of two dosage regimens. *J Am Coll Cardiol* 1990;15: 915.

60. Eleff SM, Borel C, Bell WR, et al: Acute management of intracranial hemorrhage in patients receiving thrombolytic therapy. Case reports. *Neurosurgery* 1990;26:876.

61. Kirschenbaum JM, Flaherty JT, Bahr RD, et al: Coronary thrombolysis with low dose synergistic combinations of prourokinase and recombinant tissue plasminogen activator. *Circulation* 1990;82(suppl III):III-537.

62. GUSTO Clinical Trial Protocol.

63. Grines CL, Nissen SE, Booth DC, et al: A prospective, randomized trial comparing combination half dose t-PA with streptokinase to full dose t-PA in acute myocardial infarction. Preliminary report. *J Am Coll Cardiol* 1990;15:4A.

64. Althouse R, Maynard C, Cerqueira MD, et al: The Western Washington Myocardial Infarction Registry and Emergency Department tissue plasminogen activator treatment trial. *J Am Coll Cardiol* 1990;66:1298.

65. Bassand J-P, Cassagnes J, Machecourt J, et al: A multicenter double-blind trial aimed at comparing the efficiency and safety of alteplase and anistreplase in acute myocardial infarction. *Circulation* 1990;82(suppl III):III-665.

66. Anderson JL, Karagounis L, Allen A, et al: Older age and elevated blood pressure are risk factors for intracerebral hemorrhage after thrombolysis. *J Am Coll Cardiol* 1991;68:166.

67. O'Connor CM, Meese R, MacKrell J, et al: Reduced hemorrhagic complications following APSAC therapy in acute myocardial infarction by withholding heparin. *J Am Coll Cardiol* 1992;19:91A.

68. Tranchesi B, Caramelli B, Gegara O, et al: Efficacy and safety of ridogrel versus aspirin in coronary thrombosis with alteplase for myocardial infarction. *J Am Coll Cardiol* 1992;19:92A.

69. Wall TC, Califf RM, George BS, et al: Accelerated plasminogen activator dose regimens for coronary thrombolysis. *J Am Coll Cardiol* 1992;19:482.

70. von Essen R, Neuhaus K-L, Markreiter M, et al: Double bolus of r-PA in the dosage finding. Results of the GRECO-II-Study. *J Am Coll Cardiol* 1992;19:274A.

71. Neuhaus K-L, von Essen R, Tebbe U, et al: Improved thrombolysis in acute myocardial infarction with front-loaded administration of alteplase: results of the rt-PA-APSAC Patency Study (TAPS). *J Am Coll Cardiol* 1992;19:885.

72. Cherng W-J, Chiang C-W, Kuo C-T, et al: A comparison between intravenous streptokinase and tissue plasminogen activator with early intravenous heparin in acute myocardial infarction. *Am Heart J* 1992;123:841.

73. Carney RJ, Murphy GA, Brandt TR, et al: Randomized angiographic trial of recombinant tissue-type plasminogen activator (alteplase) in myocardial infarction. *J Am Coll Cardiol* 1992;20:17.

74. Weisberg LA: The fluid blood level in intracranial hematoma due to anticoagulant medication. *J Neurol Neurosurg Psychiatry* 1987;50:1076.

75. Gorelick PB, Parik M, McDonald L: Intracoronary streptokinase and fatal cerebellar hemorrhage. *Ill Med J* 1987;171:28.

76. Proner J, Rosenblum BR, Rothman A: Ruptured arteriovenous malformation complicating thrombolytic therapy with tissue plasminogen activator. *Arch Neurol* 1990;47:105.

77. Da Silva VF, Bormanis J: Intracerebral hemorrhage after combined anticoagulant-thrombolytic therapy for myocardial infarction: two case reports and a short review. *Neurosurgery* 1992;30:943.

78. Ramsay DA, Penswick JL, Robertson DM: Fatal streptokinase-induced intracerebral hemorrhage in cerebral amyloid angiopathy. *Can J Neurol Sci* 1990;17:336.

79. Pendlebury WW, Iole ED, Tracy RP, et al: Intracerebral hemorrhage related to cerebral amyloid angiopathy and t-PA treatment. *Ann Neurol* 1991;29:210.

80. Kase CS: Intracranial hemorrhage after coronary thrombolysis with tissue plasminogen activator. In: Hacke W, del Zoppo GJ, Hirschberg M, eds: *Thrombolytic Therapy in Acute Ischemic Stroke.* Berlin: Springer-Verlag, 1991:75.

81. Sloan MA, del Zoppo GJ, Brott TG: Thrombolysis and stroke. In: Julian DG, Kubler W, et al, eds: *Thrombolysis in Cardiovascular Disease.* New York: Marcel-Dekker, 1989:361.

82. Sloan MA, Price TR: Intracranial hemorrhage following thrombolytic therapy for acute myocardial infarction. *Semin Neurol* 1991;11:385.

83. Sloan MA, Gore JM: Ischemic stroke and intracranial hemorrhage follow-

ing thrombolytic therapy for acute myocardial infarction. A risk-benefit analysis. *Am J Cardiol* 1992;69:21A.

84. Sloan MA: Stroke associated with thrombolytic therapy for acute myocardial infarction. *Heart Dis Stroke* 1992;1:287.

85. Pfeiffer MA, Moyé LA, Braunwald E, et al: Selection bias in the use of thrombolytic therapy in acute myocardial infarction. *JAMA* 1991;266:528.

86. Urokinase-Pulmonary Embolism Trial: Morbidity and mortality. *Circulation* 1973;58(suppl II):47–48, 66–72.

87. Urokinase-Pulmonary Embolism Trial. *JAMA* 1974;242:1606.

88. Berridge DC, Makin GS, Hopkinson BR: Local low dose intra-arterial thrombolytic therapy: the risk of stroke or major haemorrhage. *Br J Surg* 1989;76:1230.

89. Sussman BJ, Fitch TSP: Thrombolysis with fibrinolysin in cerebral arterial occlusion. *JAMA* 1958;167:1705.

90. Herndon RM, Meyer JS, Johnson JF, et al: Treatment of cardiovascular thrombosis with fibrinolysin. *Am J Cardiol* 1960;30:540.

91. Clarke RL, Clifton EE: The treatment of cerebrovascular thrombosis and embolism with fibrinolytic agents. *Am J Cardiol* 1960;30:546.

92. Meyer JS, Herndon RM, Gotch F: Therapeutic thrombolysis. In: Millikan CH, Seikert W, Whisnant JP, eds: *Cerebral Vascular Disease: Third Princeton Conference*. New York: Grune & Stratton, 1961:160.

93. Atkin N, Nitzberg S, Dorsey J: Lysis of intracerebral thromboembolism with fibrinolysin: Report of a case. *Angiology* 1964;15:436.

94. Brooks J, Davis D, Devivo G: Blood hypercoagulability in acute cerebrovascular syndromes: its control with urokinase therapy. *J Lab Clin Med* 1970;76:879.

95. Larcan A, Laprevote-Heully MC, Lambert H, et al: Indications de thrombolytique au cours des accidents vasculaires cérébraux thrombosants traités pars ailleurs par OMB (ZATA). *Therapie* 1977;32:259.

96. Malinovsky NN, Kozlov VA: Embolism of the cerebral arteries: In: *Anticoagulant and Thrombolytic Therapy in Surgery*. St. Louis: CV Mosby, 1979: 239.

97. Labauge A, Bland J-M, Salvaing P, et al: Traitment fibrinolytique et anticoagulant dans 37 cas d'occlusions arterielles: cervicocerebrales d'origin thromboembolique. In: *Proceedings of the Fifth International Congress on Thromboembolism, Bologna, Italy, 1978*. Pisa: Quaderni della Coagulazione, 1980:362.

98. Abe T, Kasawa M, Naito I, et al: Clinical evaluation for efficacy of tissue culture urokinase (TCUK) on cerebral thrombosis by means of multicenter double-blind study. *Blood Vessels* 1981;12:321.

99. Abe T, Kazawa M, Naito I, et al: Clinical effect of urokinase (60,000 U/d) on cerebral infarction: Comparative study by means of multicenter double-blind test. *Blood Vessels* 1981;12:342.

100. Zeumer H, Hacke W, Kolmann HL, et al: Lokale fibrinolyse bei basilaristhrombose. *Dtsch Med Wochenschr* 1982;107:728.

101. Zeumer H, Hacke W, Ringelstein EB: Intra-arterial thrombolysis in verte-brobasilar thromboembolic disease. *Am J Neuroradiol* 1983;4:401.

102. Nenci GG, Gresele P, Taramelli M, et al: Thrombolytic therapy for throm-boembolism of vertebrobasilar artery. *Angiology* 1983;34:561.

103. Miyakawa T: The cerebral vessels and thrombosis. *Rinsho Ketseuki* 1984; 25:1018.

104. Zeumer H, Hundgen R, Ferbert A, et al: Local intra-arterial fibrinolytic therapy in inaccessible internal carotid occlusion. *Neuroradiology* 1984; 76:315.

105. Zeumer H: Vascular recanalization techniques in interventional neurora-diology. *J Neurol* 1985;231:287.

106. Atarashi J, Otomo E, Araki G, et al: Clinical utility of urokinase in the treatment of acute stage of cerebral thrombosis: multicenter double-blind study in comparison with placebo. *Clin Eval* 1985;13:659.

107. Otomo E, Araki G, Itoh E, et al: Clinical efficacy of urokinase in the treat-ment of cerebral thrombosis: multicenter double-blind study in compari-son with placebo. *Clin Eval* 1985;13:711.

108. Bruckmann H, Ferbert A, del Zoppo GJ, et al: Acute vertebrobasilar thrombosis: angiologic-clinical comparison and therapeutic implications. *Acta Radiologica* 1986;369(suppl):38.

109. Koudstaal PJ, Stibbe J, Vermeulen M: Fatal ischemic brain oedema after early thrombolysis with tissue plasminogen activator in acute stroke. *Br Med J* 1988;297:1571.

110. Henze TH, Breer A, Tebbe U, et al: Lysis of basilar artery occlusion with tissue plasminogen activator. *Lancet* 1987;2:1391.

111. del Zoppo GJ, Ferbert A, Otis S, et al: Local intra-arterial fibrinolytic therapy in acute carotid territory stroke. *Stroke* 1988;19:307.

112. del Zoppo GJ: Thrombolysis: new concepts in the treatment of stroke. In: Hennerici M, Sitzer G, Weger H-D, eds: *Carotid Artery Plaques*. Basel: S Karger, 1988:242.

113. Hacke W, Zeumer H, Ferbert A, et al: Intraarterial fibrinolytic therapy improves outcome in patients with acute vertebrobasilar occlusive dis-ease. *Stroke* 1988;19:1216.

114. Mori E, Tabuchi M, Yoshida T, et al: Intracarotid urokinase with thrombo-embolic occlusion of the middle cerebral artery. *Stroke* 1988;19:802.

115. Otomo E, Tohgi H, Hirai T, et al: Clinical efficacy of AK-124 (tissue plas-minogen activator) in the treatment of cerebral thrombosis: study by means of multicenter double-blind comparison with urokinase. *Yakuri To Chiryo* 1988;16:3775.

116. Theron J, Courtheoux P, Casasco A, et al: Local intraarterial fibrinolysis in carotid territory. *Am J Neuroradiol* 1989;10:753.

117. Buteux G, Jubault V, Suisse A, et al: Local recombinant tissue plasmino-gen activator to clear cerebral artery thrombosis developing soon after surgery. *Lancet* 1988;1:1143.

118. Brückmann H, Ferbert A: Putamenal haemorrhage after recanalization

of an embolic MCA occlusion treated with tissue plasminogen activator. *Neuroradiology* 1989;31:95.

119. Olinger CP, Brott TG, Barsan WG, et al: Use of ancrod in acute or progressive ischemic cerebral infarction. *Ann Emerg Med* 1988;17:1208.

120. Zeumer H, Freitag H-J, Grzyska U, et al: Interventional neuroradiology: local intraarterial fibrinolysis in acute vertebrobasilar occlusion: Technical developments and recent results. *Neuroradiology* 1989;31:336.

121. Terashi A, Kobayashi Y, Katayama Y, et al: Clinical effects and basic studies of thrombolytic therapy on cerebral thrombosis. *Semin Thromb Hemost* 1990;16:236.

122. Ikeda S, Muraishi K: Intra-arterial urokinase infusion therapy for the superacute intracranial major artery occlusion. *Stroke* 1990;21(suppl I): I-95.

123. Hennerici M, for the German t-PA-Stroke Study Group: Fibrinolysis of intracranial arteries. *Stroke* 1990;21(suppl I):I-129.

124. Abe T, Terashi A, Tohgi H, et al: Clinical efficacy of intravenous administration of SM-9527 (t-PA) in cerebral thrombosis. *Clin Eval* 1990;18:39.

125. Asplund K, Carlberg B: Thrombolysis in stroke: timing of recanalization and its clinical consequences. In: Hacke W, del Zoppo GJ, Hirschberg M, eds: *Thrombolytic Therapy in Acute Ischemic Stroke.* Berlin: Springer-Verlag, 1991:46.

126. Hacke W: Intraarterial urokinase plasminogen activator and streptokinase in carotid and vertebrobasilar territory stroke: clinical outcome. In: Hacke W, del Zoppo GJ, Hirschberg M, eds: *Thrombolytic Therapy in Acute Ischemic Stroke.* Berlin: Springer-Verlag, 1991:131.

127. Mori E: Fibrinolytic recanalization therapy in acute cerebrovascular thromboembolism. In: Hacke W, del Zoppo GJ, Hirschberg M, eds: *Thrombolytic Therapy in Acute Ischemic Stroke.* Berlin: Springer-Verlag, 1991: 137.

128. Mori E, Yoneda Y, Tabuchi M, et al: Intravenous recombinant tissue plasminogen activator in acute carotid artery territory stroke. *Neurology* 1992;42:976.

129. von Kummer R, Forsting M, Sartor K, et al: Intravenous recombinant tissue plasminogen activator in acute stroke. In: Hacke W, del Zoppo GJ, Hirschberg M, eds: *Thrombolytic Therapy in Acute Ischemic Stroke.* Berlin: Springer-Verlag, 1991:161.

130. von Kummer R, Forsting M, Hutschenreuter M, et al: Angiography in acute stroke due to occlusions of intracerebral arteries before and after treatment with intravenous recombinant tissue plasminogen activator. *Stroke* 1990;21(suppl I):I-94.

131. von Kummer R, Hacke W: Safety and efficacy of intravenous tissue plasminogen activator and heparin in acute middle cerebral artery stroke. *Stroke* 1992;23:646.

132. Yamaguchi T, Hayakama T, Kikuchi H, et al: Thrombolytic therapy in embolic and thrombotic cerebral infarction: a cooperative study. In: Hacke

W, del Zoppo GJ, Hirschberg M, eds: *Thrombolytic Therapy in Acute Ischemic Stroke.* Berlin: Springer-Verlag, 1991:168.

133. Matsumoto K, Satoh K: Topical intraarterial urokinase infusion for acute stroke. In: Hacke W, del Zoppo GJ, Hirschberg M eds: *Thrombolytic Therapy in Acute Ischemic Stroke.* Berlin: Springer-Verlag, 1991:207.

134. Möbius E, Berg-Dammer E, Kühne D, et al: Local thrombolytic therapy in acute basilar artery occlusion: experience with 18 patients. In: Hacke W, del Zoppo GJ, Hirschberg M, eds: *Thrombolytic Therapy in Acute Ischemic Stroke.* Berlin: Springer-Verlag, 1991:213.

135. Pfeiffer G, Thayssen G, Arlt A, et al: Vertebrobasilar occlusion: outcome with and without local intraarterial fibrinolysis. In: Hacke W, del Zoppo GJ, Hirschberg M, eds: *Thrombolytic Therapy in Acute Ischemic Stroke.* Berlin: Springer-Verlag, 1991:216.

136. Biniek R, Ringelstein EB, Brückmann H, et al: Recanalization of acute middle cerebral artery occlusion monitored by transcranial Doppler sonography. In: Hacke W, del Zoppo GJ, Hirschberg M, eds: *Thrombolytic Therapy in Acute Ischemic Stroke.* Berlin: Springer-Verlag, 1991:221.

137. Pilz P, Ladurner G, Griebnitz E: Neuropathological findings after thrombolytic therapy in acute ischemic stroke. In: Hacke W, del Zoppo GJ, Hirschberg M, eds: *Thrombolytic Therapy in Acute Ischemic Stroke.* Berlin: Springer-Verlag, 1991:224.

138. Siepmann G, Müller-Jensen M, Goossens-Merkt H, et al: Local intraarterial fibrinolysis in acute middle cerebral atery occlusion. In: Hacke W, del Zoppo GJ, Hirschberg M, eds: *Thrombolytic Therapy in Acute Ischemic Stroke.* Berlin: Springer-Verlag, 1991:240.

139. Herdescheé D, Limburg U, Hijdra A, et al: Recombinant tissue plasminogen activator in two patients with basilar artery occlusion. *J Neurol Neurosurg Psychiatry* 1991;54:71.

140. Herdescheé D, Limburg M, Hijdra A, et al: Treatment of acute ischemic stroke with recombinant tissue plasminogen activator: evaluation with regional cerebral blood flow single photon emission computed tomography. In: Hacke W, del Zoppo GJ, Hirschberg M, eds: *Thrombolytic Therapy in Acute Ischemic Stroke.* Berlin: Springer-Verlag, 1991:244.

141. Wildemann B, von Kummer R, Hutschenreuter M, et al: Basilar artery occlusion associated with protein C deficiency: successful treatment using recombinant tissue plasminogen activator infusion. In: Hacke W, del Zoppo GJ, Hirschberg M, eds: *Thrombolytic Therapy in Acute Ischemic Stroke.* Berlin: Springer-Verlag, 1991:255.

142. Hamann G, Haass A, Pindur G, et al: Prourokinase therapy in stroke. In: Hacke W, del Zoppo GJ, Hirschberg M, eds: *Thrombolytic Therapy in Acute Ischemic Stroke.* Berlin: Springer-Verlag, 1991:262.

143. The rt-PA/Acute Stroke Study Group: An open safety/efficacy trial of rt-PA in acute thromboembolic stroke: final report. *Stroke* 1991;22:153.

144. del Zoppo GJ, Poeck K, Pessin MS, et al: Recombinant tissue plasminogen activator in acute thrombotic and embolic stroke. *Ann Neurol* 1992;32:78.

145. Brott TG, Haley EC, Levy DE, et al: Urgent therapy for stroke. Part I. Pilot study of tissue plasminogen activator administered within 90 minutes. *Stroke* 1992;23:632.

146. Haley EC, Levy DE, Brott TG, et al: Urgent therapy for stroke. Part II. Pilot study of tissue plasminogen activator administered 91-180 minutes from onset. *Stroke* 1992;23:641.

147. Haley EC, for the TPA Bridging Study Group: Pilot randomized trial of tissue plasminogen activator in acute ischemic stroke. *Neurology* 1992; 42(suppl 3):203.

148. Sperling B, Overgaard K, Videbk C, et al: Evaluation of thrombolytic therapy in acute ischemic stroke with pre- and posttreatment rCBF measurements. Presented at the Second International Symposium on Thrombolytic Therapy for Acute Stroke, San Diego, May, 1992.

149. Brucker B, Laich E, Bhm-Jurkovic H, et al: Relation of thrombolytic reperfusion and of collateral circulation to outcome in patients suffering cerebral main artery-occlusion. Presented at the Second International Symposium on Thrombolytic Therapy for Acute Stroke, San Diego, May, 1992.

150. Wardlaw JM, Warlow CP: A meta-analysis of all published data on the use of thrombolytic drugs to treat acute ischaemic stroke. Presented at the Second International Symposium on Thrombolytic Therapy for Acute Stroke, San Diego, May, 1992.

151. Levy DE, Brott T, Haley EC, et al: Factors associated with intracranial hematoma (ICH) in acute stroke patients treated with tissue plasminogen activator. Presented at the Second International Symposium on Thrombolytic Therapy for Acute Stroke, San Diego, May, 1992.

152. Okada Y, Sadoshima S, Nakane H, et al: Early computed tomographic findings for thrombolytic therapy in patients with acute brain embolism. *Stroke* 1992;23:20.

153. Fodstad H, Nilsson IM: Coagulation and fibrinolysis in blood and cerebrospinal fluid after aneurysmal subarachnoid hemorrhage. Effect of tranexamic acid (AMCA). *Acta Neuro Chir* 1987;56:25.

154. Yoshida Y, Ueki S, Takahashi A: Intrathecal irrigation with urokinase in ruptured cerebral aneurysm cases. Basic studies and clinical application. *Neuro Med Chir* 1985;24:987.

155. Alksne JF, Branson PJ, Bailey M: Modification of experimental post-subarachnoid hemorrhage vasculopathy with intracisternal plasmin. *Neurosurgery* 1986;19:20.

156. Alksne JF, Branson PJ, Bailey M: Modification of experimental post-subarachnoid vasculopathy with intracisternal plasmin. *Neurosurgery* 1988; 23:335.

157. Findlay JM, Weir BKA, Steinke D, et al: Effect of intrathecal thrombolytic therapy on subarachnoid clot and chronic vasospasm in a primate model of SAH. *J Neurosurg* 1988;69:723.

158. Findlay JM, Weir BKA, Kanamaru K, et al: Intrathecal fibrinolytic therapy after subarachnoid hemorrhage: dosage study in a primate model and review of the literature. *Can J Neurol Sci* 1989;16:28.

159. Findlay JM, Weir BKA, Gordon P, et al: Safety and efficacy of intrathecal thrombolytic therapy in a primate model of cerebral vasospasm. *Neurosurgery* 1989;24:491.

160. Seifert V, Eisert WG, Stolke D, et al: Efficacy of single intracisternal injection of recombinant tissue plasminogen activator to prevent delayed cerebral vasospasm after experimental subarachnoid hemorrhage. *Neurosurgery* 1989;25:590.

161. Findlay JM, Weir BKA, Kanamaru et al: The effect of timing of intrathecal fibrinolytic therapy on cerebral vasospasm in a primate model of subarachnoid hemorrhage. *Neurosurgery* 1990;26:201.

162. Brinker T, Seifert V, Stolke D: Effect of intrathecal fibrinolysis on cerebrospinal fluid absorption after experimental subarachnoid hemorrhage. *J Neurosurgery* 1991;74:784.

163. Shiobara R, Kawase T, Toya S, et al: "Scavenger surgery" for subarachnoid hemorrhage. II. Continuous ventriculocisternal perfusion using artificial cerebrospinal fluid with urokinase. In: Auer LM, ed: *Timing of Aneurysm Surgery.* Berlin: Walter de Gruyter, 1985:365.

164. Mizoi K, Yoshimoto T, Fujiwara S, et al: Prevention of vasospasm by clot removal and intrathecal bolus injection of tissue-type plasminogen activator. Preliminary report. *Neurosurgery* 1991;28:807.

165. Findlay JM, Weir BKA, Kassell NF, et al: Intracisternal recombinant tissue plasminogen activator after aneurysmal subarachnoid hemorrhage. *J Neurosurg* 1991;75:181.

166. Zabramski JM, Spetzler RF, Lee KS, et al: Phase I trial of tissue plasminogen activator for the prevention of vasospasm in patients with aneurysmal subarachnoid hemorrhage. *J Neurosurg* 1991;75:189.

167. Öhman J, Servo A, Heiskanen O: Effect of intrathecal fibrinolytic therapy on clot lysis and vasospasm in patients with aneurysmal subarachnoid hemorrhage. *J Neurosurg* 1991;75:197.

168. Stolke D, Seifert V: Single intracisternal bolus of recombinant tissue plasminogen activator in patients with aneurysmal subarachnoid hemorrhage: preliminary assessment of efficacy and safety in an open clinical study. *Neurosurgery* 1992;30:877.

169. Segal R, Dujovny M, Nelson D, et al: Local urokinase treatment for spontaneous intracerebral hematoma. *Clin Res* 1982;30:412A.

170. Matsumoto K, Hondo H: CT-guided stereotactic evaluation of hypertensive intracerebral hematomas. *J Neurosurg* 1984;61:440.

171. Niizuma H, Suzuki J: Stereotactic aspiration of putamenal hemorrhage using a double track aspirator technique. *Neurosurgery* 1988;22:432.

172. Narayan RJ, Narayan TM, Katz DA, et al: Lysis of intracranial hematomas with urokinase in a rabbit model. *J Neurosurg* 1985;62:580.

173. Itakura T, Komai N, Nadai E, et al: Stereotactic evacuation of hypertensive intracerebral hematoma using plasminogen activator. American Association of Neurological Surgeons, Dallas, TX, May 3–7, 1987.

174. Niizuma H, Otsuki T, Johkura H, et al: CT-guided stereotactic aspiration

of intracerebral hematoma: result of a hematoma-lysis method using urokinase. *Appl Neurophysiol* 1985;48:427.

175. Pang D, Sclabassi RJ, Horton JA: Lysis of intraventricular blood clot with urokinase in a canine model. Part I: canine intraventricular blood cast model. *Neurosurgery* 1986;19:540.

176. Pang D, Sclabassi RJ, Horton JA: Lysis of intraventricular blood clot with urokinase in a canine model. Part II: in vivo safety study of intraventricular urokinase. *Neurosurgery* 1986;19:547.

177. Pang D, Sclabassi RJ, Horton JA: Lysis of intraventricular blood clot with urokinase in a canine model. Part III: effects of intraventricular urokinase on clot lysis and posthemorrhagic hydrocephalus. *Neurosurgery* 1986;19:553.

178. Kaufmann HH, Schochet S, Koss W, et al: Efficacy and safety of tissue plasminogen activator. *Neurosurgery* 1987;20:403.

179. Mohadjer M, Eggert R, May J, et al: CT-guided stereotactic fibrinolysis of spontaneous and hypertensive cerebellar hemorrhage: long-term results. *J Neurosurg* 1990;73:217.

180. Kaufmann HH: Stereotactic aspiration with fibrinolytic and mechanical assistance. In: Kaufmann HH, ed: *Intracerebral Hematomas*. New York: Raven Press, 1992:181.

181. Todo T, Usui M, Takakura K: Treatment of severe intraventricular hemorrhage by intraventricular infusion of urokinase. *J Neurosurg* 1991;74:81.

182. Kanaya H, Kuroda K: Development in neurosurgical approaches to hypertensive intracerebral hemorrhage in Japan. In: Kaufmann HH, ed: *Intracerebral Hematomas*. New York: Raven Press, 1992:197.

183. Findlay JM, Weir BKA, Stollery DE: Lysis of intraventricular hematoma with tissue plasminogen activator. *J Neurosurg* 1991;74:803.

184. Alexander LF, Yamamoto Y, Ayoubi S, et al: Efficacy of tissue plasminogen activator in the lysis of thrombosis of the cerebral venous sinus. *Neurosurgery* 1990;76:559.

185. Spitzer K, Freitag J, Thei A, et al: Thrombolytic therapy in cerebral sinus thrombosis: a case report. In: Hacke W, del Zoppo GJ, Hirschberg M, eds: *Thrombolytic Therapy in Acute Ischemic Stroke*. Berlin: Springer-Verlag, 1991:251.

186. Higashida RT, Helmer E, van Halbach V, et al: Direct thrombolytic therapy for superior sagittal sinus thrombosis. *Am J Neuroradiol* 1989;10:4.

187. Scott JA, Pascuzzi RM, Hall PV, et al: Treatment of dural sinus thrombosis with local urokinase infusion. *J Neurosurg* 1988;68:284.

188. Korbmacher G, Ringelstein EB: Risk and benefit of anticoagulation in patients with acute hemispheric infarctions: preliminary results of a prospective study. In: Poeck K, Ringelstein EB, Hacke W, eds: *New Trends in Diagnosis and Management of Stroke*. Berlin: Springer-Verlag, 1987:103.

189. Weisberg LA, Stazio A, Shamsnia M, et al: Nontraumatic parenchymal brain hemorrhages. *Medicine (Baltimore)* 1990;69:277.

190. Hart RG, Easton JD: Hemorrhagic infarcts. *Stroke* 1986;17:586.

191. Fisher CM, Adams RD: Observations on brain embolism with special reference to hemorrhagic infarction. In: Furlan AJ, ed: *The Heart and Stroke*. Berlin: Springer-Verlag, 1987:17.

192. Cerebral Embolism Task Force: Cardiogenic brain embolism. The second report of the Cerebral Embolism Task Force. *Arch Neurol* 1989;46:727.

193. Ogata J, Yutani C, Imakita M, et al: Hemorrhagic infarct of the brain without a reopening of the occluded arteries in cardioembolic stroke. *Stroke* 1989;20:876.

194. Okada Y, Yamaguchi T, Minematsu K, et al: Hemorrhagic transformation in cerebral embolism. *Stroke* 1989;20:598.

195. Bogousslavsky J, Regli F, Uske A, et al: Early spontaneous hematoma in cerebral infarct: is primary cerebral hemorrhage over diagnosed? *Neurology* 1991;41:837.

196. Mutlu N, Berry RG, Alpers BJ: Massive cerebral hemorrhage. *Arch Neurol* 1963;8:644.

197. Kase CS: Intracerebral hemorrhage: nonhypertensive causes. *Stroke* 1986;17:590.

198. Chaitman BR, Thompson B, Wittry MD, et al: The use of tissue plasminogen activator for acute myocardial infarction in the elderly: results from the Thrombolysis in Myocardial Infarction Phase I Open-Label Studies, and the Thrombolysis in Myocardial Infarction Phase II Pilot Study. *J Am Coll Cardiol* 1989;14:1159.

199. Cragg DR, Friedman HZ, Bonema JD, et al: Outcome of patients with acute myocardial infarction who are ineligible for thrombolytic therapy. *Ann Intern Med* 1991;115:173.

200. Weaver WD, Litwin PE, Martin JS, et al: Effect of age on use of thrombolytic therapy and mortality in acute myocardial infarction. *J Am Coll Cardiol* 1991;18:657.

201. Grines CL, DeMaria AL: Optimal utilization of thrombolytic therapy for acute myocardial infarction: concepts and controversies. *J Am Coll Cardiol* 1990;16:223.

202. Muller DMW, Topol EJ: Selection of patients with acute myocardial infarction for thrombolytic therapy. *Ann Intern Med* 1990;113:949.

203. Kennedy JW: Expanding the use of thrombolytic therapy for acute myocardial infarction (editorial). *Ann Intern Med* 1990;113:907.

204. Gurwitz JH, Goldberg RJ, Gore JM: Coronary thrombolysis for the elderly? *JAMA* 1991;263:1720.

205. Krumholz HM, Pasternak RC, Weinstein MC, et al: Cost effectiveness of thrombolytic therapy with streptokinase in elderly patients with suspected acute myocardial infarction. *N Engl J Med* 1992;327:7.

206. Hendra TJ, Marshall AJ: Increased prescription of thrombolytic treatment to elderly patients with suspected acute myocardial infarction associated with audit. *Br Med J* 1992;304:423.

207. Califf RM, Fortin DF, Tenaglia AN, et al: Clinical risks of thrombolytic therapy. *Am J Cardiol* 1992;69:12A.

208. Feit F, Breed J, Anderson JL, et al: A randomized, placebo-controlled, trial

of tissue plasminogen activator in elderly patients with acute myocardial infarction. *Circulation* 1990;82(suppl III):III-666.

209. Caplan LR: Intracerebral hemorrhage revisited. *Neurology* 1988;38:624.

210. Burke AM, Greenberg JH, Sladky J, et al: Regional variations in cerebral perfusion during acute hypertension. *Neurology* 1987;37:94.

211. Thrombolytic therapy in thrombosis: a National Institutes of Health Consensus Development Conference. *Ann Intern Med* 1980;73:141.

212. Althouse RH, Weaver WD, Kennedy JW: Transient elevation of diastolic blood pressure in acute myocardial infarction: a contraindication to thrombolytic therapy. *Circulation* 1987;76(suppl IV):IV-306.

213. Braunwald E, Knatterud GL, Passamani ER, et al: Announcement of protocol change in thrombolysis in myocardial infarction trial (letter). *J Am Coll Cardiol* 1987;9:467.

214. Braunwald E, Knautterud GL, Passamani E, et al: Update from the Thrombolysis in Myocardial Infarction trial (letter). *J Am Coll Cardiol* 1987;10:970.

215. Collen D: Designing thrombolytic agents: focus on safety and efficacy. *Am J Cardiol* 1992;69:71A.

216. Sobel BE, Collen D: Questions unresolved by the Third International Study of Infarct Survival. *Am J Cardiol* 1992;70:385.

217. Tanswell P, Tebbe U, Neuhaus K-L, et al: Pharmacokinetics and fibrin specificity of alteplase during accelerated infusions in acute myocardial infarction. *J Am Coll Cardiol* 1992;19:1071.

218. Vaughan DE, Braunwald E: Front-loaded accelerated infusions of tissue plasminogen activator: putting a better foot forward. *J Amer Coll Cardiol* 1992;19:1076.

219. Sane DC, Califf RM, Topol EJ, et al: Bleeding during thrombolytic therapy for acute myocardial infarction: mechanisms and management. *Ann Intern Med* 1989;111:1010.

220. Gimple LW, Gold HK, Leinbach RC, et al: Correlation between template bleeding times and spontaneous bleeding during treatment of acute myocardial infarction with recombinant tissue type plasminogen activator. *Circulation* 1989;80:581.

221. Hirsch DR, Goldhaber SZ: The bleeding time: its potential utility among patients receiving thrombolytic therapy. *Am Heart J* 1990;119:158.

222. Kiyomoto A, Sasaki Y, Odawara A, et al: Inhibition of platelet aggregation by diltiazem. *Circ Res* 1983;52(suppl I):I-115.

223. Mehta J: Influence of calcium-channel blockers on platelet function and arachidonic acid metabolism. *Am J Cardiol* 1985;55(suppl):158B.

224. Califf RM, Topol EJ, Kereiakes DJ, et al: Cardiac resuscitation should not be a contraindication to thrombolytic therapy for myocardial infarction (abstract). *Circulation* 1988;78(suppl II):II-127.

225. Scholz KM, Tebbe U, Herrmann C, et al: Frequency of complications of cardiopulmonary resuscitation after thrombolysis during acute myocardial infarction. *J Am Coll Cardiol* 1992;69:724.

226. Sherry S: Dissimilar systemic and local adverse effects of thrombolytic therapy. *Am J Cardiol* 1988;61:1344.

227. Marder VJ, Sherry S: Thrombolytic therapy: current status. *N Engl J Med* 1988;318:1512.

228. Bovill E, Stump D, Tracy R, et al: Dose response relationship of rt-PA infusion to induction of systemic fibrinogenolysis in the thrombolysis in myocardial infarction (TIMI) trial (abstract). *Blood* 1987;70:367a.

229. Bovill EG, Terrin ML, Stump DC, et al: Hemorrhagic events during therapy with recombinant tissue-type plasminogen activator, heparin, and aspirin for acute myocardial infarction. Results of the Thrombolysis in Myocardial Infarction (TIMI), Phase II Trial. *Ann Intern Med* 1991;115:256.

230. Rao AK, Pratt C, Burke A, et al: Thrombolysis in Myocardial Infarction (TIMI) trial-Phase I. Hemorrhagic manifestations and changes in plasma fibrinogen and the fibrinolytic system in patients treated with recombinant tissue plasminogen activator and streptokinase. *J Am Coll Cardiol* 1988;11:1.

231. Collen D, Bounameaux H, DeCock F, et al: Analysis of coagulation and fibrinolysis during intravenous infusion of recombinant human tissue type plasminogen activator in patients with acute myocardial infarction. *Circulation* 1986;73:511.

232. Stump DC, Topol EJ, Chen AB, et al: Monitoring of hemostasis parameters during coronary thrombolysis with recombinant tissue type plasminogen activator. *Thromb Haemost* 1985;59:133.

233. Stump DC, Taylor FB, Nesheim ME, et al: Pathological fibrinolysis as a cause of clinical bleeding. *Semin Thromb Hemost* 1990;16:260.

234. Lawler CM, Bovill EG, Stump DC, et al: Fibrin fragment D-Dimer and fibrinogen B-b peptides in plasma as markers of clot lysis during thrombolytic therapy in acute myocardial infarction. *Blood* 1990;76:1341.

235. Tracy RP, Bovill EG: Fibrinolytic parameters and hemostatic monitoring: identifying and predicting patients at risk for major hemorrhagic events. *Am J Cardiol* 1992;69:52A.

236. Adelman B, Michelson AD, Loscalzo J: Plasmin effect on platelet glycoprotein Ib-von Willebrand factor interactions. *Blood* 1985;65:32.

237. Stricker RB, Wang D, Shiu DT, et al: Activation of plasminogen by tissue plasminogen activator on normal and thromboasthenic platelets: effect of surface proteins and platelet aggregation. *Blood* 1986;68:278.

238. Loscalzo J, Vaughan DE: Tissue plasminogen activator promotes platelet disaggregation in plasma. *J Clin Invest* 1987;79:1749.

239. Vaughan DE, Kirschenbaum JM, Loscalzo J: Streptokinase-induced antibody-mediated platelet aggregation: a potential cause of clot propagation in vivo. *J Am Coll Cardiol* 1988;11:1343.

240. Terres W, Umnus S, Mathey DG, et al: Effects of streptokinase, urokinase, and recombinant tissue plasminogen activator on platelet aggregability and stability of platelet aggregates. *Cardiovasc Res* 1990;24:471.

241. Fitzgerald DJ, Cabella F, Roy I, et al: Marked platelet activation in vivo

after intravenous streptokinase in patients with acute myocardial infarction. *Circulation* 1988;77:142.

242. Fitzgerald DJ, Hanson M, FitzGerald GA: Attenuation of the thrombolytic response to urokinase by platelets is minimal. *Circulation* 1989;80(suppl II):II-422.

243. Coller BS: Platelets and thrombolytic therapy. *N Engl J Med* 1990;332:33.

244. Collen D: Coronary thrombolysis: streptokinase or recombinant tissue plasminogen activator? *Ann Intern Med* 1990;112:529.

245. Vaughan DE, Declerck PJ, de Mol M, et al: Recombinant plasminogen activator inhibitor-I reverses the bleeding tendency associated with combined administration of tissue-type plasminogen activator and aspirin in rabbits. *J Clin Invest* 1989;84:586.

246. White HD: GISSI-2 and the heparin controversy. *Lancet* 1990;336:297.

247. Steering Committee: Final report on the aspirin component of the ongoing Physicians Health Study. *N Engl J Med* 1989;321:129.

248. Rosenblum B: Pathophysiology of arteriovenous malformations: recent advances in analysis and therapy. In: Rosenblum B, ed: *State of the Art Reviews in Neurosurgery: Cerebral and Spinal Arteriovenous Malformations*. Philadelphia: Hanley-Belfus, 1988:1.

249. Vinters HV: Cerebral amyloid angiopathy. A critical review. *Stroke* 1987;18:311.

250. Kalyan-Raman UP, Kalyan-Raman K: Cerebral amyloid angiopathy causing intracranial hemorrhage. *Ann Neurol* 1984;16:321.

251. Okazaki H, Regan TJ, Campbell RJ: Clinical pathologic studies of primary cerebral amyloid angiopathy. *Mayo Clin Proc* 1979;54:22.

252. Vonsattel JP, Hedley-Whyte ET, Ropper AH, et al: Coincidence of fibrinoid necrosis with amyloid angiopathy as the cause of cerebral hemorrhage. *J Neuropathol Exp Neurol* 1984;43:316.

253. Powers JM, Schlaepfer WW, Willingham MC, et al: An immunoperoxidase study of senile cerebral amyloidosis with pathogenetic considerations. *J Neuropathol Exp Neurol* 1981;40:598.

254. Charcot JM, Bouchard C: Nouvelles recherches sur la pathogénie de l'hémorragie cérébrale. *Arch Physiol Norm Pathol* 1868;1:110.

255. Green FHK: Miliary aneurysms in the brain. *J Pathol Bacteriol* 1930;33:71.

256. Ross Russell RW: Observations on intracerebral aneurysms. *Brain* 1963;86:425.

257. Cole FM, Yates P: Intracerebral microaneurysms and small cerebrovascular lesions. *Brain* 1967;90:759.

258. Cole FM, Yates PO: The occurrence and significance of intracerebral micro-aneurysms. *J Pathol Bacteriol* 1967;30:393.

259. Fisher CM: Cerebral military aneurysms in hypertension. *Am J Pathol* 1971;66:313.

260. Fisher CM: Pathological observations in hypertensive cerebral hemorrhage. *J Neuropathol Exp Neurol* 1971;30:536.

261. Cole FM, Yates PO: Pseudoaneurysms in relationship to massive cerebral hemorrhage. *J Neurol Neurosurg Psychiatry* 1967;30:61.

262. Takebayashi S, Kaneko M: Electron microscopic studies of ruptured arteries in hypertensive intracerebral hemorrhage. *Stroke* 1983;14:28.

263. Takebayashi S: Ultrastructural morphometry of hypertensive medial damage in lenticulostriate and other arteries. *Stroke* 1985;16:449.

264. Rosenblum WI: Miliary aneurysms and "fibrinoid" degeneration of cerebral blood vessels. *Human Pathol* 1977;8:133.

265. Wakai S, Nagai M: Histological verification of micro-aneurysms as a cause of cerebral hemorrhage in surgical specimens. *J Neurol Neurosurg Psychiatry* 1989;52:595.

266. Bayle ALJ: Traité des maladies du cerveau et de ses membranes. *Maladies Mentales*. Paris: Gabon, 1826.

267. Labadie EL: Fibrinolysis in the formation and growth of chronic subdural hematomas: In: Sawaya R, ed: *Fibrinolysis and the Central Nervous System*. Philadelphia: Hanley-Belfus, 1990:141.

268. Labadie EL, Glover D: Local alterations of hemostatic-fibrinolytic mechanisms in reforming subdural hematomas. *Neurology* 1975;25:669.

269. Ito H, Yamamoto S, Komai T, et al: Role of local hyperfibrinolysis in the etiology of chronic subdural hematoma. *J Neurosurg* 1976;45:26.

270. Ito H, Komai T, Yamamoto S: Fibrinolytic enzyme in the lining walls of chronic subdural hematoma. *J Neurosurg* 1978;48:197.

271. Weir B, Gordon P: Factors suffering coagulation: fibrinolysis in chronic subdural fluid collections. *J Neurosurg* 1985;58:242.

272. Skinner JR, Phillips SJ, Zeff RH, et al: Immediate coronary bypass following failed streptokinase infusion in evolving myocardial infarction. *Thorac Cardiovasc Surg* 1984;87:567.

273. Harker LA, Malpass TW, Branson HE, et al: Mechanism of abnormal bleeding in patients undergoing cardiopulmonary bypass: acquired transient platelet dysfunction associated with selective (alpha) granule release. *Blood* 1980;56:824.

274. Kereiakes DJ, Topol EJ, George BS, et al: Emergency coronary artery bypass surgery preserves global and regional left ventricular function after intravenous tissue plasminogen activator therapy for acute myocardial infarction. *J Am Coll Cardiol* 1988;11:899.

275. Harker LA: Bleeding after cardiopulmonary bypass: *N Engl J Med* 1986; 314:1446.

276. Salzman EW, Weinstein MJ, Weintraub RM, et al: Treatment with desmopressin acetate to reduce blood loss after cardiac surgery. *N Engl J Med* 1986;314:1402.

277. Cerebral Embolism Study Group: Cardioembolic stroke, early anticoagulation, and brain hemorrhage. *Arch Intern Med* 1987;147:636.

278. Jorgensen L, Torvik A: Ischemic cerebrovascular diseases in an autopsy series, part 2. Prevalence, location, pathogenesis and clinical course of cerebral infarcts. *J Neuro Sci* 1969;9:285.

279. Furlan AJ, Cavalier SJ, Hobbs RE, et al: Hemorrhage and anticoagulation after nonseptic embolic brain infarction. *Neurology* 1982;32:280.
280. Koller RL: Recurrent embolic cerebral infarction and anticoagulation. *Neurology* 1982;32:283.
281. Weisberg LA: Nonseptic cardiogenic cerebral embolic stroke: Clinical-CT correlations. *Neurology* 1985;35:896.
282. Lodder J, van der Lugt PJM: Evaluation of the risk of immediate anticoagulant treatment in patients with embolic stroke of cardiac origin. *Stroke* 1983;14:42.
283. Cerebral Embolism Study Group: Immediate anticoagulation of embolic stroke: a randomized trial. *Stroke* 1983;14:68.
284. Hakim AM, Ryder-Cooke A, Melanson D: Sequential computerized tomographic appearance of strokes. *Stroke* 1983;14:893.
285. Cerebral Embolism Study Group: Immediate anticoagulation of embolic stroke: brain hemorrhage and management options. *Stroke* 1984;15:779.
286. Lodder J: CT-detected hemorrhagic infarction: relation with the size of the infarct and the presence of midline shift. *Acta Neurol Scand* 1984;70: 329.
287. Fisher M, Zito JL, Siva A, et al: Hemorrhagic infarction: a clinical and CT study. *Stroke* 1984;15:192.
288. Shields RW, Laureno R, Lachman T, et al: Anticoagulant-related hemorrhage in acute cerebral embolism. *Stroke* 1984;15:426.
289. Hornig CR, Dorndorf W, Agnoli AL: Hemorrhagic cerebral infarction: a prospective study. *Stroke* 1986;17:179.
290. Lodder J, Krijne-Kubat B, Broekman J: Cerebral hemorrhagic infarction at autopsy: cardiac embolism cause and the relationship to the cause of death. *Stroke* 1986;17:626.
291. Ott BR, Zamani A, Kleefied J, et al: The clinical spectrum of hemorrhagic infarction. *Stroke* 1986;17:630.
292. Hart RG, for the Cerebral Embolism Study Group: Timing of hemorrhagic transformation of cardioembolic stroke. In: Stober T, Schimrigk K, Ganten D, et al, eds: *Central Nervous System Control of the Heart*. Boston: Martinus Nijhoff, 1986:229.
293. Hart RG, Tegeler CH: Hemorrhagic infarction on CT in the absence of anticoagulant therapy. *Stroke* 1986;17:558.
294. Sherman DB, Hart RG, for the Cerebral Embolism Study Group: Brain hemorrhage in embolic stroke. In: Stober R, Schimrigk K, Ganten D, et al, eds: *Central Nervous System Control of the Heart*. Boston: Martinus Nijhoff, 1986:249.
295. Laureno R, Shields RW, Narayan T: The diagnosis and management of cerebral embolism and hemorrhagic infarction with sequential computerized cranial tomography. *Brain* 1987;110:93.
296. Fisher CM, Adams RD: Observations on brain embolism with special reference to the mechanism of hemorrhagic infarction. *J Neuropathol Exp Neurol* 1951;10:92.
297. Beghi E, Bogliun G, Cavaletti G, et al: Hemorrhagic infarction: risk fac-

tors, clinical and tomographic features, and outcome. A case-control study. *Acta Neurol Scand* 1989;80:226.

298. Lodder J, Krijne-Kuhat B, van der Lugt PJM: Timing of autopsy-proven hemorrhagic infarction with reference to cardioembolic stroke. *Stroke* 1988;19:1482.

299. Pessin MS, del Zoppo GJ, Estol CJ: Thrombolytic agents in the treatment of stroke. *Clin Neuropharmacol* 1990;13:271.

300. del Zoppo GJ, Pessin MS, Mori E, et al: Thrombolytic intervention in acute thrombotic and embolic stroke. *Semin Neurol* 1991;11:368.

301. Zivin JA: A perspective on the future of thrombolytic stroke therapy. In: Ginsberg MD, Dietrich WD, eds: *Cerebrovascular Diseases*. New York: Raven Press, 1989:33.

302. Pessin MS: Hemorrhagic transformation in the natural history of acute embolic stroke. In: Hacke W, del Zoppo GJ, Hirschberg M, eds: *Thrombolytic Therapy in Acute Ischemic Stroke*. Berlin: Springer-Verlag, 1991:67.

303. Bozzoa L, Angeloni U, Bastianello, et al: Early angiographic and CT findings in patients with hemorrhagic infarction in the distribution of the middle cerebral artery. *Am J Neuroradiol* 1991;12:1115.

304. Pessin MS, Teal PA, Caplan LR: Hemorrhagic infarction: guilt by association? *Am J Neuroradiol* 1991;12:1123.

305. Faris AA, Hardin CA, Poser CM: Pathogenesis of hemorrhagic infarction of the brain. *Arch Neurol* 1963;9:468.

306. Bruetman ME, Fields WS, Crawford ES, et al: Cerebral hemorrhage in carotid artery surgery. *Arch Neurol* 1963;9:458.

307. Caplan LR, Skillman J, Ojemann R, et al: Intracerebral hemorrhage following carotid endarterectomy: a hypertensive complication? *Stroke* 1978; 9:457.

308. Sundt TM, Sharbrough FW, Piepgras DG, et al: Correlation of cerebral blood flow and electroencephalographic changes during carotid endarterectomy with results of surgery and hemodynamics of cerebral ischemia. *Mayo Clin Proc* 1981;56:533.

309. Petito CK: Early and late mechanisms of increased vascular permeability following experimental cerebral infarction. *J Neuropathol Exp Neurol* 1979;38:222.

310. Garcia JH: Experimental ischemic stroke: a review. *Stroke* 1983;14:5.

311. Kamijyo Y, Gureia JM, Cooper J: Temporary regional cerebral ischemia in the cat: a model of hemorrhagic and subcortical infarction. *J Neuropathol Exp Neurol* 1977;36:338.

312. Garcia JH, Lowry SL, Briggs L, et al: Brain capillaries expand and rupture in areas of ischemia and reperfusion. In: Reivich M, Hurtig ML, eds: *Cerebrovascular Diseases*. New York: Raven Press, 1983:169.

313. Globus JH, Epstein JA: Massive cerebral hemorrhage: spontaneous and experimentally induced. *J Neuropathol Exp Neurol* 1953;12:107.

314. Laurent JP, Molinari GF, Oakley JC: Primate model of cerebral hematoma. *J Neuropathol Exp Neurol* 1976;35:560.

315. Saku Y, Choki J, Waki R, et al: Hemorrhagic infarct induced by arterial

hypertension in cat brain following middle cerebral artery occlusion. *Stroke* 1990;21:589.

316. Horowitz SG, Zito JL, Donnarumma R, et al: Computed tomographic-angiographic findings within the first five hours of cerebral infarction. *Stroke* 1991;22:1245.

317. Lyden PD, Zivin JA, Soll M, et al: Intracerebral hemorrhage after experimental embolic infarction. Anticoagulation. *Arch Neurol* 1987;44:848.

318. Centeno RS, Hackney DB, Rothrock JR: Streptokinase clot lysis in acute occlusion of the cranial circulation: study in rabbits. *Am J Neuroradiol* 1985;6:589.

319. Zivin JA, Fisher M, DeGirolami U, et al: Tissue plasminogen activator reduces neurological damage after cerebral embolism. *Science* 1985;320: 1289.

320. del Zoppo GJ, Copeland BR, Waltz TA, et al: The beneficial effect of intra-carotid urokinase on acute stroke in a baboon model. *Stroke* 1986;17:638.

321. Slivka A, Pulsinelli W: Hemorrhagic complications of thrombolytic therapy in experimental stroke. *Stroke* 1987;18:1148.

322. Watson BD, Prado R, Dietrich MD, et al: Mitigation of evolving cortical infarction in rats by recombinant tissue plasminogen activator following photochemically induced thrombosis. In: Raichle ME, Powers WJ, eds: *Cerebrovascular Diseases*. New York: Raven Press, 1987:317.

323. Kissel P, Chehrazi B, Seibert JA, et al: Digital and angiographic quantification of blood flow dynamics in embolic stroke treated with tissue-type plasminogen activator. *J Neurosurg* 1987;67:399.

324. Hirschberg M, Hofferberth B: Rapid fibrinolysis at different time intervals in a canine model of acute stroke. *Stroke* 1987;18(suppl I):292.

325. Hirschberg M, Hofferberth B: Thrombolytic therapy with urokinase and prourokinase in a canine model of acute stroke. *Neurology* 1987;37(suppl I):I-133.

326. Papadopoulos SM, Chandler WF, Salamat MS, et al: Recombinant human tissue-type plasminogen activator therapy in acute thromboembolic stroke. *J Neurosurg* 1987;67:394.

327. Penar LP, Greer CA: The effect of intravenous tissue-type plasminogen activator in a rat model of embolic cerebral ischemia. *Yale J Biol Med* 1987;60:233.

328. Chehrazi BB, Siebert AJ, Hein I, et al: Evaluation of tissue plasminogen activator (t-PA) in embolic stroke. *Stroke* 1988;19(suppl I):33.

329. DeLey G, Weyne J, Demeester G, et al: Experimental thromboembolic stroke studied by positron emission tomography: immediate versus delayed reperfusion by fibrinolysis. *J Cereb Blood Flow Metab* 1988;8:539.

330. del Zoppo GJ, Copeland BR, Hacke W, et al: Intracerebral hemorrhage following rt-PA infusion in a primate stroke model. *Stroke* 1988;19(suppl I):134.

331. Lyden P, Zivin JA, Clark WM, et al: t-PA-mediated thrombolysis and intracerebral hemorrhage after MCA occlusion. *Neurology* 1988;38(suppl I):I-148.

332. Phillips DA, Davis MA, Fisher M: Selective embolization and clot dissolution with t-PA in the internal carotid artery circulation of the rabbit. *Am J Neuroradiol* 1988;9:899.

333. Phillips DA, Fisher M, Smith TW, et al: The safety and angiographic efficacy of tissue plasminogen activator in a cerebral embolization model. *Ann Neurol* 1988;23:391.

334. Zivin JA, Lyden PD, DeGirolami U, et al: Tissue plasminogen activator: reduction of neurologic damage after experimental embolic stroke. *Arch Neurol* 1988;45:387.

335. Zivin JA: Therapy of embolic stroke with tissue plasminogen activator plus a glutamate antagonist. *Neurology* 1989;37(suppl I):I-372.

336. Phillips DA, Fisher M, Smith TW, et al: The effects of a new tissue plasminogen activator analogue, Fb-Fb-CF, on cerebral reperfusion in a rabbit embolic stroke model. *Ann Neurol* 1989;25:281.

337. Lyden PD, Zivin JA, Clark W, et al: Tissue plasminogen activator-mediated thrombolysis of cerebral emboli and its effect on hemorrhagic infarction in rabbits. *Neurology* 1989;39:703.

338. DeLey G, Weyne G, Demeester G, et al: Streptokinase treatment versus calcium overload blockade in experimental thromboembolic stroke. *Stroke* 1989;20:357.

339. Fisher M, Phillips DA, Smith TW, et al: Delayed treatment with a t-PA analog in an embolic stroke model. *Stroke* 1989;20(suppl I):154.

340. Chehrazi BB, Siebert JA, Hein L, et al: Differential effect of t-PA induced thrombolysis in the CNS and systemic arteries. *Stroke* 1989;20(suppl I): 153.

341. Clark WM, Madden KP, Zivin JA, et al: Intracerebral hemorrhage: TPA versus streptokinase thrombolytic therapy. *Neurology* 1989;39(suppl I): I-183.

342. del Zoppo GJ, Copeland BR, Anderchele K, et al: Hemorrhagic transformation following tissue plasminogen activator in experimental cerebral infarction. *Stroke* 1990;21:596.

343. Lyden PD, Madden KP, Clark WM, et al: Incidence of cerebral hemorrhage after antifibrinolytic treatment for embolic stroke in rabbits. *Stroke* 1990;21:1589.

344. Benes V, Zabramski JM, Boston M, et al: Effect of intra-arterial antifibrinolytic agents on autologous arterial emboli in the cerebral circulation of rabbits. *Stroke* 1990;21:1594.

345. Bednar MM, McAuliffe T, Raymond S, et al: Tissue plasminogen activator reduces brain injury in a rat model of thromboembolic stroke. *Stroke* 1990; 21:1705.

346. Hirschberg M, Klemens B, Hacke W: Usefulness of intravenous thrombolytic therapy with single chain urokinase-type plasminogen activator in a model of acute stroke. *Stroke* 1990;21(suppl I):I-106.

347. Fisher M, Phillips DA, Davis MA, et al: Delayed treatment with a t-PA analogue and streptokinase in a rabbit embolism stroke model. *Stroke* 1990;21(suppl I):I-135.

348. Clark W, Madden K, Lyden P, et al: Experimental cerebral hemorrhagic risk of aspirin or heparin therapy with t-PA thrombolysis. *Neurology* 1991;41(suppl I):386.

349. Carter PL: Modification of brain ischemia due to embolic stroke by tissue-type plasminogen activator with and without heparin in a rabbit model. Presented at the Second International Symposium on Thrombolytic Therapy for Acute Stroke, San Diego, May, 1992.

350. Carter LP, Guthkelch AN, Orozco J, et al: Influence of tissue plasminogen activator and heparin on cerebral ischemia in a rabbit model. *Stroke* 1992; 23:883.

351. Overgaard K, Sereghy T, Boysen G, et al: Reduction of infarct volume and mortality by thrombolysis with rt-PA in an embolic stroke model. *Stroke* 1992;23:1167.

352. Molinari GF: Clinical relevance of experimental stroke models. In: Price TR, Nelson E, eds: *Cerebrovascular Diseases: Eleventh Princeton Conference.* New York: Raven Press, 1979:19.

353. Molinari GF: Experimental models of ischemic stroke. In: Barnett HJM, Mohr JP, Stein BM, et al, eds: *Stroke: Pathophysiology, Diagnosis and Management.* New York: Churchill-Livingstone, 1986:57.

354. Moossy J: Morphologic validation of ischemic stroke models. In: Price TR, Nelson E, eds: *Cerebrovascular Diseases: Eleventh Princeton Conference.* New York: Raven Press, 1979:3.

355. Waltz AG: Comparative pathophysiology of ischemic stroke models: an evaluation. In: Price TR, Nelson E, eds: *Cerebrovascular Diseases. Eleventh Princeton Conference.* New York: Raven Press, 1979:11.

356. Molinari GF: Thrombolytic therapy in ischemic stroke: relevance and limitations of animal models. In: Hacke W, del Zoppo GJ, Hirschberg M, eds: *Thrombolytic Therapy in Acute Ischemic Stroke.* Berlin: Springer-Verlag, 1991:105.

357. Sloan MA: Thrombolytic therapy in experimental focal cerebral ischemia. In: Sawaya R, ed: *Fibrinolysis and the Central Nervous System.* Philadelphia: Hanley and Belfus, 1990:177.

358. del Zoppo GJ: Relevance of focal cerebral ischemia models. Experience with fibrinolytic agents. *Stroke* 1990;21(suppl IV):IV-155.

359. Hirschberg M: Update on animal model experience with recombinant tissue plasminogen activator. In: Hacke W, del Zoppo GJ, Hirschberg M, eds: *Thrombolytic Therapy in Acute Ischemia Stroke.* Berlin: Springer-Verlag, 1991:114.

360. Brott T: Thrombolytic therapy for stroke. *Cerebrovasc Brain Metab Rev* 1991;3:91.

361. Brott T: Thrombolytic therapy. *Neurol Clin* 1992;10:219.

362. Gomez CR, Burger SK, Puricelli M, et al: Early computed tomography demonstration of cerebral infarction does not correlate with clinical outcome. *J Stroke Cerebrovasc Dis* 1992;2:146.

363. Fisher CM, Kistler JP, Davis JM: Relation of cerebral vasospasm to sub-

arachnoid hemorrhage visualized by computerized tomographic scanning. *Neurosurgery* 1980;6:1.

364. Kistler JP, Crowell RW, Davis KR, et al: The relation of cerebral vasospasm to the extent and location of subarachnoid blood visualized by CT scan. A prospective study. *Neurology* 1983;33:424.

365. Findlay JM, Macdonald RL, Weir BKA: Current concepts of pathophysiology and management of cerebral vasospasm following aneurysmal subarachnoid hemorrhage. *Cardiovasc Brain Metab Rev* 1991;3:336.

366. Macdonald RL, Weir BKA: A review of hemoglobin and the pathogenesis of cerebral vasospasm. *Stroke* 1991;22:971.

Chapter 7

Intracranial Hemorrhage Due to Neoplasms

Lisa M. DeAngelis, MD

Hemorrhage into cerebral neoplasms is uncommon and represents an unusual cause of intracranial hemorrhage. Most tumor-related hemorrhages result in an intraparenchymal hematoma; less commonly, cerebral neoplasms can cause subarachnoid (SAH) or subdural hemorrhage (SDH). Hemorrhage into a previously diagnosed intracerebral tumor may prove a therapeutic but rarely a diagnostic problem. However, hemorrhage is often the first unequivocal indicator of a pre-existing neoplasm, and may be difficult to distinguish from the more common causes of intracerebral hemorrhage (ICH), such as hypertension. The patient's clinical history or radiographic studies may suggest the presence of an underlying neoplasm which would require subsequent pathologic confirmation. Tumor-related hemorrhage warrants a different therapeutic approach and carries a different prognosis from spontaneous or traumatic ICH.

Throughout this chapter and the literature cited in the references, a brain tumor-associated hemorrhage represents a macroscopic hemorrhage producing a significant blood clot. On pathologic specimens many tumors have necrotic foci which permit leakage of small amounts of blood or have microscopic extravasation of red blood cells into neighboring tissue.[1] This degree of microscopic hemorrhage is not associated with clinical or radiographic abnormalities and is not considered a tumor-related hemorrhage in this discussion. Likewise, all forms of intracranial hemorrhage (parenchymal, subarachnoid, and subdural) can occur in patients with systemic cancer who have thrombocytopenia or a coagulopathy, but not direct tumor infiltration of the nervous system. The hemorrhagic complications of systemic cancer independent of intratumoral hemorrhage are not the subject of this chapter, but are discussed in detail by Grauss et al.[2]

Epidemiology

Neoplasms account for only 0.8% to 9.0% of all nontraumatic ICHs in large series (Table 1).[3-8] The relatively high incidence (9.0%) of neoplastic hemor-

From Feldmann E (ed). *Intracerebral Hemorrhage*. Armonk, NY: Futura Publishing Company, Inc., © 1994.

Table 1
Incidence of Intracerebral Hemorrhage Due To Brain Tumor (BT)

Reference	Author	Year	# BT bleeds/ # all bleeds	Percentage
3	Mutlu et al	1963	2/225	0.8
4	Luessenhop et al	1967	2/130	1.5
5	Bitoh et al	1984	3/119	2.5
6	Wakai et al	1992	2/50	4.0
7	Little et al	1979	10/172	5.8
8	McCormick & Rosenfield	1973	13/144	9.0

rhage reported by McCormick and Rosenfield may be partly attributed to a high incidence of metastatic brain tumors in their population, which accounted for the majority of their tumor-related intracranial hemorrhages.[8]

Subarachnoid and subdural hemorrhage are even less commonly caused by neoplasms. Locksley et al reported on the cooperative study of subarachnoid hemorrhage (SAH) in 1966, and found that only 0.4% of all SAHs could be attributed to intracranial neoplasms, half from primary brain tumors and half from metastatic tumors.[9] When examining SAH not attributed to aneurysms or arteriovenous malformations (AVMs), tumors still accounted for only 1.3% of SAHs. Subdural hemorrhage (SDH) secondary to neoplasm occurs almost exclusively in patients with metastatic disease and is rarely associated with primary brain tumors.[10,11] Both solid tumors, particularly breast and prostate carcinoma, and hematologic malignancies can infiltrate the dura and lead to hemorrhage.

Hemorrhage occurs in only 1% to 8% of all brain tumors (Table 2), but the

Table 2
Incidence of Hemorrhage into Brain Tumors According to Histologic Type of Neoplasm

	Oldberg[12] (n = 31/832)	Wakai et al[11] (n = 94/1861)	Kondziolka et al[1] (n = 49/905)	Scott[13] (n = 8/590)	Drake & McGee[14] (n = 18/236)	Bitoh et al[5] (n = 3/497)	Manganiello[15] (n = 7/183)	Globus & Sapirstein[16] (n = 9/94)
All BT‡	—	5.0	5.4	1.3	7.6	0.6	—	9.6
All Gliomass‡	3.7	4.4	—	—	—	—	3.8	12.2
astrocytoma	1.1	4.9†	10.9	—	—	—	2.5	—
anaplastic astro	5.4		6.1	—	—	—	6.2	—
GBM	5.6	7.8	6.4	—	—	—	5.5	—
oligodendro	10.3	7.0	14.3*	—	—	—	—	—
medulloblastoma	2.3	1.6	0	—	—	—	—	0
ependymoma	0	8.8	0	—	—	—	8.0	0
Meningiomas	—	1.3	0.5	—	—	—	—	0
Pituitary Tumors	—	15.8	—	—	—	—	—	0
Metastases	—	2.9	6.1	—	—	—	—	9.4

Legend: BT = brain tumor; Astro = astrocytoma; GBM = glioblastoma multiforme; oligodendro = oligodendroglioma.

† incidence is a combination of astrocytoma and anaplastic astrocytoma.

* 29.2% incidence in mixed oligo-astrocytomas.

‡ numbers in the table relfect percent of tumors in that category that bled.

propensity for hemorrhage varies greatly among the different types of neoplasms.[1,5,11–16] Among the astrocytomas, the grade of malignancy is directly related to the risk of tumor-induced hemorrhage, and the malignant gliomas account for the majority of brain tumor-associated hemorrhage. Hemorrhage is seen in 5% to 8% of all glioblastomas multiforme and malignant astrocytomas, but in only 1% to 2% of benign astrocytomas. Despite the fact that the majority of oligodendrogliomas are histologically benign, the oligodendroglioma also has a high incidence of hemorrhage (7% to 14%).[1,11,12] Because this is an uncommon tumor, oligodendrogliomas account for a small fraction of tumor-associated hemorrhages, but almost all series note its high incidence of bleeding. Intracranial hemorrhage has been reported with meningiomas, but is very unusual.[1,11,17–19] It has been seen with intraventricular meningiomas, tumors located over the convexity, and in the cerebellopontine angle. Hemorrhage does not appear to be associated with any particular histologic variant of meningioma and has usually been reported with pathologically benign lesions, although this may be due to the rarity of malignant meningiomas.

Pituitary tumors are also benign intracranial malignancies which bleed. Hemorrhage into pituitary adenomas occurs fairly often, but is not always associated with the clinical syndrome of pituitary apoplexy.[20,21] The incidence of hemorrhage into pituitary tumors is about 17%, but only 55% of these patients had an acute episode that suggested bleeding. The remaining 45% were asymptomatic due to the small size of the hemorrhage. The relatively high incidence of clinically silent hematomas into pituitary tumors has been appreciated only since the development of computed tomography (CT) and magnetic resonance (MR) scanning.

Metastatic brain tumors cause ICH, but the overall incidence has not been as well studied as it has for primary brain tumors. Although brain metastases from any primary can bleed, specific tumors have a definite predilection to hemorrhage. Melanoma, renal carcinoma, and choriocarcinoma metastases bleed frequently. However, the most common cause of a hemorrhagic metastatic brain tumor is non-small cell lung cancer, both because of the high incidence of bronchogenic carcinoma in the general population and the tendency for this tumor to metastasize to the brain.[1,11,22,23]

Although total numbers were small, Kondziolka et al found that 35.7% (5 of 14) of melanomatous brain metastases were hemorrhagic; 3.5% of metastatic adenocarcinomas and anaplastic carcinomas had macroscopic hemorrhage, but no hemorrhages were associated with metastatic squamous cell carcinoma.[1] In a CT scan-based study, Weisberg[24] reported that 40% of metastatic melanomas had evidence of hemorrhage, 70% of renal carcinomas, and only 5% of bronchogenic carcinomas. Lung cancer, however, accounted for 40% of hemorrhagic brain metastases, with melanoma representing 40% and renal 20%.[24] Mandybur[22] reported a series of 15 patients with hemorrhagic metastatic brain tumors. Eight had bronchogenic carcinoma, three had choriocarcinoma, and there was one patient each with renal, epidermoid of the larynx, malignant carcinoid, and testicular carcinoma.[22] Since melanoma represents a significant proportion of primaries in all other reports, its absence here was unusual.

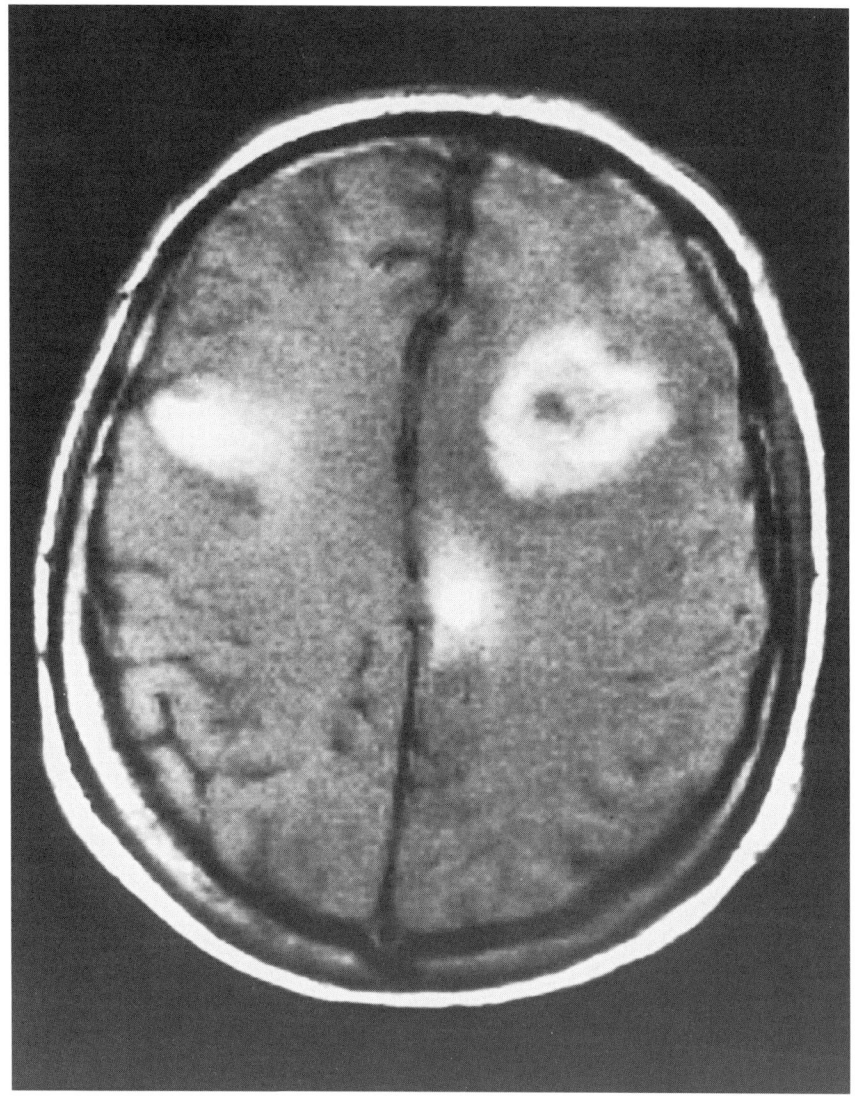

Figure 1: Pregadolinium T_1 weighted MR scan showing multiple hyperintense lesions due to hemorrhage into brain metastases from melanoma.

Unlike primary brain tumors, brain metastases are multiple in half of patients. Furthermore, particular types of tumors tend to produce multiple metastatic brain deposits as opposed to single lesions. For example, melanoma produces multiple metastases in 60% of patients (Figure 1).[25] Several authors have noted that hemorrhage may develop in multiple metastatic brain tumors simultaneously, particularly those that arise from melanoma, choriocarcinoma, and renal carcinoma (Figures 1 and 2).[22-24] Therefore, any patient who presents

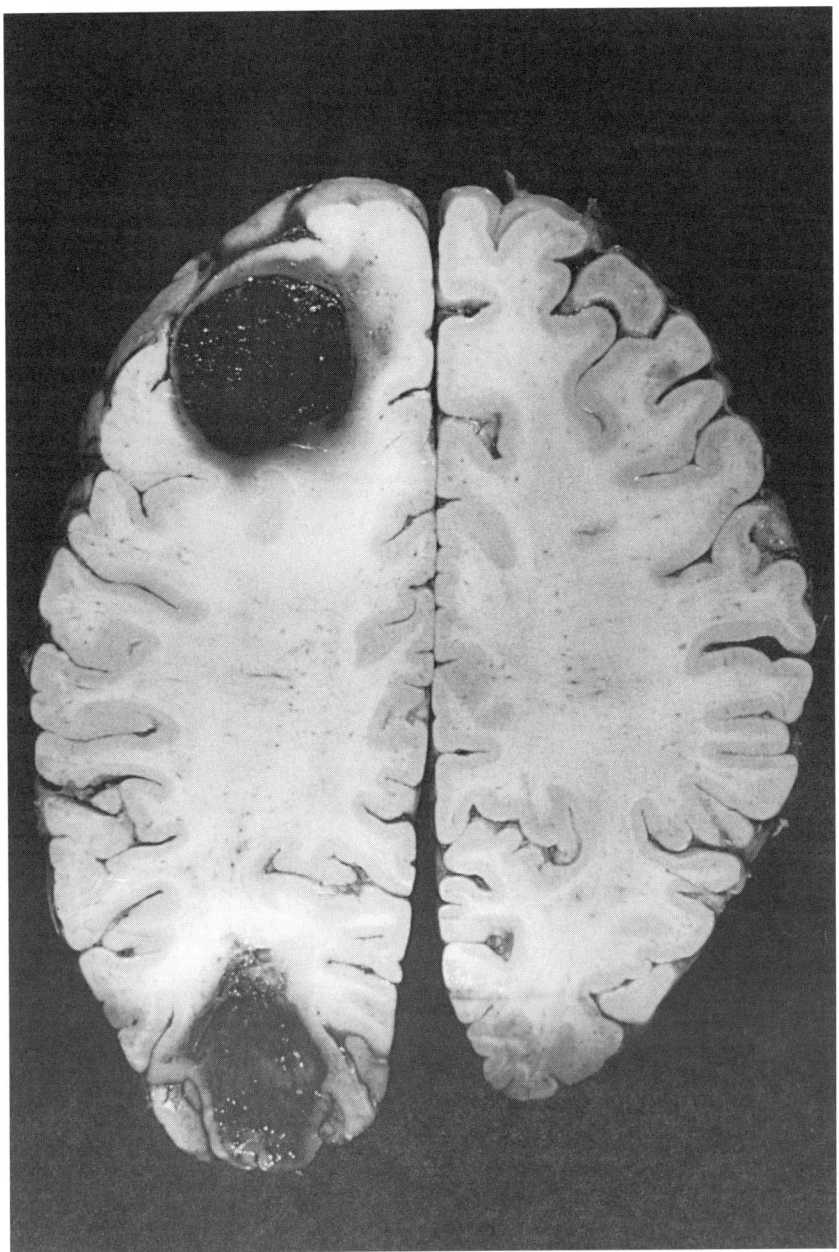

Figure 2: Gross autopsy specimen demonstrating simultaneous hemorrhage into two melanomatous cerebral metastases.

with multiple concurrent parenchymal cerebral hemorrhages should be suspect for intracranial metastases, particularly from these primaries.

Hemorrhage into a neoplasm is primarily determined by the nature of the underlying tumor. The risk of hemorrhage does not appear to be significantly affected by other more common risk factors for intracranial hemorrhage. Trauma does not increase the risk of neoplastic hemorrhage.[14-16] Although hypertension is an important risk factor for ICH, it does not appear to increase the risk for tumor-related intracranial bleeding.[1,8,14] Coagulopathy is a known risk for the development of intracranial bleeding, particularly in patients with systemic cancer, but coagulopathy rarely contributes to intratumoral hemorrhage, even in patients with brain metastases.[1,2] Most neoplastic hemorrhages occur in the absence of coagulopathy. Likewise, patients with brain tumors can be safely anticoagulated for thrombotic complications without risking an increased incidence of ICH unless anticoagulation is excessive.[26,27]

Pathogenesis

The mechanism of intratumoral hemorrhage is not clear, but several histologic features of malignant neoplasms may explain their tendency to bleed. A growing neoplasm develops new blood vessels to keep pace with its expansion. Often, tumors are more vascular than the organ from which they arose, producing an angiographic blush, a feature which is used to diagnose malignancies. All intracranial malignant neoplasms contain vasculature which is distinctly different from normal cerebral blood vessels. Primary brain tumors have neovessels which are immature, fenestrated, and lack tight junctions, making them more permeable than normal.[28-30] These neovessels permit greater penetration of plasma and, in some cases, passage of red blood cells through the vascular channel into the surrounding brain parenchyma has been identified pathologically. Therefore, these vessels are more vulnerable and predispose to hemorrhage.

There are three patterns of capillary growth seen in brain tumors: axial, retiform, and glomeruloid. Tumors often contain more than one type of capillary, but only the retiform capillary is significantly associated with tumor-related hemorrhage. Retiform capillaries take a convoluted and tortuous course through tumor tissue. They are plentiful in gliomas, and their presence correlates with the tendency of a tumor to bleed, particularly in malignant gliomas.[30] However, retiform vessels are also common in oligodendrogliomas where they have a tendency to calcify. Calcification further increases the risk of hemorrhage, which may explain the high incidence of hematomas in this otherwise benign brain tumor. Whether calcified vessels have a greater tendency to bleed because of increased vascular fragility or reduced mechanical support from surrounding tissue is unknown. The vascular predisposition to hemorrhage in other benign tumors, such as the meningioma, is poorly defined, although abnormal, thin walled blood vessels have been identified pathologically in regions of hemorrhage in meningiomas.[17,18] Metastatic brain tumors develop blood vessels similar to those of their primary site, explaining the variability of neoplastic hemorrhage among the different types of metastases. However, the specific features of these vessels which lead to hemorrhage are poorly understood.

In addition to containing abnormal vessels, both malignant gliomas and metastatic brain tumors can invade vessel walls and further compromise vascular integrity. This has been demonstrated both angiographically and pathologically.[31–33] The incidence of vascular infiltration by tumor is probably underestimated since a large hematoma may destroy an infiltrated vessel so it is not identified at angiography or autopsy. Furthermore, tumors tend to involve small blood vessels below angiographic resolution and, therefore, vascular invasion may not be appreciated on radiographic studies.

Tumor necrosis is an additional feature which may lead to hemorrhage. Necrosis of underlying tumor tissue, its vasculature, and loss of structural support for the remaining peripheral viable tumor can increase the risk of neoplastic hemorrhage. Necrosis is a hallmark of glioblastoma multiform and is occasionally seen in metastatic lesions, contributing to the high incidence of tumor-related hemorrhage in these particular neoplasms.[1]

The development of neoplastic aneurysms is occasionally responsible for hemorrhage in association with an intracranial tumor, usually a metastasis. Aneurysms have been associated with a variety of tumor types including choriocarcinoma, bronchogenic carcinoma, atrial myxoma, and malignant glioma.[33–35] Clinical presentation was that of an ICH. Angiograms demonstrated single or multiple peripheral aneurysms associated with an intra-axial mass. Pathologically, tumor invades the vessel wall producing a focal aneurysmal dilitation with eventual rupture. Patients with metastatic disease were thought to develop the aneurysm when a tumor embolus lodged within the vessel and grew. Although unusual, neoplastic aneurysms are important because they may require surgical repair in addition to treatment of the underlying neoplasm and hematoma.

Clinical Presentation

The clinical presentation of intratumoral hemorrhage can be indistinguishable from spontaneous ICH of a more typical etiology, such as hypertension. However, the presence of an underlying structural lesion may result in a more varied clinical presentation. Intratumoral hemorrhage can produce a stroke-like syndrome of rapid onset, with the abrupt appearance of lateralizing signs or profound impairment of consciousness and a rapidly devastating clinical course. Intratumoral bleeding can also produce subacute neurologic signs that develop over a period of days to weeks, and may even be asymptomatic with hemorrhage discovered on radiographic studies.[1,5,11,13,24,36–38] The proportion of patients who present with acute, subacute, or clinically silent intratumoral hemorrhage varies among different series and depends upon the means of diagnosing intratumoral hematoma used in each study. Older, autopsy-based series will be skewed towards large hemorrhages which produced rapid symptoms and death, whereas a CT/MR scan-based study will detect small and asymptomatic hemorrhages.

Stroke-like presentation, including lateralizing signs and abrupt change in level of alertness, occurs in 24% to 67% of patients,[11,13,22,24,38] and 25% to 54% of all patients present in coma.[7,13,39] Progressive development of neurologic signs over a period of several days occurs in 33% to 62% of patients. Most series do not report asymptomatic patients, but Wakai et al[11] reported that 42% of their patients with neoplastic hemorrhage had no symptoms suggestive of sudden bleeding and were considered asymptomatic. Presumably these patients had neurologic symptoms which brought them to medical attention, but they were not defined.[11]

In patients with an abrupt onset, there may be clinical clues which suggest an underlying mass lesion prior to the acute bleeding episode. A history of segmental signs or headache antedating the acute ictus should suggest the presence of a pre-existing structural lesion which requires further investigation. In Little et al's series, 8 of 13 (62%) patients had pre-existing neurologic symptoms and signs referable to an intracranial mass before the onset of hemorrhage, but no patient in Weisberg's series had symptoms prior to hemorrhage.[7,24,38] In our experience at Memorial Sloan-Kettering Cancer Center, most patients with an acute intratumoral hemorrhage have neurologic symptoms prior to bleeding, but they are often mild, and careful questioning of family members may be required to elicit them.

Pituitary apoplexy is a specific clinical syndrome which is often, but not always, due to hemorrhage into a pituitary adenoma. Pituitary apoplexy is characterized by sudden headache, visual impairment, and ophthalmoplegia often accompanied by vomiting and meningeal signs. Clinically it may be confused with aneurysmal rupture and SAH.[20,21] Diagnosis requires the identification of hemorrhage into a seller mass, but not all patients with a hemorrhagic pituitary mass have the apoplectic syndrome, and "apoplexy" is reserved for those with clinical symptoms.[40]

Diagnosis

The diagnosis of ICH, spontaneous or tumor related, is made by CT or MR scan. In the patient who presents with the rapid development of lateralizing signs and diminished level of alertness, a CT or MR scan should be obtained promptly. Like intracerebral hematoma from any cause, intratumoral hemorrhage appears as a hyperdense lesion on precontrast CT scan.[23,24,38] Hemorrhage has a variable appearance on MR images depending upon the time interval between the onset of hemorrhage and the scan. Hemorrhage is usually hyperintense on T_1 and T_2 weighted MR images, but may be hypointense on either sequence depending upon its evolutionary stage.[41] Furthermore, mixed signal intensity can be seen, particularly in tumor-related hemorrhage, and hemorrhagic tumors appear to progress from one MR stage to the next more slowly than spontaneous intracerebral hematomas, presumably because of continued low-grade bleeding within the neoplasm. The MR characteristics of cerebral hemorrhage are discussed in detail in Chapter 12, and apply to intratumoral as well as spontaneous ICH.

There are, however, unique radiographic features which suggest an underlying tumor as opposed to a spontaneous hematoma. In general, tumors, particularly malignant neoplasms, enhance after the administration of IV contrast for CT scan or gadolinium for magnetic resonance imaging (MRI). This enhancement may still be seen after intratumoral hemorrhage (Figure 3).[23,24,38] In Weisberg's patients with primary or metastatic cerebral neoplasms that bled, all had significant enhancement on the postcontrast CT scan.[24,38] While a large hemorrhage may destroy the underlying tumor and temporarily obliterate any enhancement, this is unusual. Intracerebral hemorrhage may itself lead to enhancement, but this occurs after several days to weeks, and is not present on the initial scan where enhancement is often prominent in tumor-associated hemorrhage.[42] Therefore, after an abrupt ictus due to an ICH, the demonstration of significant contrast enhancement on an initial CT or MR scan should strongly suggest the presence of an underlying tumor. Other lesions besides tumors which cause cerebral hemorrhage, such as an AVM, may enhance after contrast administration, but the pattern of enhancement often permits a specific diagnosis. Enhancement of an AVM typically demonstrates the serpiginous vessels of the lesion itself, whereas neoplastic enhancement is usually nodular, diffuse, or ring enhancing throughout the tissue adjacent to the hemorrhage and does not have vascular characteristics.

In addition to enhancement, the presence of significant or widespread edema on an acute scan after intracranial hemorrhage also suggests the presence of an underlying neoplasm, since edema from hemorrhage does not occur acutely. Location of the hematoma may also suggest neoplasm, since tumors tend to occur in different regions of the brain than the typical locations of traumatic or hypertensive hemorrhage.[23,38] Primary brain tumors are usually located in the hemispheric white matter, and metastases tend to occur at the gray-white junction. Tumor-related hemorrhages would predominate in these locations, unlike the deep basal ganglia location of hypertensive hemorrhages or frontal and temporal polar regions for traumatic hemorrhages (Table 3).

Table 3
Features Suggesting Tumor in Patients with Intracerebral Hemorrhage (ICH)

A. *Clinical*
    1. History of neurologic symptoms prior to bleeding episode
B. *Radiographic*
    1. Mixed MR signal intensity within an ICH
    2. Contrast enhancement on CT/MR scan after an acute ICH
    3. Significant edema around an acute ICH
    4. Tumor-related ICH is located in hemispheric white matter

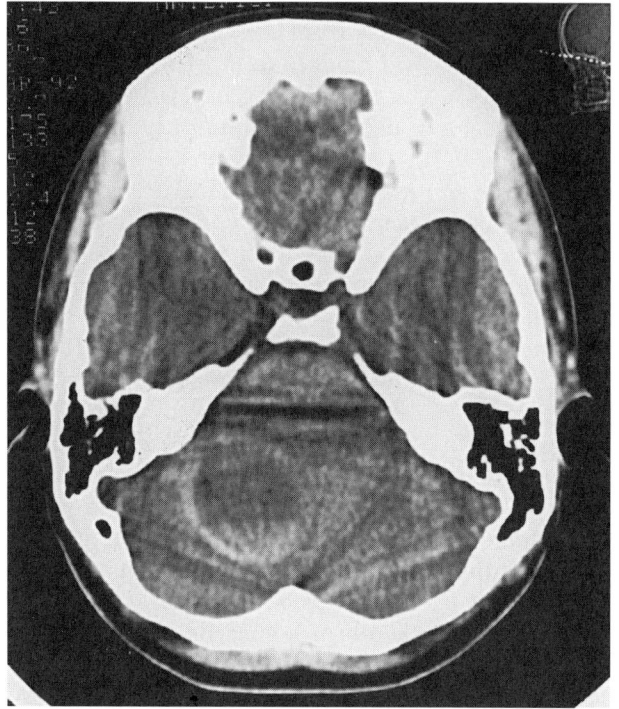

Figure 3A

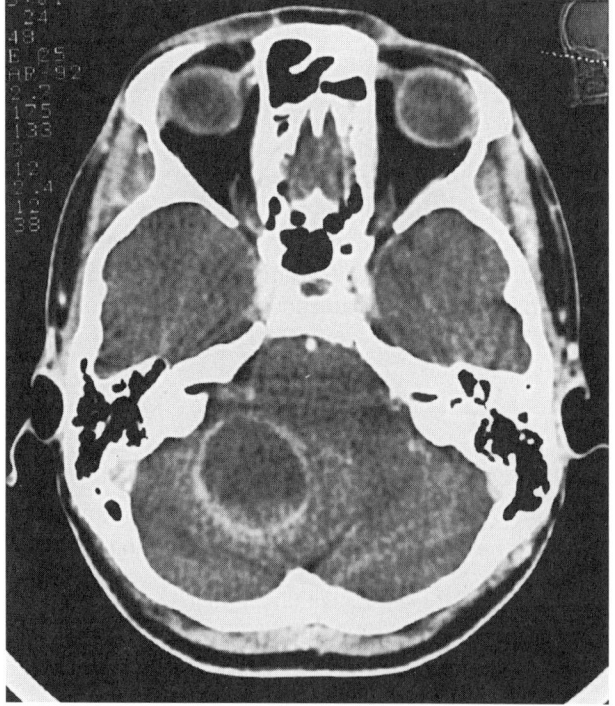

Figure 3B

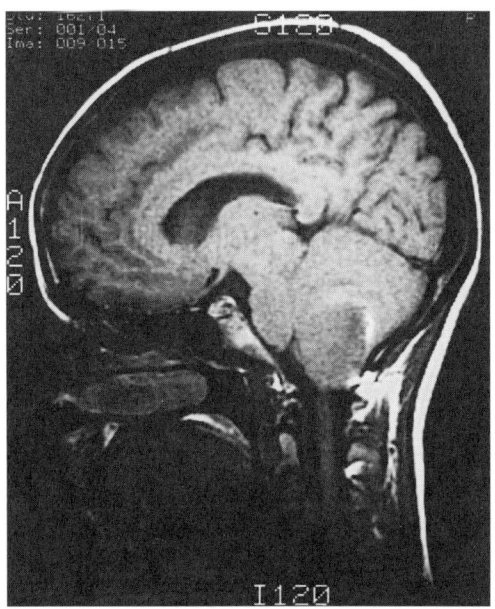

Figure 3C

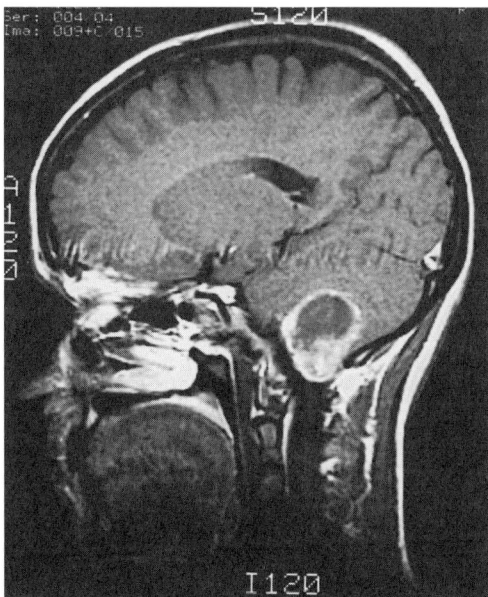

Figure 3D

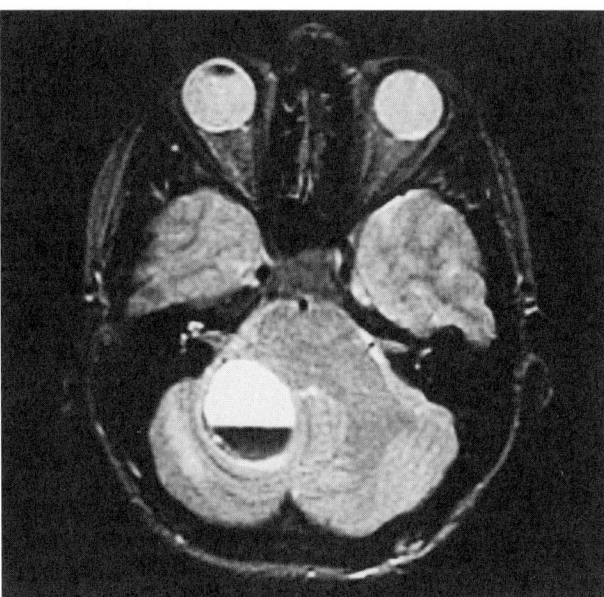

Figure 3E

Figure 3: Simultaneous CT and MR scans on a patient with a hemorrhagic oligodendroglioma. Pre- **(A)** and postcontrast **(B)** CT scans demonstrating a hyperdense lesion which enhances around the periphery; a hematocrit level is apparent on both images. Pre-**(C)** and postgadolinium **(D)** MR images of the same patient. Less hyperintensity is appreciated on the pregadolinium MR scan than on the precontrast CT, but more prominent enhancement is apparent after gadolinium. The T_2 weighted image **(E)** demonstrates that the lesion is hyperintense except for the hematocrit level which is hypointense.

Treatment

The treatment for neoplastic hemorrhage is primarily directed against the underlying tumor and includes symptomatic and definitive therapies. Symptomatic management includes the use of corticosteroids and anticonvulsants. Corticosteroids are very helpful in the management of peritumoral edema, and can produce rapid clinical improvement in patients with both primary and secondary neoplasms.[43] While steroids have no established efficacy in patients with spontaneous supratentorial hemorrhage, patients with neoplastic hemorrhage will benefit from corticosteroids since there is often established vasogenic edema from the underlying tumor.[44] Treatment of edema is important since it will reduce the total mass produced by tumor, hematoma, and edema, and permit the institution of definitive surgical and medical therapy.

Anticonvulsants are used for patients who present with seizures as a manifestation of their tumor. Acute hemorrhage can cause seizures, and may be the explanation for the high incidence of seizures (50%) in patients with brain metastases from melanoma.[45] Although no prospective study has been performed, retrospective data have failed to establish efficacy of prophylactic anticonvulsants in patients with brain tumors, even in those with melanomatous cerebral metastases.[46,47] In addition, anticonvulsants have a high incidence of side effects. Therefore, we do not routinely use prophylactic anticonvulsants for patients with cerebral neoplasms. There are, however, situations in which patients may benefit from prophylactic medication. Patients with large intratumoral hematomas associated with significant mass effect may benefit from a short course of anticonvulsants until definitive therapy can be undertaken to remove or reduce the hemorrhage and tumor. This might prevent clinical deterioration caused by the increase in intracranial pressure associated with a generalized seizure in a patient who is already markedly compromised. Once definitive therapy is undertaken, the prophylactic anticonvulsants can be discontinued.

Definitive treatment includes surgery, cranial irradiation, and chemotherapy. Complete resection is the goal for most primary brain tumors, and the presence of a large hemorrhage will often mandate urgent surgery if significant mass effect is caused by the combined volume of tumor and blood.[48] When intratumoral hemorrhage is the presentation of a neoplasm, surgery is often necessary for diagnosis, even if a complete resection cannot be achieved. Surgery usually results in clinical improvement, and in emergent situations will get the patient out of immediate danger. The clinical stability achieved with surgery permits the patient to receive further treatment with radiotherapy and chemotherapy which are usually effective, but neither produces immediate amelioration of symptoms.

Patients with hemorrhagic brain metastases may also benefit from surgery, even if there is more than one lesion. Single brain metastases should be resected whether they are hemorrhagic or not.[49] Patients with multiple brain metastases who have a single large hemorrhagic lesion, or a hemorrhagic mass in a critical location, or a hemorrhagic tumor which is responsible for disabling clinical symptoms may all benefit from extirpation of that hemorrhagic tumor. This approach is applicable to patients with brain metastases from any primary source. However, many of the tumors which commonly cause hemorrhagic brain metastases respond poorly to medical treatment. Melanoma and renal carcinoma are relatively radio- and chemoresistant neoplasms, and patients with these tumors should always be considered for surgical therapy, including the resection of multiple lesions (two or, rarely, three metastases), since radiotherapy is not likely to produce a meaningful or durable response.

Cranial irradiation is the mainstay of nonsurgical treatment for patients with primary and metastatic brain tumors. Regardless of whether the tumor presented with intracranial hemorrhage, the appropriate course of cranial radiotherapy for that particular neoplasm should be administered. Radiation may be postoperative in the case of all primary brain tumors and those metastases which are resected, or it may be the primary treatment for patients with multiple brain metastases or tumor in a critical area (ie, brainstem) that cannot be approached surgically. Although some authors have suggested that radiotherapy predisposes to neoplastic hemorrhage, there are no data to support this supposition, and cranial irradiation should not be delayed in patients with hemorrhagic tumors.

Stereotactic radiosurgery or brachytherapy with I^{125} implants has been used for patients with recurrent malignant gliomas and with metastatic brain tumors.[50-52] Either of these techniques can be used in a patient with a prior history of tumor-related hemorrhage. In the presence of a large hematoma, tumor margins may be difficult to define for radiosurgery, and brachytherapy would be contraindicated until the blood resolves. However, small hematomas would not prevent stereotactic radiosurgery. Both of these radiotherapy techniques deliver high doses of irradiation to circumscribed regions of tumor, sparing the surrounding normal brain. They are particularly useful for treatment of relatively radioresistant lesions such as melanoma metastases, which respond to doses of radiation that are dangerous when delivered by external beam therapy.

Chemotherapy is based upon the pathology of the underlying neoplasm, and its use is not restricted by the presence of an intratumoral hemorrhage. Chemotherapy is used in the adjuvant setting for patients with oligodendrogliomas and malignant gliomas, but not for patients with astrocytomas or meningiomas.[53,54] Brain metastases are not usually treated with chemotherapy, but particular types of metastatic lesions are uniquely chemosensitive. These include breast and small cell lung cancer, neither of which commonly cause cerebral hemorrhage. Choriocarcinoma, however, has a high incidence of ICH and is exquisitely sensitive to systemic chemotherapy.[55]

Prognosis

The prognosis of a hemorrhagic neoplasm is primarily determined by the prognosis of the underlying malignancy. Subacute or radiographic hemorrhage which does not significantly affect the patient's clinical status does not change the expected prognosis from that of an identical nonhemorrhagic tumor. Hemorrhage affects prognosis when the patient suffers an acute neurologic deterioration as a consequence of bleeding into the tumor. In all series, patients who present in coma or with acute, severe neurologic signs have a poor prognosis, typically surviving only days to weeks after the acute event.[2,7,11,13,16,20–22,37] In these patients, short survival occurs even with vigorous therapy, including early surgical extirpation, presumably as a consequence of the neurologic damage caused by herniation due to the rapid rise in intracranial pressure from the hematoma. Even the occasional patient who recovers from an acute ictus often succumbs within several months.[13]

Despite the poor prognosis of many patients with intratumoral hemorrhage, the widespread use of CT and MR scanning has demonstrated the broad clinical spectrum of neoplastic hemorrhage, and many patients will enjoy prolonged survival with appropriate surgical and medical therapy. The presence of an hemorrhage within an intracranial neoplasm should not, in and of itself, alter the therapeutic approach to a minimally or moderately symptomatic patient, and will not significantly affect prognosis.

References

1. Kondziolka D, Bernstein M, Resch L, et al: Significance of hemorrhage into brain tumors: clinicopathological study. *J Neurosurg* 1987;67:852.
2. Graus F, Rogers LR, Posner JB: Cerebrovascular complications in patients with cancer. *Medicine* 1985;64:16.
3. Mutlu N, Berry RG, Alpers BJ: Massive cerebral hemorrhage: clinical and pathological correlations. *Arch Neurol* 1963;8:644.
4. Luessenhop AJ, Shevlin WA, Ferrero AA, et al: Surgical management of primary intracerebral hemorrhage. *J Neurosurg* 1967;27:419.
5. Bitoh S, Hasegawa H, Ohtsuki H, et al: Cerebral neoplasms initially presenting with massive intracerebral hemorrhage. *Surg Neurol* 1984;22:57.
6. Wakai S, Kumakura N, Nagai M: Lobar intracerebral hemorrhage: a clinical, radiographic, and pathological study of 29 consecutive operated cases with negative angiography. *J Neurosurg* 1992;76:231.
7. Little JR, Dial B, Belanger G, et al: Brain hemorrhage from intracranial tumor. *Stroke* 1979;10:283.
8. McCormick WF, Rosenfield DB: Massive brain hemorrhage: a review of 144 cases and an examination of their causes. *Stroke* 1973;4:946.
9. Locksley HB, Sahs AL, Sandler R: Report of the cooperative study of intracranial aneurysms and subarachnoid hemorrhage. *J Neurosurg* 1966;24:1034.
10. Minette SE, Kimmel DW: Subdural hematoma in patients with systemic cancer. *Mayo Clin Proc* 1989;64:637.
11. Wakai S, Yamakawa K, Manaka S, et al: Spontaneous intracranial hemor-

rhage caused by brain tumor: its incidence and clinical significance. *Neurosurgery* 1982;10:437.

12. Oldberg E: Hemorrhage into gliomas: a review of eight hundred and thirty-two consecutive verified cases of glioma. *Arch Neurol Psychiat* 1933;30:1061.

13. Scott M: Spontaneous intracerebral hematoma caused by cerebral neoplasms: report of eight verified cases. *J Neurosurg* 1975;42:338.

14. Drake CG, McGee D: Apoplexy associated with brain tumours. *Can Med Assoc J* 1961;84:303.

15. Manganiello LOJ: Massive spontaneous hemorrhage in gliomas: a report of seven verified cases. *J Nerv Ment Dis* 1949;110:277.

16. Globus JH, Sapirstein M: Massive hemorrhage into brain tumor: its significance and probable relationship to rapidly fatal termination and antecedent trauma. *JAMA* 1942;120:348.

17. Modesti LM, Binet EF, Collins GH: Meningiomas causing spontaneous intracranial hematomas. *J Neurosurg* 1976;45:437.

18. Nakao S, Sato S, Ban S, et al: Massive intracerebral hemorrhage caused by angioblastic meningioma. *Surg Neurol* 1977;7:245.

19. Goran A, Ciminello VJ, Fisher RG: Hemorrhage into meningiomas. *Arch Neurol* 1965;13:65.

20. Cardoso ER, Peterson EW: Pituitary apoplexy: a review. *Neurosurgery* 1984;14:363.

21. Wakai S, Fukushima T, Teramoto A, et al: Pituitary apoplexy: its incidence and clinical significance. *J Neurosurg* 1981;55:187.

22. Mandybur TI: Intracranial hemorrhage caused by metastatic tumors. *Neurology* 1977;27:650.

23. Gildersleeve N Jr, Koo AH, McDonald CJ: Metastatic tumor presenting as intracerebral hemorrhage: report of 6 cases examined by computed tomography. *Radiology* 1977;124:109.

24. Weisberg LA: Hemorrhagic metastatic intracranial neoplasms: clinical-computed tomographic correlations. *Comput Radiol* 1985;9:105.

25. Delattre JY, Krol G, Thaler HT, et al: Distribution of brain metastases. *Arch Neurol* 1988;45:741.

26. Ruff RL, Posner JB: Incidence and treatment of peripheral venous thrombosis in patients with glioma. *Ann Neurol* 1983;13:334.

27. Choucair AK, Silver P, Levin VA: Risk of intracranial hemorrhage in glioma patients receiving anticoagulant therapy for venous thromboembolism. *J Neurosurg* 1987;66:357.

28. Hirano A, Matsui T: Vascular structures in brain tumors. *Human Pathol* 1975;6:611.

29. Weller RO, Foy M, Cox S: The development and ultrastructure of the microvasculature in malignant gliomas. *Neuropathol Appl Neurobiol* 1977;3:307.

30. Liwnicz BH, Wu SZ, Tew JM Jr: The relationship between the capillary structure and hemorrhage in gliomas. *J Neurosurg* 1987;66:536.

31. Leeds NE, Rosenblatt R: Arterial wall irregularities in intracranial neoplasms. *Radiology* 1972;103:121.

32. Cowen RL, Siqueira EB, George E: Angiographic demonstration of a glioma involving the wall of the anterior cerebral artery. *Radiology* 1970;97:577.
33. New PFJ, Price DL, Carter B: Cerebral angiography in cardiac myxoma. *Radiology* 1970;96:335.
34. Seigle JM, Caputy AJ, Manz HJ, et al: Multiple oncotic intracranial aneurysms and cardiac metastasis from choriocarcinoma: case report and review of the literature. *Neurosurgery* 1987;20:39.
35. Ho K-L: Neoplastic aneurysm and intracranial hemorrhage. *Cancer* 1982; 50:2935.
36. Barker CS: Peripheral cerebral aneurysm associated with a glioma. *Neuroradiology* 1992;34:30.
37. Richardson RR, Siqueira EB, Cerullo LJ: Malignant glioma: its initial presentation as intracranial hemorrhage. *Acta Neurochirurgica* 1979;46:77.
38. Weisberg LA: Hemorrhagic primary intracranial neoplasms: clinical-computed tomographic correlations. *Comput Radiol* 1986;10:131.
39. Shuangshoti S, Panyathanya R, Wichienkur P: Intracranial metastases from unsuspected choriocarcinoma. *Neurology* 1974;24:649.
40. Glick RP, Tiesi JA: Subacute pituitary apoplexy: clinical and magnetic resonance imaging characteristics. *Neurosurgery* 1990;27:214.
41. Destian S, Sze G, Krol G, et al: MR imaging of hemorrhagic intracranial neoplasms. *Am J Roentgenol* 1989;152:137.
42. Wakai S, Andoh Y, Ochiai C, et al: Postoperative contrast enhancement in brain tumors and intracerebral hematomas: CT study. *J Comput Assist Tomogr* 1990;14:267.
43. Weinstein JD, Toy FJ, Jaffe ME, et al: The effect of dexamethasone on brain edema in patients with metastatic brain tumors. *Neurology* 1972;23: 121.
44. Poungvarin N, Bhoopat W, Viriyavejakui A, et al: Effects of dexamethasone in primary supratentorial intracerebral hemorrhage. *N Engl J Med* 1987; 316:1229.
45. Byrne TN, Cascino TL, Posner JB: Brain metastasis from melanoma. *J Neuro-Oncol* 1983;1:313.
46. Cohen N, Strauss G, Lew R, et al: Should prophylactic anticonvulsants be administered to patients with newly-diagnosed cerebral metastases? A retrospective analysis. *J Clin Oncol* 1988;6:1621.
47. Hagen NA, Cirrincione C, Thaler HT, et al: The role of whole brain radiotherapy following resection of cerebral metastasis from melanoma. *Neurology* 1990;40:158.
48. Wood JR, Green SB, Shapiro WR: The prognostic importance of tumor size in malignant gliomas: a computed tomographic scan study by the brain tumor cooperative group. *J Clin Oncol* 1988;6:338.
49. Patchell RA, Tibbs PA, Walsh JW, et al: A randomized trial of surgery in the treatment of single metastases to the brain. *N Engl J Med* 1990;322: 494.
50. Prados M, Leibel S, Barnett CM, et al: Interstitial brachytherapy for metastatic brain tumors. *Cancer* 1989;63:657.

51. Adler JR, Cox RS, Kaplan I, et al: Stereotactic radiosurgical treatment of brain metastases. *J Neurosurg* 1992;76:4444.

52. Gutin PH, Leibel SA, Wara WM, et al: Recurrent malignant gliomas: survival following interstitial brachytherapy with high-activity iodine-125 sources. *J Neurosurg* 1987;67:865.

53. Shapiro WR, Green SB, Burger PC, et al: Randomized trial of three chemotherapy regimes and two radiotherapy regimens in postoperative treatment of malignant glioma. *J Neurosurg* 1989;71:1.

54. Glass J, Hochberg FH, Gruber ML, et al: The treatment of oligodendrogliomas and mixed oligodendroglioma-astrocytomas with PCV chemotherapy. *J Neurosurg* 1992;76:741.

55. Weed JC, Hunter VJ: Diagnosis and management of brain metastasis from gestational trophoblastic disease. *Oncology* 1991;5:48.

Chapter 8

Vascular Malformations and Aneurysms

Barney J. Stern, MD, Agha Khan, MD

Vascular Malformations

Vascular malformations include arteriovenous malformations (AVMs), cavernous malformations, venous malformations, and capillary telangiectases.[1] Bleeding from a vascular malformation typically produces an intraparenchymal hemorrhage, at times with intraventricular extension,[2] and only in a small minority of patients does it cause a primary subarachnoid hemorrhage (SAH) (Table 1).[3] Patients suffering an intraparenchymal hemorrhage from a vascular malformation constitute approximately 6% of all patients with an intracerebral hemorrhage (ICH) and tend to be younger than individuals having an aneurysmal intraparenchymal hemorrhage.[4]

Arteriovenous Malformations

Arteriovenous malformations are the result of abnormal fetal development at approximately 3 weeks gestation.[1] The malformation is characterized by direct artery to vein communication without an intervening capillary bed.[1] The blood vessel walls contain elastin and smooth muscle cells. Brain parenchyma within an AVM is usually gliotic and nonfunctional.[1] Over 90% of AVMs are in the cerebral hemispheres. Approximately 18% are deep, and the remainder are lobar.[1] Most AVMs are sporadic, but familial AVMs occur and appear to have an autosomal dominant inheritance with incomplete penetrance.[5,6]

The annual risk of initial bleeding from an AVM is 1% to 4%.[7] Hemorrhage is the presenting feature of AVMs in approximately one half of patients, and almost two thirds of bleeds are intracerebral.[7] There is no constant relation

From Feldmann E (ed). *Intracerebral Hemorrhage*. Armonk, NY: Futura Publishing Company, Inc., © 1994.

Table 1
Clues To Suspecting a Vascular Malformation as a Cause of Intracerebral Hemorrhage

History of seizures, especially partial seizures
History of neurologic symptoms referable to a mass—chronic or subacute progressive or fluctuating course
No history of hypertension
Lobar hematoma in young, normotensive person
Pregnancy or postpartum period
Cocaine use
Family history of hemorrhagic stroke or known vascular malformation
Cranial bruit
Ocular vascular malformation
Skin vascular malformation
Calcification proximate to an intracerebral hematoma
CT scan enhancement of a lesion proximate to an intracerebral hematoma
Unexpected area of decreased CT scan density proximate to or within an acute hematoma
Indentation of otherwise smooth rim of an acute hematoma on imaging study

between the patient's level of activity and risk of hemorrhage and no characteristic clinical presentation to set apart bleeding from an AVM from other causes of intraparenchymal hemorrhage.[7] Seizures, headache, an audible bruit, progressive focal neurologic deficits, and cognitive decline can also occur.[1,7] Approximately one third of patients develop seizures before hemorrhage.[8] Intracranial hypertension is a rare complication of AVMs and may be due to increased superior sagittal sinus and cortical venous pressures.[9] Patients with posterior fossa vascular malformations can present with hemorrhage or fluctuating or progressive ataxia, weakness, and cranial nerve problems. Presenting symptoms referrable to isolated cranial nerve dysfunction, such as dizziness, are atypical.[10] The mechanisms for this varied symptomatology include unsuspected hemorrhage, mass effect, and hydrocephalus.[10]

Arteriovenous malformations typically present in the third and fourth decades,[11,12] though infants and children can be symptomatic.[13] As expected, most (71%) AVM-associated hemorrhages in patients aged 15 to 45 years are lobar, although basal ganglion, thalamic, posterior fossa, and intraventricular bleeding also occur.[14] An AVM should be suspected as the source of hemorrhage in patients less than 40 years of age who have a lobar hematoma, especially if they are normotensive and have no coagulopathy.[4] As with all ICH, the presenting features relate to its location and size.

Diagnosis of an ICH by CT scan requires a hyperdense, usually globular lesion within the brain. There can be coexistent subarachnoid and intraventricular bleeding. Mass effect can be considerable, but early in the clinical course there is little surrounding edema. Clues to the coexistence of an AVM include the presence of a comparatively large area of decreased density around the hematoma, heterogeneous densities within the hematoma, intraparenchymal calcifications, serpiginous vessels appearing with the infusion of a contrast agent, and a lobar location in a young, normotensive individual (Figure 1).

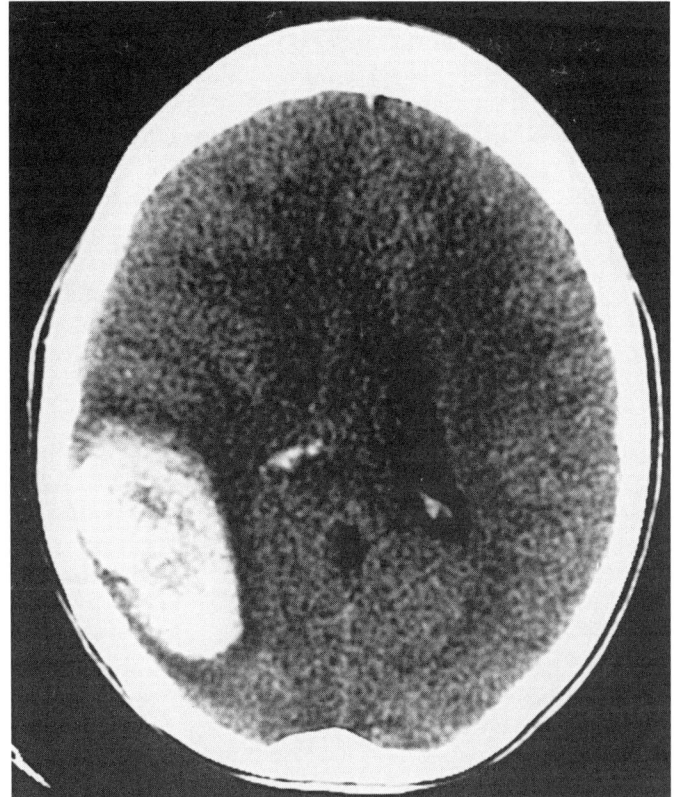

Figure 1A

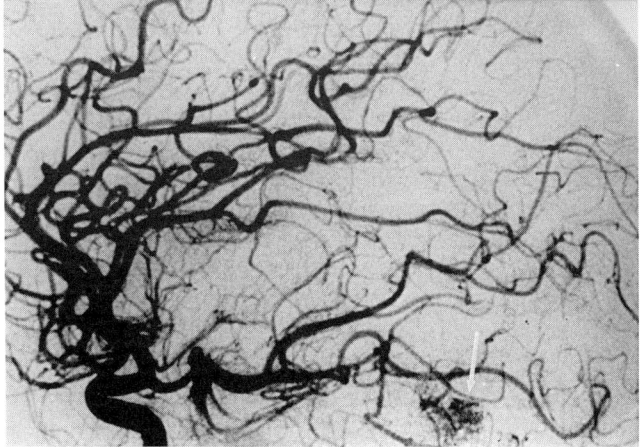

Figure 1B

Figure 1: (A) CT scan showing a parietal hematoma. Note the region of heterogenous density in hematoma. **(B)** Angiogram reveals a small arteriovenous malformation (arrow).

Magnetic resonance imaging (MRI) does not demonstrate acute hemorrhage as well as computed tomography (CT) scan,[15] as hematomas appear as isointense or hypointense masses on T_1 weighted images because of intracellular deoxyhemoglobin. Clues to the presence of an AVM include a hypointense rim surrounding a hyperintense hematoma on T_2 weighted images, suggesting a prior bleed, and areas of intraparenchymal linear or serpiginous flow-void, suggesting intravascular moving blood, in the vicinity of a hematoma. Calcifications within an AVM are not easily detected by MRI.

Angiography is the definitive diagnostic procedure for an AVM (Figure 1). Malformations less than or equal to 3 cm in diameter are more likely to bleed than larger AVMs,[16] perhaps because blood pressure in feeding arteries of small AVMs more closely approximates mean arterial pressure (91% of mean arterial pressure) than in larger AVMs (47% to 67%), thereby increasing perfusion pressure in small AVMs.[16] Hemorrhage from an AVM is also more likely if there is a central draining vein, an intranidal aneurysm, or a periventricular or intraventricular location of the AVM.[17] Other risk factors for hemorrhage include only a single draining vein, obstructed venous drainage, and isolated deep venous drainage.[18] Angiomatous change, meaning "multiple dilated cortical vessels that feed the AVM with collateral supply from arteries that do not directly supply the AVM nidus," is negatively predictive of bleeding.[17] Fifteen percent of patients with nontraumatic lobar hematomas referred for angiography at a tertiary referral hospital were found to have an AVM with angiography.[19] Normotensive patients aged 15 to 45 years with a lobar hemorrhage are particularly likely to have an AVM.[20]

Early angiography is indicated in young, normotensive individuals with a lobar hematoma. If early angiography does not reveal the source of the lobar hematoma, MRI and angiography should be performed after the mass effect of the hematoma has resolved. A false-negative study may have been caused by spontaneous, transient thrombosis of the AVM or compression of the abnormal vessels by the hematoma.[11]

Approximately 10% of patients die from an AVM hemorrhage.[12,21] The risk of rebleeding in the first year after the presenting hemorrhage is 6%. Thereafter, the annual risk of hemorrhage is 2% to 3%.[12] Patients with a coexisting AVM and aneurysm have a 7% per year risk of hemorrhage.[22]

Emergent surgical management of an AVM-associated hemorrhage is occasionally indicated. If the clinical status allows, angiography should be performed prior to surgery. If a small AVM and hematoma are in a critical life-threatening area, both can be resected during a single procedure. If the hemorrhage and AVM are large and the clinical status is tenuous, the hematoma can be decompressed and the AVM left untouched pending stabilization of the patient. If angiography was not performed prior to emergent surgery, and an AVM is found, postoperative angiography should be performed to fully define the AVM, even if a small AVM was thought to be completely resected at the time of surgery.

The elective treatment of AVMs, especially those that have bled, incorporates a multimodality approach including interventional neuroradiologic techniques (embolization), stereotactic radiotherapy, and surgery.[23] Interventional neuroradiology can obliterate an AVM or decrease its size so as to make surgery easier or permit stereotactic radiosurgery. Patients with surgically inaccessible AVMs can be treated with a combination of interventional neuroradiologic techniques or stereotactic radiotherapy. Occasionally, stereotactic radiotherapy alone can obliterate an AVM and, needless to say, surgery itself can constitute monotherapy for an AVM. Overall, multimodality therapy can obliterate an otherwise difficult to treat AVM, and thereby prevent future bleeding, in over 80% of patients.[23,24]

Cavernous Malformations

Cavernous malformations, which represent approximately 10% of vascular malformations, are made up of dilated, endothelium lined, fibrous channels. There is no smooth muscle or elastin in the vascular walls and no neural tissue between the vessels, except occasionally at the periphery of the lesion.[25] Thrombosis and calcification occur, and gliosis and hemosiderin often surround the malformation.[26,27] Most (80%) cavernous malformations occur in the hemispheres, though brainstem and intraventricular lesions are also found.[25,26] Malformations range in size from several millimeters to 4.5 cm in diameter.[25,26] The malformations can grow in size, perhaps due to "reendothelialization of hemorrhage cavities, growth of new blood vessels as part of the organization of the hematomas, and laying down of additional fibrous scar tissue."[28] Multiple malformations can occur in a single patient.[29] Cavernous malformations are evident in approximately 0.5% of consecutive MRI scans performed at a tertiary referral center.[25]

Cavernous malformations can present with autosomal dominant inheritance, with penetrance approaching 100%.[27,30] Lesions are also found in the retina and skin.[30] Hispanic patients may be at particular risk for the familial disorder.[27] Therefore, all patients with a family history of cavernous malformations should have a skin and ophthalmologic examination as well as a neuroimaging procedure (see below). Nearly 50% of patients with cavernous malformations have the familial form and are especially likely to have multiple lesions.[27]

Clinically apparent hemorrhage can occasionally arise from a cavernous malformation. Fortunately, most patients recover from a bleeding episode.[25,31] The estimated lifetime risk of clinical bleeding is 0.1% per person-year per lesion, or 0.25% per person-year.[31] Robinson et al, in a series of patients identified by the MRI presence of a malformation, report that 2 of 17 (11.8%) infratentorial malformations demonstrated hemorrhage by MRI, cerebrospinal fluid (CSF), or surgical criteria compared to 5 of 59 (8.4%) supratentorial lesions.[25] There is no apparent relationship between malformation size or age and the likelihood of hemorrhage, but females are more prone to hemorrhage.[25] Subclinical hemorrhage around the malformation is frequent, and the hemosiderin tends to enlarge over time.[25,31] A cavernous malformation can be seen in association with a venous malformation[25,29,32] and, if there has been hemorrhage, it is more likely that the cavernous malformation is the culprit (Figures 2 and 3).[32]

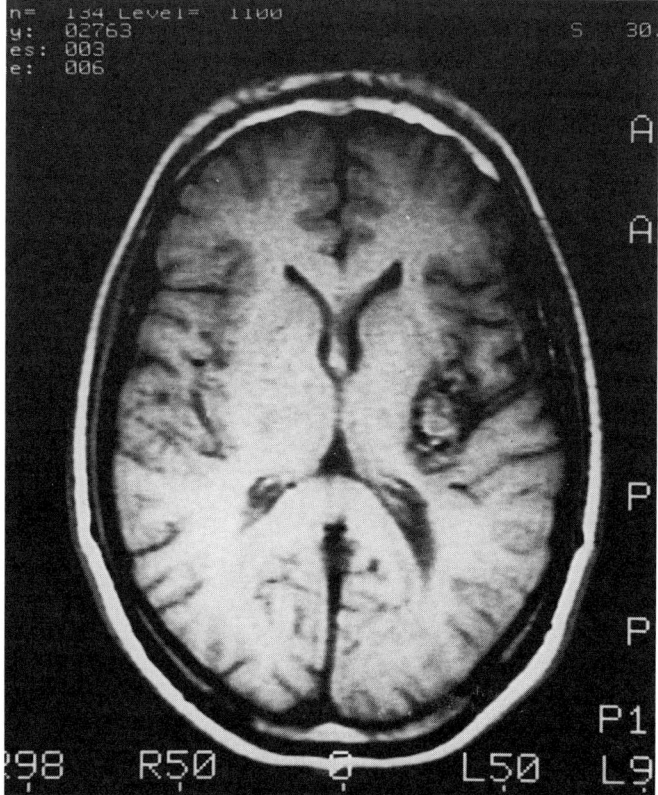

Figure 2A

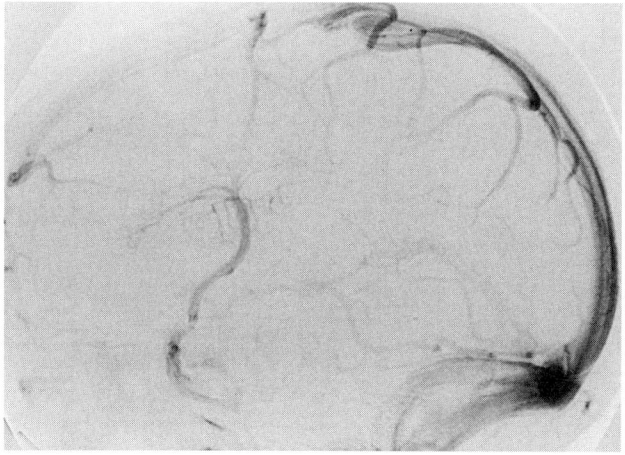

Figure 2B

Figure 2: **(A)** A T_1 weighted MRI demonstrating a cavernous malformation and an associated venous malformation. **(B)** An angiogram demonstrates the venous malformation but not the cavernous malformation. (Courtesy of Danielle Rigamonti, MD.)

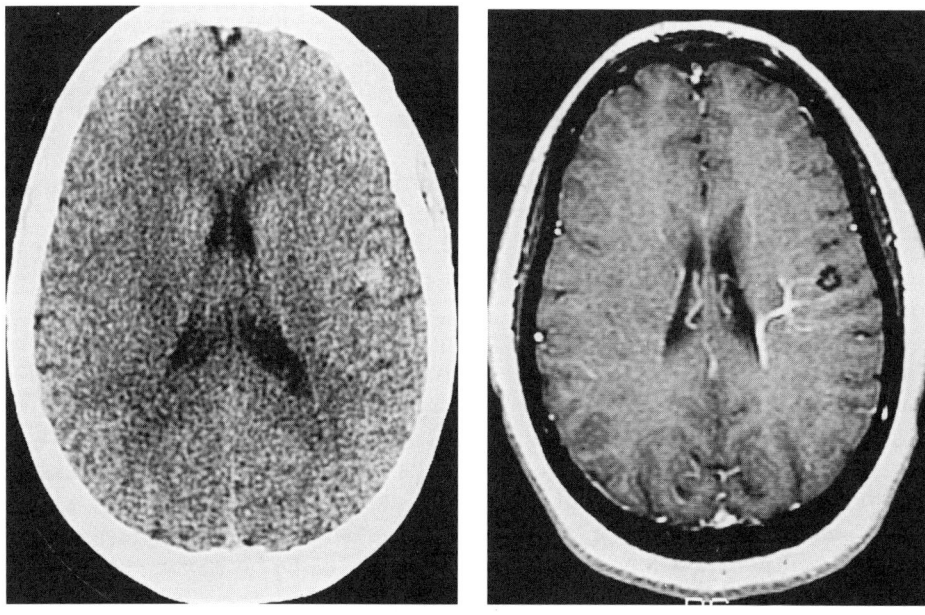

Figure 3A **Figure 3B**

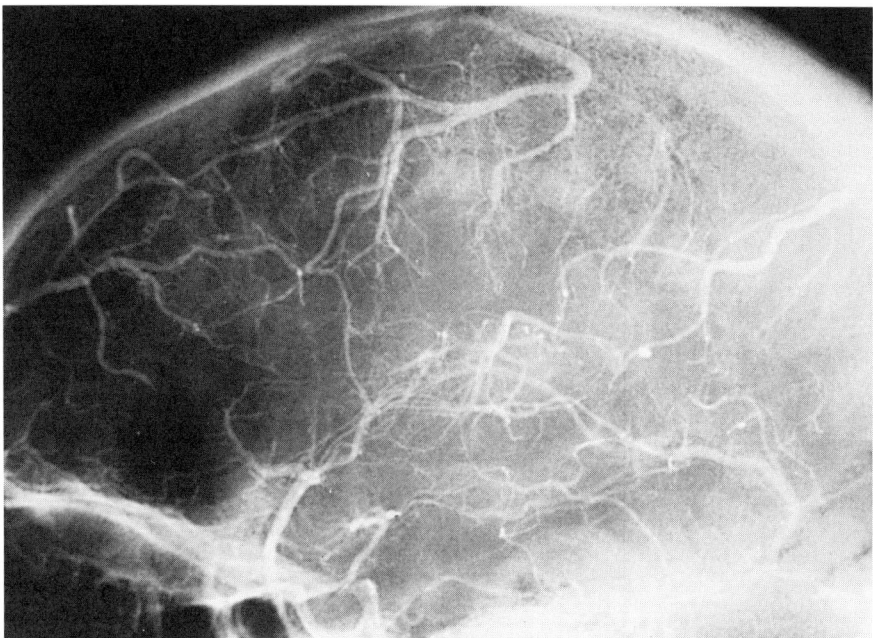

Figure 3C

Figure 3: **(A)** CT scan showing a small frontoparietal hematoma. **(B)** A contrast enhanced T_1 weighted MRI demonstrates a cavernous malformation and an associated venous malformation. **(C)** An angiogram demonstrates the venous malformation but not the cavernous malformation. (Courtesy of George Oyler, MD, PhD.)

Seizures can also be caused by a cavernous malformation.[26] Simple partial, complex partial, and generalized seizures occur[26] at a rate of 1.5% per person per year[31] and are most common with supratentorial lesions.[25] Symptoms related to the mass effect of the malformation can develop and are most likely to develop with infratentorial lesions.[25]

Computed tomography scans of cavernous malformations may demonstrate a calcified area within an enhancing lesion,[25,27,29] though in the setting of an intracerebral hematoma, calcification or enhancement can be hard to detect. In general, CT scans are not sensitive to the presence of a cavernous malformation.[27,31]

Magnetic resonance imaging is the imaging procedure of choice for visualizing cavernous malformations.[29] The malformation appears as a well-defined region with a central area of mixed signal intensity surrounded by a (black) rim of hypointensity on T_2 weighted images, representing hemosiderin.[27,29] With administration of contrast, the central area can enhance but no "feeding or draining" vessels are apparent.[31] Small malformations may appear only as "black dots" on T_2 weighted images.[27] Acute or subacute hemorrhage can be diagnosed if there is evidence of bleeding beyond the hemosiderin ring (Figure 4).[25]

Most angiographic studies do not detect a cavernous malformation. Angiographic findings include avascular mass effect, abnormal venous drainage, and a vascular blush (Figure 5).[26,27]

Surgery is appropriate therapy for malformations that have clinically bled and are accessible,[26,28,31] since rebleeding can occur at a "low," but as yet undefined rate.[25,28] However, since the risk of a fatal hemorrhage is low, some authors advocate surgery only after a recurrent bleed.[31] Stereotactic radiosurgery is of unproven value.[31] However, a stereotactic biopsy has been safely performed in a child.[28]

Venous Malformations

A venous malformation is composed entirely of veins, which are usually thickened and hyalinized and have minimal elastic tissue and smooth muscle.[33] The anomalous veins converge on a draining vein. Normal brain parenchyma is interspersed among the veins. The malformation seems to represent a congenitally anomalous venous drainage system.[34]

Venous malformations are the most common form of vascular malformation, accounting for 50% to 63% of malformations.[34] The association of a sublingual venous malformation with an ipsilateral cerebral venous malformation has been observed.[35]

The risk of hemorrhage from a venous malformation has been estimated at 0.22% per annum,[34] but only one patient in this series of 100 individuals with a venous malformation developed bleeding.[34] This finding is in contrast to other studies that demonstrate a substantially higher risk of hemorrhage,[36]

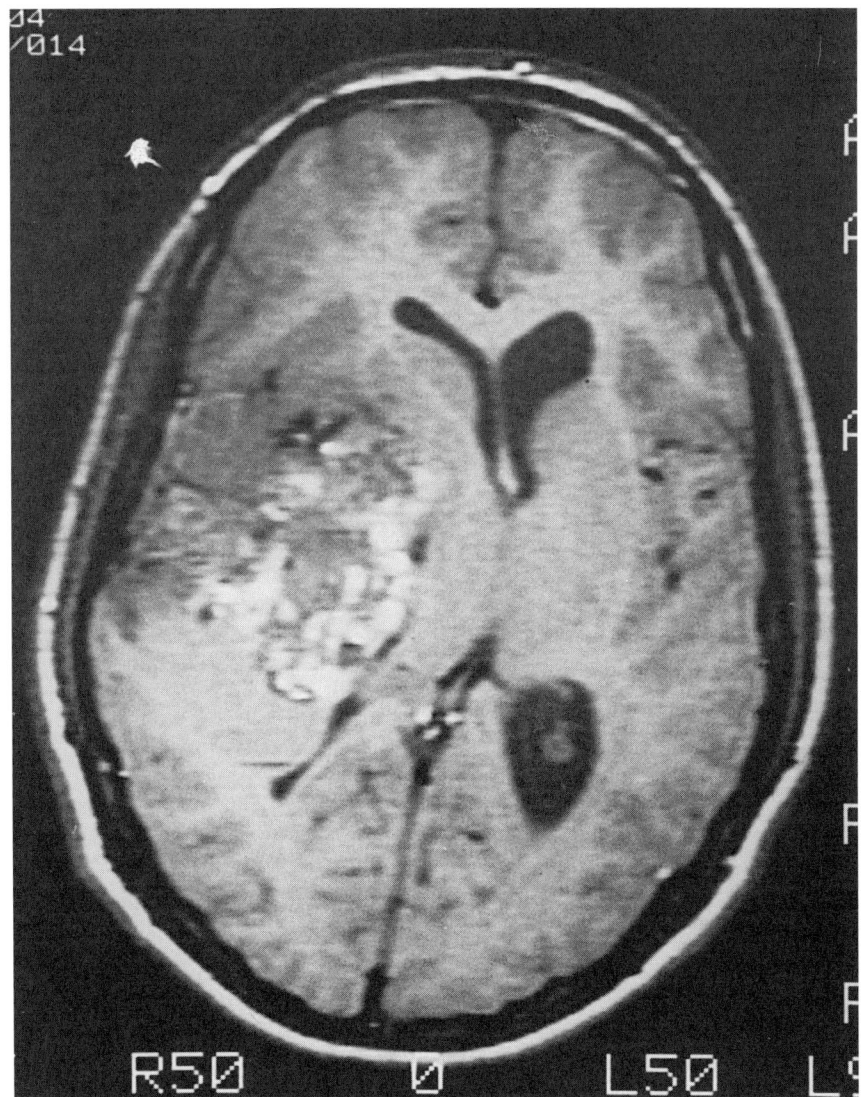

Figure 4: A T_1 weighted MRI demonstrates hemorrhage within a cavernous malformation. (Courtesy of Danielle Rigamonti, MD.)

but other reports have concentrated on a more select patient cohort.[34] Some patients can have recurrent hemorrhage.[36] Patients with a cerebellar venous malformation may be more prone to hemorrhage than patients with a supratentorial malformation.

Occasionally, seizures may also be associated with venous malformations, as can headaches and focal neurologic deficits.[34]

Venous malformations are usually not visible on an unenhanced CT scan,

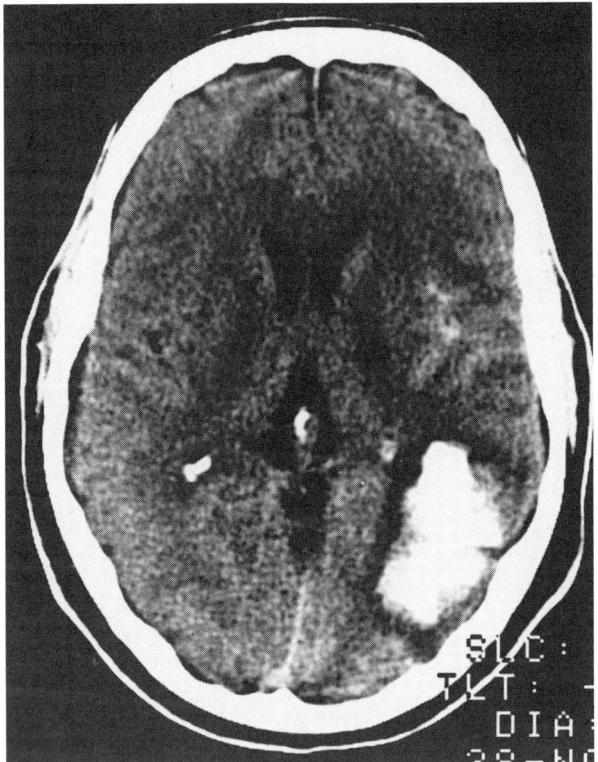

Figure 5A

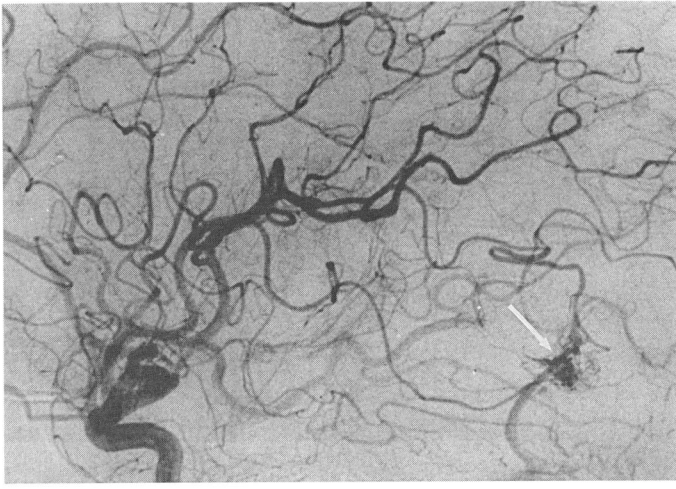

Figure 5B

Figure 5: **(A)** CT scan demonstrating a parietal hematoma in a 41-year-old man. **(B)** Angiogram revealed a vascular blush (arrow). At surgery a cavernous malformation was found. (Courtesy of Hyo Ahn, MD.)

though an area of increased density, representing the "caput medusae" is occasionally seen. With contrast enhancement, a venous malformation appears as a linear density, representing the draining vein, that merges with a dural sinus or the deep or superficial venous system. The "caput medusae" can appear as an enhancing density near the linear draining vein.[34] In the setting of an intracerebral hematoma, the malformation may become apparent with contrast administration.

Magnetic resonance imaging can reveal a venous malformation as a linear hypointense lesion on T_1 weighted images (Figure 6) that become hyperintense with contrast infusion (Figure 7). If the flow velocity is low, the linear draining vein can appear hyperintense. With enhancement, the anomalous veins may be seen emptying into the draining vein. On T_2 weighted images, a mixed hypo- and hyperintense lesion can be appreciated.[34]

The arterial phase of an angiogram is normal. In the venous phase, anomalous medullary veins converge on the "caput medusae" and empty into the central draining vein which, in turn, courses to a sinus or the deep or superficial venous system.

Given the generally benign nature of venous malformations, surgical resection is rarely indicated even if hemorrhage has occurred[37] because of the surgical risk. Since the anomalous vessels are part of the venous drainage of the brain, a hemorrhagic venous infarction can develop following resection of the

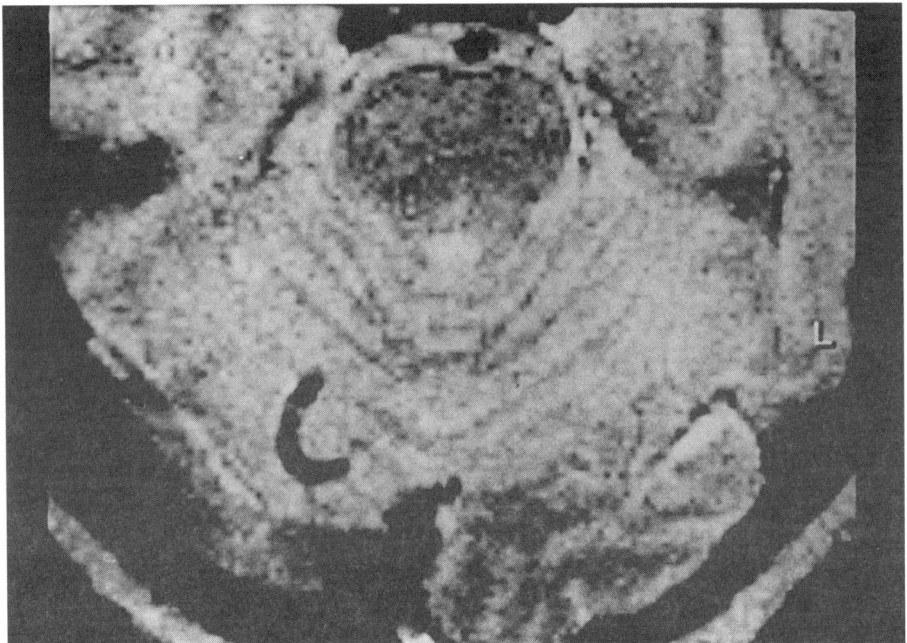

Figure 6: T_1 weighted MRI of cerebellar venous malformation. TR = 3.0 msec, TE = 80 msec. (Courtesy of Hyo Ahn, MD.)

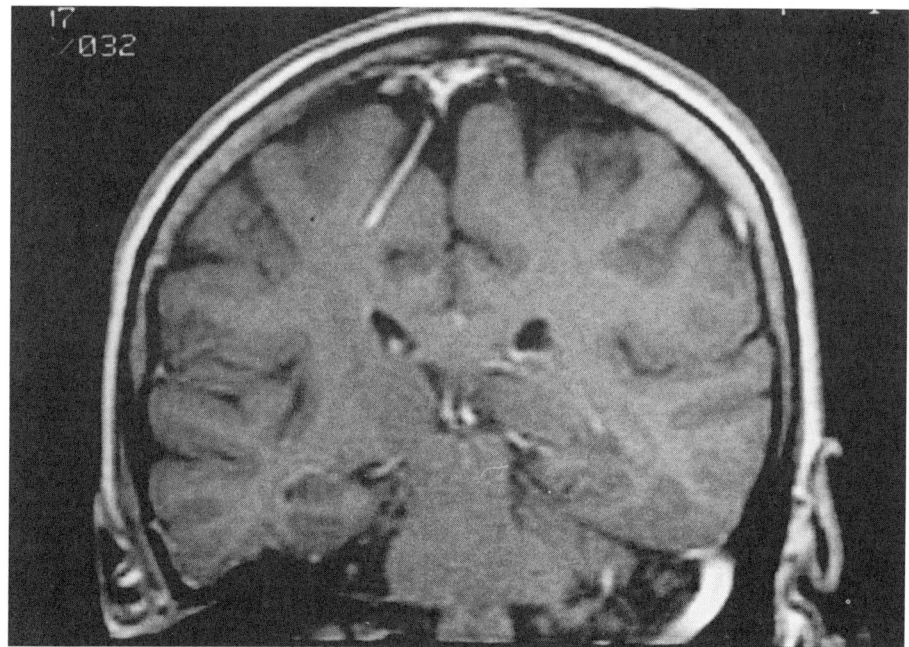

Figure 7: T$_1$ weighted, contrast enhanced MRI revealing a venous angioma.

malformation.[34,37] If the patient has had a spontaneous hemorrhage from a venous malformation and requires removal of the hematoma, it may be prudent to leave the malformation intact.[32,34] Furthermore, another lesion prone to hemorrhage, such as a cavernous malformation,[32,34] may be associated with the venous malformation and be more deserving of surgical attention.

Telangiectatic Malformations

Telangiectases are small malformations that typically consist of capillary-like structures.[7] Capillary telangiectases and cavernous malformations may represent a spectrum of the same lesion.[26] Telangiectatic malformations are thought to be clinically silent and do not have a noteworthy risk of hemorrhage.[7]

Angiographically Occult Vascular Malformations

An angiographically occult vascular malformation refers to vascular malformations that have bled but are not visualized by angiography. Occult malformations may account for up to 30% of lobar hematomas in patients with negative angiography.[38,39] A recurrent hemorrhage at the same site as the previous bleed is suggestive of an underlying malformation.[38] Occult malformations are less likely to bleed into the ventricles than are angiographically apparent AVMs.[38,39] Small AVMs, thrombosed AVMs, venous malformations, and cavernous malformations are often considered within this category.[39-42] With CT imaging of the acute hematoma, there may be a slightly hyper- or hypodense indentation of the otherwise fairly smooth perimeter of the clot, suggesting the presence of a malformation.[38] Many angiographically occult vascular malformations are found to be cavernous malformations upon histologic examination.[40] Therefore, MR imaging, especially with its ability to define cavernous malformations, is particularly important in the evaluation of patients with lobar hemorrhage and normal angiography.[43,44]

Dural Arteriovenous Malformations

Dural AVMs[45] constitute 5% to 20% of intracranial vascular malformations. They are congenital or acquired sites of arterial and venous communication within the dura mater. Intraparenchymal, as well as subarachnoid, epidural, and subdural, hemorrhage occurs in 15% of patients with dural AVMs. Lesions located about the tentorium, anterior cranial fossa, or cerebral convexities are most prone to bleed; rarely is hemorrhage associated with malformations about the transverse-sigmoid or cavernous sinuses. Angiographically demonstrable pial venous drainage, especially when associated with a venous aneurysm (varix) also predisposes to hemorrhage. Another risk factor for bleeding is venous sinus hypertension. Since the hemorrhage originates from venous structures, the damage tends to be less severe than when an arterial source causes bleeding and the mortality from such a hemorrhage is 10% to 20%.

Dural AVMs with pial venous drainage should be treated prophylactically because of their propensity to bleed (1% to 2% per year) and rebleed (1% to 2% within a month of ictus). A lesion that has bled should also be extirpated. Treatment often involves a multimodality approach combining interventional neuroradiologic (including arterial embolization and transvenous procedures) and surgical techniques. At times, a surgical or interventional radiologic procedure alone is sufficient to treat a dural AVM. Stereotactic radiosurgery may also play a role in treatment.

Pregnancy

Approximately one quarter of pregnant patients who have an intracranial hemorrhage have an AVM (Figure 8).[46] In 1974, Robinson et al reported that if a pregnant woman has an SAH, an AVM will be the source of bleeding 50% of the time.[47] They also reported that the risk of hemorrhage during pregnancy

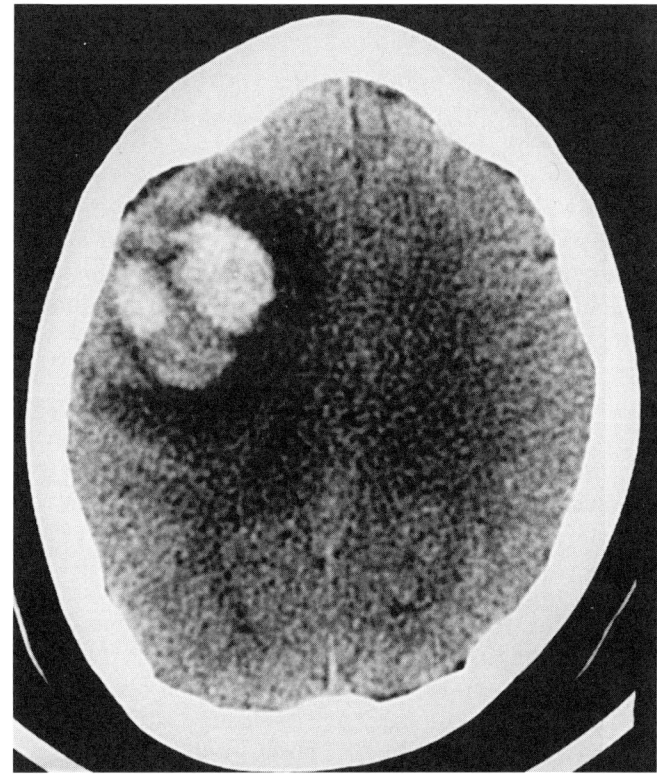

Figure 8A

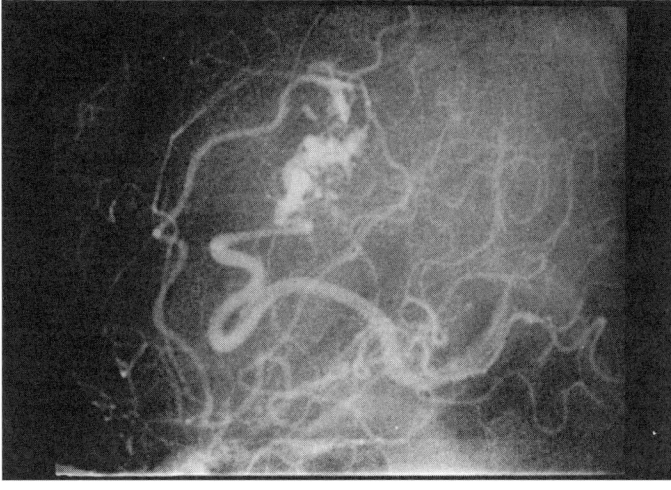

Figure 8B

Figure 8: (A) Pregnancy-associated hemorrhage from an AVM. Note irregular, heterogeneous increased density of blood on CT image. **(B)** Angiogram of underlying AVM.

to a woman with a known AVM was 87%. A primiparous woman who is not eclamptic and suffers an intraparenchymal hemorrhage during weeks 16 to 24 of pregnancy or during labor, delivery, or the early puerperium is especially likely to harbor an AVM.

In 1990, Horton et al, reviewing their data from a highly select population referred for proton beam therapy, found no increased risk for hemorrhage from an AVM during pregnancy and a 12-week postpartum period.[48] The rate of first hemorrhage for pregnant women was 0.035 per person-year (a risk of 3.5%) and for nonpregnant women was 0.031 per person-year. Furthermore, Horton et al found no stage of pregnancy or the puerperium to carry an excess risk of bleeding, whereas Dias and Sekhar found a modestly increasing risk of bleeding over the course of gestation.[46,48] To account for the discrepant results between their data and Robinson's, Horton et al stated that the "correct interpretation [of Robinson's data] is that when an AVM becomes clinically evident in association with pregnancy, a hemorrhage will be the first manifestation in 87% of cases."[48] Viewed in this manner, in Horton's series a hemorrhage was the initial manifestation of an AVM in 61% of pregnant women.[48]

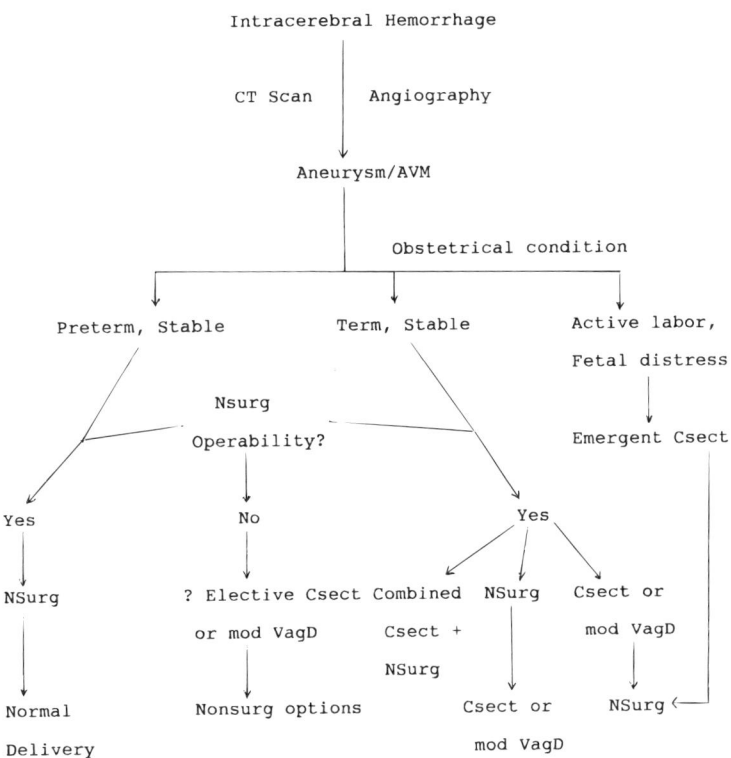

Figure 9: Approach to the pregnant patient. NSurg: neurosurgery; CSect: cesarean section; mod VagD: modified vaginal delivery; Nonsurg: nonsurgical.

In a recent series of cavernous angiomas, 2 of the 6 women with a cavernous malformation who developed clinically apparent hemorrhage did so in their first trimester of pregnancy.[25]

Garner et al noted that 39 women with a venous malformation had 68 pregnancies and deliveries without suffering a central nervous system (CNS) hemorrhage.[34] However, 2 of 9 patients with a venous malformation that bled in Malik's series were pregnant or postpartum.[36]

There are no definitive recommendations for the management of the pregnant patient with an intracranial hemorrhage.[49] The physician needs to consider both the neurosurgical status of the mother and the health of the fetus.[46] If the source of bleeding has not been obliterated, either cesarean section or vaginal delivery, with measures to minimize maternal hemodynamic stress, can be pursued. If there is fetal distress, emergent cesarean section is indicated (Figure 9).

Aneurysms

Berry aneurysms are the most common cause of aneurysmal intracerebral hematomas. Mycotic aneurysms or traumatic aneurysms can occasionally cause an intraparenchymal hematoma. Though aneurysms are usually considered a rare cause of isolated intracerebral hematoma, one third of patients suffering from aneurysmal SAH can have an associated intraparenchymal hematoma.[50]

Clinical Features

On average, a patient with an intracerebral hematoma caused by a ruptured berry aneurysm is younger than a patient with a hypertensive hematoma.[51] Although definite genetic transmission has not been proven, there is a tendency for aneurysms to occur in families.[52] Aneurysms are also more common among patients with hereditary connective tissue disorders, such as Ehlers-Danlos syndrome, pseudoxanthoma elasticum, arachnodactyly, and Marfan's syndrome.[53] Also, aneurysms occur more commonly in patients with polycystic kidney disease, coarctation of the aorta, and polyarteritis nodosa. If a patient with one of these conditions has an intracerebral hematoma, an aneurysm should be suspected and appropriate diagnostic studies pursued.

In general, aneurysms located between brain surfaces, or aneurysms that have bled a second or third time, tend to cause ICH. Aneurysms that have previously ruptured tend to develop surrounding fibrosis and adhesions. Such aneurysms, and those slowly growing in size and embedding themselves into the brain, are prone to cause intracerebral hematomas if scarring directs the jet of blood into the brain. If the hematoma is entirely intracerebral and there is no, or little, SAH, the clinical presentation will be typical of an intracerebral hematoma occurring at the site in question. Headache, vomiting, convulsions, focal neurologic signs, rapid deterioration of consciousness, and hypertension suggest the presence of an intracerebral hematoma. Patients with an isolated SAH usually have a severe onset of headache and stiff neck, and may or may not lose consciousness. In the absence of an intracerebral hematoma, focal findings in patients with a ruptured aneurysm, except for cranial nerve palsies, are usually absent. After the initial clinical evaluation, a patient who presents with these symptoms should have an immediate CT scan.

Diagnosis

A high index of suspicion that an ICH is due to a berry or mycotic aneurysm must always be maintained. The patient's age, presence of SAH, and location of the hematoma are helpful in deciding whether further neuroradiologic investigations are indicated.

Some authors believe that hemorrhage location is paramount in suggesting the diagnosis of aneurysmal ICH. Hayward and O'Reilly claim that in the absence of any clinical information, a diagnosis of either cerebral aneurysm rupture or primary ICH can be made with an accuracy of 90% based upon the CT scan alone.[54] Hemorrhage into the head of the caudate nucleus, for example, was said to be a rare but absolute indication of primary ICH, though, rarely, it can represent an aneurysmal bleed.

According to Crompton's classic observations of 103 fatal aneurysmal ruptures,[55] direct rupture into the brain, as opposed to extension via a subarachnoid hematoma, occurred from aneurysms arising from the internal carotid artery, pericallosal artery, and anterior cerebral artery. Anterior communicating artery aneurysms bleed directly into the gyrus rectus, anterolaterally into the orbital frontal lobe, or into the cavum septum pallucidum. Internal carotid and posterior communicating artery aneurysms usually bleed directly into the temporal lobe. Internal carotid artery bifurcation aneurysms bleed directly into the frontal lobe. Pericallosal and anterior cerebral artery aneurysms produce frontal lobe and interhemispheric hematomas (Table 2).

Crompton also found that 58% of the ICHs originated from a rupture of a subarachnoid hematoma secondarily into the brain. The site of origin of these subarachnoid hematomas were: interfrontal, Sylvian fissure, olfactory sulcus, supracallosal or intracingulate, and interpeduncular.[55]

The frontal and temporal lobes are common sites for an aneurysmal hematoma but an uncommon location for a hypertensive hematoma. Parietal lobe or corona radiata hematomas are uncommonly associated with aneurysms but are often seen with hypertensive hemorrhage. External capsule involvement is moderately common with aneurysmal rupture but very common with hypertensive hemorrhage. Discrete thalamic hematomas are almost always considered to be due to hypertension. Caval and callosal hematomas are almost always due to aneurysms.

Table 2
Possible Indicators of Aneurysm-Associated Hemorrhage

Location of the ICH on CT Scan	Possible Aneurysm Location
1. Gyrus rectus, cavum septum pellucidum, frontal lobe	anterior communicating artery
2. Temporal lobe	internal carotid artery (posterior communicating artery, anterior choroidal artery, and carotid bifurcation)
3. Sylvian fissure; midfrontal or temporal lobe	middle cerebral artery
4. Interhemispheric fissure/anterior frontal lobe	pericallosal artery
5. Distal middle cerebral or posterior cerebral artery territory hemorrhage	mycotic aneurysm
6. Caudate nucleus, basal ganglia	typically hypertensive; rarely aneurysmal

Aside from location, the CT scan appearance of the hematoma itself caused by aneurysms or hypertension is not always similar.[56] A lenticular-shaped hematoma in the Sylvian fissure, a flame-shaped hematoma in the basal frontal lobe (Figure 10), and a hematoma of the cavum, gyrus rectus, or temporal lobe (Figure 11) should alert the clinician to the possibility of a ruptured aneurysm. If a giant aneurysm has caused an ICH, one is likely to see the aneurysm lumen and calcification of the aneurysm wall on a CT scan (Figure 12).

Prognosis/Treatment

If a hematoma is small and there is little associated SAH, the prognosis is good compared to individuals with pure SAH. When an intracerebral hematoma due to an aneurysm is larger than 3 cm in diameter, the patient's prognosis is adversely affected.[57]

Angiography is required to establish that an intracerebral hematoma has been caused by a ruptured aneurysm. A definitive treatment plan should then be established. Currently there is no role for MR angiography in acute ICH when there is a reasonable suspicion of an aneurysm.

With improved, modern anesthesia and state-of-the-art neurosurgical technology, it is becoming apparent that overall patient survival and long-term prognosis is improved by early and definitive surgical treatment of aneurysms. In a patient with an aneurysmal intracerebral hematoma, the treatment plan should include evacuation of a large hematoma and definitive resection of the causative aneurysm. More and more surgeons are aggressively treating patients with profound neurologic deficits (Hunt and Hess grade IV and V patients). Patients who present in grade IV or V and harbor an intracerebral

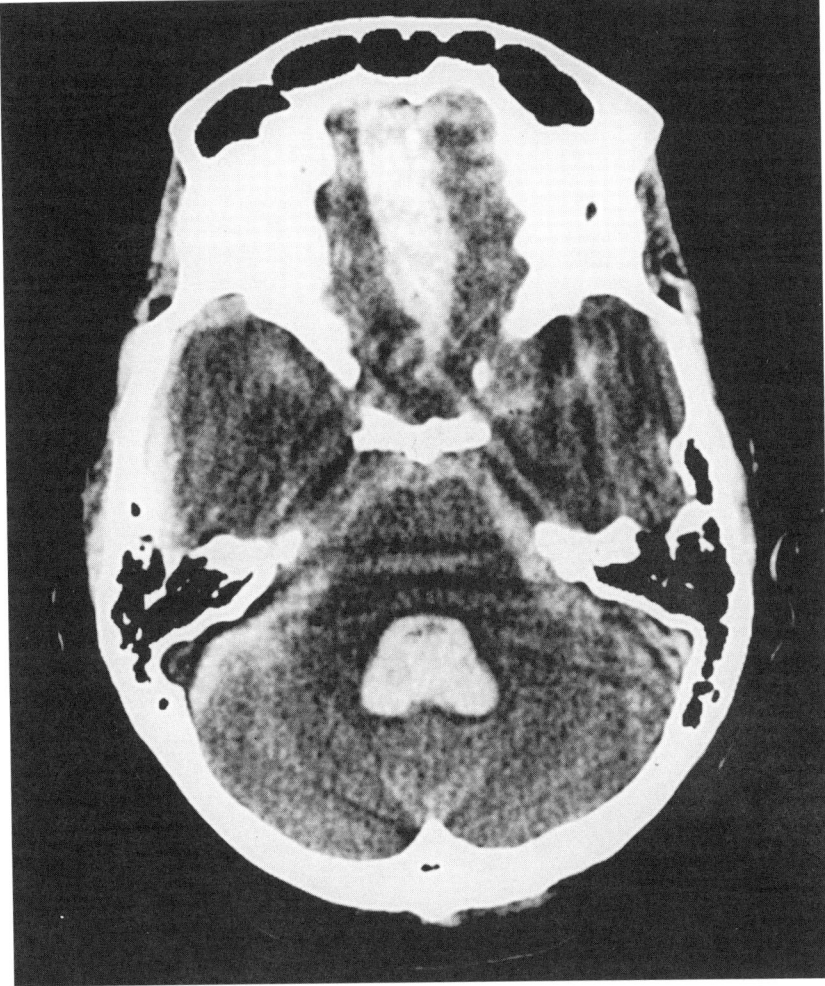

Figure 10: CT scan demonstrating an interhemispheric hematoma originating from an anterior communicating artery aneurysm.

hematoma due to a ruptured aneurysm are now candidates for aggressive neurosurgical decompression and clipping of the aneurysm.[58] Samson and Batjer recommend that no patient with a poor clinical grade who harbors an intracranial hematoma greater than 3 cm diameter should be denied early and definitive operation on the basis of poor neurologic function unless brain death has occurred.[59] The poor clinical status of these patients is attributed to the large intraparenchymal mass lesion. Prompt removal may result in dramatic and early improvement of neurologic function.[60] Brandt and associates showed that early and aggressive treatment of apparently moribund patients with an aneurysmal intracerebral hematoma enjoyed an acceptable clinical outcome.[61] De-

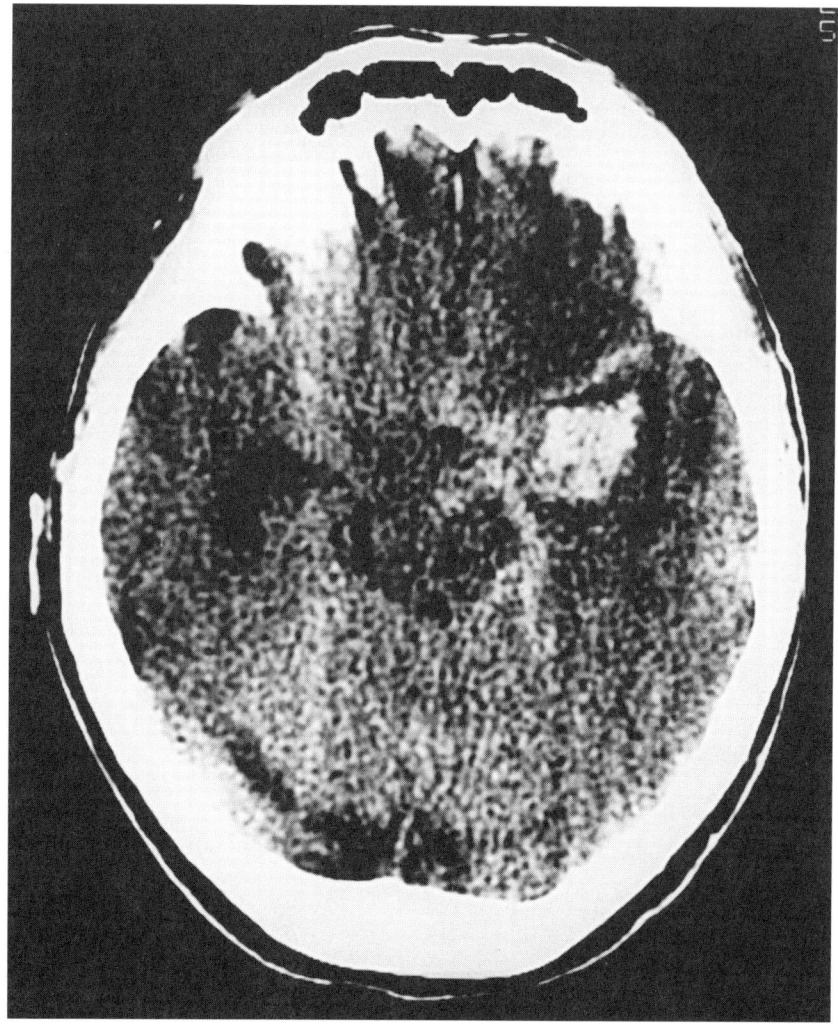

Figure 11: CT scan showing an intraparenchymal and SAH originating from a middle cerebral artery aneurysm.

compression of the hematoma without definitive treatment of the ruptured aneurysm is discouraged because fatal rehemorrhages are common after such an approach.[60]

Mycotic Aneurysm

Intraparenchymal hematoma caused by mycotic aneurysm rupture is rare. The hemorrhages are typically located in the distribution of the distal middle cerebral artery,[62–64] and there is usually an associated history of subacute bacte-

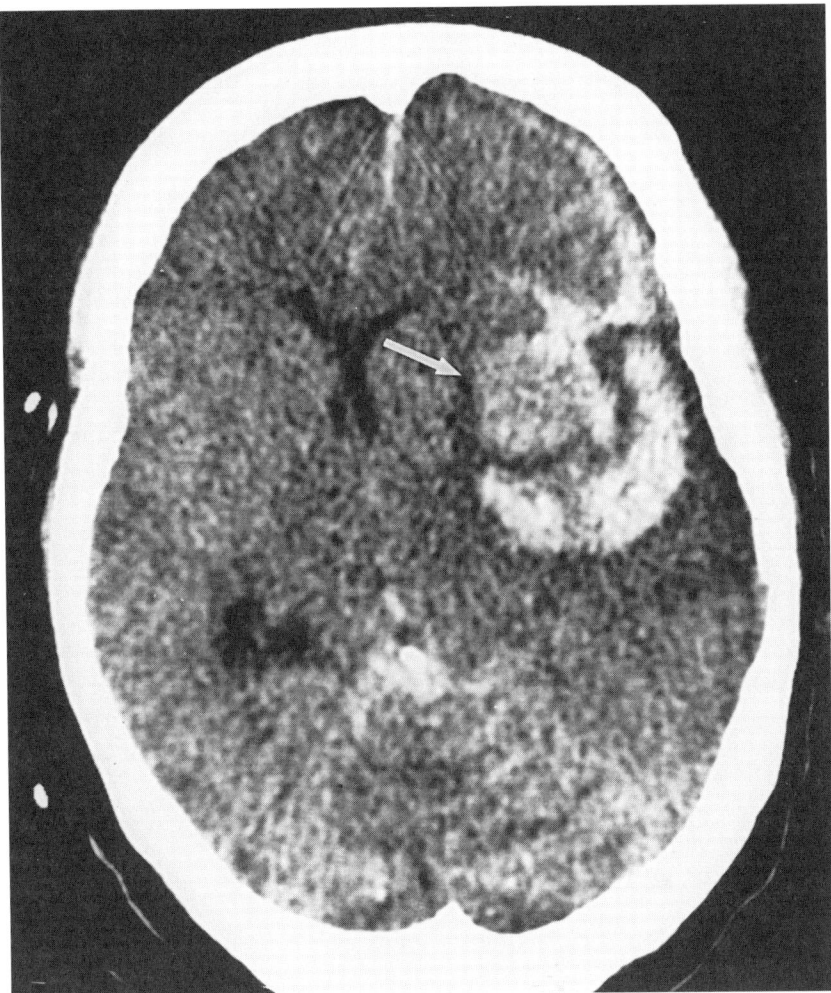

Figure 12: CT scan showing a giant middle cerebral artery aneurysm (arrow) with intraparenchymal and SAH. (Courtesy of Hyo Ahn, MD.)

rial endocarditis. Rarely, rupture of a mycotic aneurysm is the presenting feature of endocarditis. If the hematoma is the result of a ruptured mycotic aneurysm, obliteration of the aneurysm and evacuation of the hematoma is probably indicated if the aneurysm is surgically accessible.[65] If there are multiple aneurysms, or if the aneurysm is not surgically approachable, antibiotic treatment alone is appropriate.[63] The response to treatment is monitored by serial angiography.

Pregnancy

Eclampsia is a common cause of SAH or ICH during pregnancy.[49] However, the incidence of aneurysmal rupture is higher than expected during pregnancy.

Principles of diagnosis and treatment of an aneurysm during pregnancy are the same as mentioned in earlier parts of this chapter (Figure 9). The pregnancy should be managed according to standard obstetrical principles.[49]

Summary

When a patient presents with an ICH, the CT scan should be reviewed to determine whether the hematoma could be the result of an intracranial aneurysm. If appropriate, an angiogram should be performed to search for an aneurysm. If an aneurysm is found by angiography, an aggressive surgical approach toward the aneurysm and the intracerebral hematoma is warranted, even for the patient with severe neurologic compromise. With comprehensive, aggressive care the outcome of patients is improved.

References

1. Stein BM, Wolpert SM: Arteriovenous malformations of the brain. I: current concepts and treatment. *Arch Neurol* 1980;37:1.
2. Nagata S, Matsushima T, Fujii K, et al: Lateral ventricular arteriovenous malformations: natural history and surgical indications. *Acta Neurochir (Wien)* 1991;112:37.
3. Aoki N: Do intracranial arteriovenous malformations cause subarachnoid haemorrhage? Review of computed tomography features of ruptured arteriovenous malformations in the acute stage. *Acta Neurochir (Wien)* 1991; 112:92.
4. Schutz H, Bodeker R-H, Damian M, et al: Age-related spontaneous intracerebral hematoma in a German community. *Stroke* 1990;21:1412.
5. Snead OC III, Acker JD, Morawetz R: Familial arteriovenous malformation. *Ann Neurol* 1979;5:585.
6. Alberts MJ: Genetic aspects of cerebrovascular disease. *Stroke* 1991;22: 276.
7. Mohr JP, Stein BM, Hilal SK: Arteriovenous malformations. *Handbook Clin Neurol* 1989;10:361.
8. Murphy MJ: Long-term follow-up of seizures associated with cerebral arteriovenous malformations. Results of therapy. *Arch Neurol* 1985;42:477.
9. Chimowitz MI, Little JR, Awad IA, et al: Intracranial hypertension associated with unruptured cerebral arteriovenous malformations. *Ann Neurol* 1990;27:474.
10. Silber MH, Sandok BA, Ernest F IV: Vascular malformations of the posterior fossa. Clinical and radiologic features. *Arch Neurol* 1987;44:965.
11. Kase CS: Intracerebral hemorrhage: non-hypertensive causes. *Stroke* 1986; 17:590.

12. Wilkins RH: Natural history of intracranial vascular malformations: a review. *Neurosurgery* 1985;16:421.

13. Kelly JJ, Mellinger JF, Sundt TM Jr: Intracranial arteriovenous malformations in childhood. *Ann Neurol* 1978;3:338.

14. Toffol GJ, Biller J, Adams HP Jr: Nontraumatic intracerebral hemorrhage in young adults. *Arch Neurol* 1987;44:483.

15. Special Report from the National Institute of Neurological Disorders and Stroke. Classification of cerebrovascular diseases III. *Stroke* 1990;21:637.

16. Spetzler RFF, Hargraves RW, McCormick PW, et al: Relationship of perfusion pressure and size to risk of hemorrhage from arteriovenous malformations. *J Neurosurg* 1992;76:918.

17. Marks MP, Lane B, Steinberg GK, et al: Hemorrhage in intracerebral arteriovenous malformations: angiographic determinants. *Radiology* 1990;176:807.

18. Miyasaka Y, Yada K, Ohwada T, et al: An analysis of the venous drainage system as a factor in hemorrhage from arteriovenous malformations. *J Neurosurg* 1992;76:239.

19. Loes DJ, Smoker WRK, Biller J, et al: Nontraumatic lobar intracerebral hemorrhage: CT/angiographic correlation. *AJNR* 1987;8:1027.

20. Toffol GJ, Biller J, Adams HP Jr, et al: The predicted value of arteriography in nontraumatic intracerebral hemorrhage. *Stroke* 1986;17:881.

21. Graf CJ, Perret GE, Torner JC: Bleeding from cerebral arteriovenous malformations as part of their natural history. *J Neurosurg* 1983;58:331.

22. Brown RD, Wiebers DO, Forbes GS: Unruptured intracranial aneurysms and arteriovenous malformations: frequency of intracranial hemorrhage and relationship of lesions. *J Neurosurg* 1990;73:859.

23. Lunsford LD, Kondziolka D, Flickinger JC, et al: Stereotactic radiosurgery for arteriovenous malformations of the brain. *J Neurosurg* 1991;75:512.

24. Vinuela F, Dion JE, Duckwiler G, et al: Combined endovascular embolization and surgery in the management of cerebral arteriovenous malformations: experience with 101 cases. *J Neurosurg* 1992;75:856.

25. Robinson JR, Awad IA, Little JR: Natural history of the cavernous angioma. *J Neurosurg* 1991;75:709.

26. Farmer J-P, Cosgrove GR, Villemure J-G, et al: Intracerebral cavernous angiomas. *Neurology* 1988;38:1699.

27. Rigamonti D, Hadley MN, Drayer BP, et al: Cerebral cavernous malformations. Incidence and familial occurrence. *N Engl J Med* 1988;319:343.

28. Scott RM, Barnes P, Kupsky W, et al: Cavernous angiomas of the central nervous system in children. *J Neurosurg* 1992;76:38.

29. Requena I, Arias M, Lopez-Ibor L, et al: Cavernomas of the central nervous system: clinical and neuroimaging manifestations in 47 patients. *J Neurol Neurosurg Psychiat* 1991;54:590.

30. Dobyns WB, Michels VV, Groover RV, et al: Familial cavernous malformations of the central nervous system and retina. *Ann Neurol* 1987;21:578.

31. Del Curling O Jr, Kelly DL Jr, Elster AD, et al: An analysis of the natural history of cavernous angiomas. *J Neurosurg* 1991;75:702.

32. Rigamonti D, Spetzler RF: The association of venous and cavernous malformations. Report of four cases and discussion of the pathophysiological, diagnostic, and therapeutic implications. *Acta Neurochir (Wien)* 1988;92:100.

33. McCormick WF: The pathology of vascular ("arteriovenous") malformations. *J Neurosurg* 1966;24:807.

34. Garner TB, Del Curling O Jr, Kelly DL Jr, et al: The natural history of intracranial venous angiomas. *J Neurosurg* 1991;75:715.

35. Branch CE Jr, Kunath AM, Buscemi JH: Sublingual venous angioma. Marker of intracranial lesion? *Arch Neurol* 1981;38:259.

36. Malik GM, Morgan JK, Boulos RS, et al: Venous angiomas: an underestimated cause of intracranial hemorrhage. *Surg Neurol* 1988;30:350.

37. Biller J, Toffol GJ, Shea JF, et al: Cerebellar venous angiomas. A continuing controversy. *Arch Neurol* 1985;42:367.

38. Wakai S, Ueda Y, Inoh S, et al: Angiographically occult angiomas: a report of thirteen cases with an analysis of the cases documented in the literature. *Neurosurgery* 1985;17:549.

39. Lobato R, Rivas JJ, Gomez PA, et al: Comparison of the clinical presentation of symptomatic arteriovenous malformations (angiographically visualized) and occult vascular malformations. *Neurosurgery* 1992;31:331.

40. Tung H, Giannotta SL, Chadrasoma PT, et al: Recurrent intraparenchymal hemorrhages from angiographically occult vascular malformations. *J Neurosurg* 1990;73:174.

41. Lobato RD, Perez C, Rivas JJ, et al: Clinical, radiological, and pathological spectrum of angiographically occult intracranial vascular malformations. Analysis of 21 cases and review of the literature. *J Neurosurg* 1988;68:518.

42. Bitoh S, Hasegawa H, Fujiwara M, et al: Angiographically occult vascular malformations causing intracranial hemorrhage. *Surg Neurol* 1982;17:35.

43. Ogilvy CS, Heros RC, Ojemann RG, et al: Angiographically occult arteriovenous malformations. *J Neurosurg* 1988;59:350.

44. Kilpatrick TJ, Davis SM, Tress BM, et al: Lateral tegmental pontine haemorrhage due to vascular malformations. *Cerebrovasc Res* 1991;1:108.

45. King WA, Martin NA: Intracerebral hemorrhage due to dural arteriovenous malformations and fistulae. *Neurosurg Clin North Am* 1992;3:577.

46. Dias MS, Sekhar LN: Intracranial hemorrhage from aneurysms and arteriovenous malformations during pregnancy and the puerperium. *Neurosurgery* 1990;27:855.

47. Robinson JL, Hall CS, Sedzimir CB: Arteriovenous malformations, aneurysms, and pregnancy. *J Neurosurg* 1974;41:63.

48. Horton JC, Chambers WA, Lyons SL, et al: Pregnancy and the risk of hemorrhage from cerebral arteriovenous malformations. *Neurosurgery* 1990;27:867.

49. Stern BJ: Cerebrovascular disease and pregnancy. In: Goldstein PJ, Stern BJ, eds: *Neurological Disorders of Pregnancy*. 2nd Ed. Mount Kisco, NY: Futura Publishing, 1992:51.

50. Kendall BE, Lee BC, Claviera E: Computerized tomography and angiography in subarachnoid hemorrhage. *Br J Radiol* 1976;49:483.

51. Stehbens WE: Aneurysms and anatomical variations of cerebral arteries. *Arch Pathol* 1963;75:45.

52. Shinton R, Palsingh J, Williams B: Cerebral haemorrhage and berry aneurysm: evidence from a family for a pattern of autosomal dominant inheritance. *J Neurol Neurosurg Psychiat* 1991;54:838.

53. Dixon JM: Angioid streaks and pseudoxanthoma elasticum with aneurysm of the internal carotid artery. *Am J Opthalmol* 1951;34:1322.

54. Hayward RD, O'Reilly GVA: Intracerebral hemorrhage: accuracy of computerized transverse axial scanning in predicting the underlying aetiology. *Lancet* 1976;i:1.

55. Crompton MR: Intracerebral hematoma complicating ruptured cerebral berry aneurysm. *J Neurol Neurosurg Psychiat* 1962;25:378.

56. Weir B: *Aneurysms Affecting the Nervous System*. Baltimore: Williams & Wilkens, 1987:234.

57. Sacco RL, Wolf PA, Bharucha NE, et al: Subarachnoid and intracerebral hemorrhage: natural history, prognosis and precursive factors in the Framingham study. *Neurology* 1984;34:847.

58. Benoit BG, Cochrane DD, Durity F, et al: Clinical radiological correlates in intracerebral hematomas due to aneurysmal rupture. *Can J Neurol Sci* 1981:409.

59. Samson D, Batjer HH: Intracerebral hematomas secondary to ruptured aneurysms and intracranial vascular malformations. In: Kaufman HH, ed: *Intracerebral Hematomas*. New York: Raven Press, 1992:75.

60. Yasargil MG: *Microneurosurgery II. Clinical Considerations, Surgery of the Intracranial Aneurysms and Results*. Stuttgart: George Thieme Verlag, 1984.

61. Brandt L, Sonesson B, Ljunggren B, et al: Ruptured middle cerebral artery aneurysm with intracerebral hemorrhage in younger patients appearing moribund: emergency operation? *Neurosurgery* 1987;20:925.

62. Hart RG, Kagan-Hallet K, Joerns SE: Mechanisms of intracranial hemorrhage in infective endocarditis. *Stroke* 1987;18:1048.

63. Salgado AV: Central nervous system complications of infective endocarditis. *Stroke* 1991;22:1461.

64. Masuda J, Yutani C, Waki R, et al: Histopathological analysis of the mechanisms of intracranial hemorrhage complicating infective endocarditis. *Stroke* 1992;23:843.

65. Brust JCM, Dickinson PCT, Hughes JEO, et al: The diagnosis and treatment of cerebral mycotic aneurysms. *Ann Neurol* 1990;27:238.

Chapter 9

Ethanol

Philip B. Gorelick, MD, Michael A. Kelly, MD

Ethyl alcohol is a clear, colorless, hydroxylated aliphatic hydrocarbon that is consumed by millions of Americans annually. It is estimated that 18 million Americans are alcohol abusers or alcoholics.[1,2] Alcoholism is an important cause of death,[3] and alcohol contributes substantially to accidental deaths, suicides, homicides, general hospital admissions, emergency room admissions, and outpatient office visits.[4] It is estimated that the annual economic cost of alcohol abuse and alcoholism will rise to $150 billion in 1995.[5] While about 65% of Americans drink alcohol, only a relatively small percentage (about 7%) of the population is identified as being at high risk for the multiple dangers of heavy alcohol abuse.[6] Given the availability of alcohol, the large numbers of persons adversely affected, and the economic impact, alcoholism and alcohol-related health problems[7] merit careful surveillance and continued research efforts to facilitate a better understanding of biomedical, genetic, and health policy aspects.[8]

Alcohol is well known for its damaging effects to the liver, pancreas, gastrointestinal tract, heart, and developing fetus. In addition, alcohol may be linked to various cancers, hypertension, disruption of male reproductive function, and bone disease.[9] With acute alcohol intoxication there may be a spectrum of nervous system manifestations that include excitational and disinhibited behavior, impaired coordination and motor performance, stupor, and coma. With chronic alcohol abuse there are abstinence syndromes, nutritional diseases, and disorders associated with hepatic dysfunction.[10,11] Recently, stroke has been added to the list of neurologic complications associated with alcohol use.[12,13]

In this chapter we will describe the role of alcohol in the etiology of intracerebral hemorrhage (ICH). We will review the epidemiology of alcohol-related ICH, its pathophysiology, clinical features, and treatment.

Supported in part by National Institute on Aging Award 1R01 AG10102-01 and the MR Bauer Foundation.
From Feldmann E (ed). *Intracerebral Hemorrhage*. Armonk, NY: Futura Publishing Company, Inc., © 1994.

Epidemiology

Historical Perspective

The history of the recognition of alcohol consumption as a possible risk factor for stroke is provocative. As early as 1725, Sedgwick made reference to the possibility that alcohol was a risk factor for stroke.[14] However, it was not until the 1950s and 1960s that this association was again emphasized. Pakkenberg[15] and Balow et al[16] suggested that alcohol ingestion might predispose to ischemic stroke, especially in young adults. The next wave of studies originated in Finland in the 1970s and early 1980s. Hillbom and Kaste captured the attention of the epidemiologic community when they published a series of articles that linked ischemic brain infarction in young adults and adolescents with occasional ethanol intoxication, and in middle-aged women and young men with both occasional alcohol intoxication and regular heavy drinking.[17–19] Furthermore, alcohol intoxication was linked not only to ischemic stroke but to subarachnoid hemorrhage (SAH).[20] Although these studies were criticized for methodologic weaknesses, they brought about substantial interest in the possible association between alcohol and stroke, and stimulated further research.

One of the more striking features of Hillbom and Kaste's reports was the fact that predominantly young adults were affected. In concordance with this finding, Walbran and colleagues[21] noted in an autopsy study that cerebral infarction occurred more commonly at an earlier age in alcoholics than nonalcoholics. In a controlled retrospective study, Lee[22] found that a history of excessive alcohol intake was significantly more frequent among normotensive cerebrovascular thrombosis index cases under 50 years of age than controls, and Taylor and Coombs-Orme[23] reported that alcohol consumption within 24 hours of hospitalization was more common in stroke patients 50 years of age or younger than in matched hospital controls.

Additional support for the hypothesis that alcohol might be a risk factor for stroke emanated from the Yugoslavia Heart Study,[24] where those with the most frequent alcohol consumption were at highest risk of death from stroke. Furthermore, the Honolulu Heart Study[25,26] provided epidemiologic evidence that alcohol consumption was associated with fatal and nonfatal intracranial hemorrhage but not thromboembolic strokes. Given these epidemiologic observations, by 1984 the Stroke Council's Subcommittee on Risk Factors and Stroke listed alcohol as a "less well-documented" risk factor for stroke.[27] A similar conclusion was arrived at by the World Health Organization Task Force on Stroke and Other Cerebrovascular Disorders.[28]

Synthesis and Overview of Epidemiologic Studies

Review of select epidemiologic studies suggests that alcohol consumption is a risk factor for intracranial hemorrhage.[29] In a cohort study of residents of a rural community located in Shikoku Island, Japan, Tanaka et al[30] reported that high alcohol intake was a risk factor for cerebral hemorrhage but was not a risk factor for cerebral infarction. Kagan et al[26] observed an association between alcohol intake and cerebral hemorrhage among Japanese men living in Hawaii. Furthermore, in a follow-up study of this cohort of Japanese men, Donahue et al[31] found that intracranial hemorrhage increased monotonically with increased alcohol intake. This was true for both ICH and SAH, but the effect was greatest for SAH. Several other studies have suggested that alcohol consumption increased the risk for intracranial hemorrhage,[32,33] and reduction in alcohol consumption may be associated with reduction in risk of subsequent hemorrhagic stroke.[31]

In a thoughtful and comprehensive review, Camargo[34] analyzed the epidemiologic findings from 62 observational studies that were published in the English literature regarding moderate alcohol intake (less than 5 standard drinks or 60 g ethanol per day) and stroke. For ICH or SAH, he concluded that there was a positive linear association between *customary* (usual) moderate alcohol consumption and the relative risk of stroke in most population groups. However, among predominantly black populations, there was a paucity of study data from which to draw a firm conclusion about the relationship between *customary* moderate alcohol consumption and ICH or SAH. In addition, there was insufficient data from which to draw a conclusion about the relationship between *recent* (acute) alcohol consumption and hemorrhagic stroke among diverse or homogenous racial or ethnic populations.

In contradistinction, for ischemic stroke a J-shaped curve described the relationship between *customary* moderate alcohol consumption and stroke among predominantly white populations. Little if any association was found among Japanese and black populations.[34] Similar to hemorrhagic stroke, there was insufficient data from which to draw a substantial conclusion about *recent* alcohol consumption and ischemic stroke among diverse or homogeneous racial or ethnic populations. Thus, ischemic stroke, like coronary heart disease, may follow an epidemiologic pattern of excess risk at high levels of customary alcohol consumption, but "protection" from ischemia at moderate levels of alcohol consumption for some populations.

Status of Other Risk Factors for Intracerebral Hemorrhage

Most studies have shown that hypertension is the leading risk factor for ICH.[35-37] Furthermore, hypertensive ICH is often associated with left ventricular hypertrophy.[38] Age appears to be a risk factor in some reports[38]; however, additional study is needed to substantiate its role. Street drugs such as cocaine, amphetamines, "Ts and Blues," and phencyclidine; anticoagulants; cerebral amyloid; and possibly aspirin have also been associated with ICH.[39] Other studies have shown that low serum cholesterol, high serum cholesterol, low intake of animal fat and protein, and high levels of uric acid and proteinuria may be predictors of ICH.[40,41] Orientals appear to be at high risk of ICH, as may some blacks.[35] The role of cigarette smoking, seasonal pattern, diabetes mellitus, and obesity need to be clarified.[42]

Status of Other Risk Factors for Subarachnoid Hemorrhage

The incidence of SAH rises with age, but this rise with age appears less marked than for other stroke subtypes. Thus, the young carry a disproportionate burden. In some studies age-specific rates are higher among women than men, suggesting the possibility that these differences could relate to the effects of female hormones.[43–45] Hypertension is the most widely accepted risk factor for SAH, yet the evidence to support this association is somewhat limited.[45] Several studies have shown that current and former users of oral contraceptives are at risk for SAH.[46,47] Current heavy smokers, women smokers, smokers who exercise, and those smoking and using oral contraceptives also appear to be at greater risk for SAH.[45,48,49] Other factors that may be associated with SAH include street drugs, coarctation of the aorta, polycystic kidney disease, Marfan's syndrome, pseudoxanthoma elasticum, Ehler-Danlos syndrome, familial factors, fibromuscular dysplasia, arteriovenous malformation, atherosclerosis, and moya-moya disease.[45]

Pathophysiology

Heavier alcohol consumption is related to higher hospitalization rates for hemorrhagic cerebrovascular disease.[50] What are the pathophysiologic mechanisms by which alcohol-associated intracranial hemorrhage may occur?

Alcohol might potentiate or contribute to intracranial hemorrhage in several ways.[9,13] Hypertension is a risk factor for both ICH and SAH , and may be more prevalent among alcohol users.[51] Klatsky et al[52] found that men and women consuming three or more drinks per day had higher systolic and diastolic blood pressures as compared to nondrinkers and those taking two or fewer drinks per day. In addition, there was a higher prevalence of blood pressure greater than or equal to 160/95 mm Hg among those consuming three or more drinks per day. These findings have been substantiated in other studies as well.[53,54] Blood pressure changes may be most extreme during withdrawal from alcohol, and blood pressure elevation could be explained by increased plasma levels of cortisol, renin, aldosterone, arginine vasopressin, and heightened adrenergic activity after alcohol ingestion.[51] With abstinence from alcohol, blood pressure may return to normal.[45] Caplan has postulated that abrupt, significant elevation of systemic blood pressure with an increase in blood flow might be an important factor in the pathogenesis of ICH.[55] Such events could occur in association with alcohol ingestion or withdrawal.

Alcohol might also contribute to intracranial hemorrhage by affecting the coagulation mechanism. For example, in alcoholics with cirrhosis there are decreased circulating levels of clotting factors produced by the liver, excessive fibrinolysis, laboratory evidence of disseminated intravascular coagulation, and qualitatively abnormal fibrinogens.[56,57] Furthermore, thrombocytopenia may accompany alcohol use and could underlie or potentiate intracranial hemorrhage.[58] Alcohol also has a direct action on cerebral vascular smooth muscle, causing vasospasm,[59] which could potentiate the vasospasm of aneurysmal SAH.

Alcohol might also contribute to ischemic stroke via several mechanisms. These include cardiac arrhythmias and cardiac wall motion abnormalities that might be associated with alcoholic cardiomyopathy or "holiday heart syndrome,"[60,61] induction of hypertension,[52] enhancement of platelet aggregation,[58,62] activation of the clotting cascade,[63] and reduction of cerebral blood flow.[64] Furthermore, users of alcohol who smoke may have elevated blood levels of fibrinogen and other clotting factors, enhanced platelet aggregation, increased blood viscosity, vasoconstriction, and hastening of atherogenesis which could contribute to ischemic stroke.[65–67] On the other hand, moderate alcohol consumption could protect against ischemic stroke, as prostacyclin and fibrinolytic activity are augmented, and the concentration of low-density lipoproteins may be depressed and high-density lipoproteins may be elevated.[57,68,69]

Clinical Features

Based on the above discussion of pathophysiologic mechanisms, it is clear that alcohol affects the coagulation system, platelets, and the cardiovascular system in key ways that could underlie unique clinical features of alcohol-associated ICH. Furthermore, several studies have shown that alcohol may influence the distribution and severity of atherosclerosis.[70,71] What have clinical studies taught us about features of ICH associated with alcohol consumption?

Niizuma et al[72] evaluated liver function and coagulation parameters in 117 patients with spontaneous ICH. There were 68 men and 49 women. Key laboratory findings included: 1) liver dysfunction was more common among men than women, and this finding could be explained by differences in alcohol consumption; and 2) the number of thrombocytes and fibrinogen concentrations were lower, primarily in men with elevated concentrations of glutamic oxaloacetic transaminase, glutamic pyruvic transaminase, or elevated gamma-globulin fraction. Furthermore, six patients rebled, and all were men and heavy alcohol consumers with liver dysfunction. Fibrinogen concentration was low in 4 of these 6 men. Two showed thrombocytopenia and one showed a prolonged prothrombin time. The authors concluded that liver dysfunction produced a state in which hemorrhage occurred more readily, and that this hemorrhagic tendency might be a causal factor for spontaneous ICH. Interestingly, in this series the frequency of hypertension was slightly higher among women, while liver dysfunction was more common among men. Several other studies have concluded that spontaneous ICH may be associated with liver cirrhosis, and that such brain hemorrhage may be extensive.[73–75]

In a second report, Niizuma et al[76] studied the influence of liver dysfunction on volume of putaminal hemorrhage in 141 patients with spontaneous hemorrhage. Overall, hematomas were larger in men, regular alcohol consumers, those with liver dysfunction, and those with low platelet counts. The authors concluded that the volume of hematoma in such patients was large and that this reflected the fact that almost all the alcohol consumers were men and most had liver dysfunction. Niizuma et al[76] underscored liver dysfunction as a possible risk factor for ICH and emphasized that the presence of thrombocytopenia, decreased concentrations of coagulation factors, and hyperfibrinolysis retarded hemostasis and resulted in the formation of large hematomas.

Monforte et al[77] studied the role of high ethanol consumption, hypertension, liver disease, cigarette smoking, and coagulation disorder in a case-control study of 24 young and middle-aged patients with ICH. After controlling for possible confounding factors, high ethanol consumption and hypertension were the only independent risk factors for ICH. Furthermore, the hemorrhages found in cases with high ethanol intake were more commonly located in the cerebral lobes than in the typical location of hypertensive hematomas, the basal ganglia. The authors concluded that chronic, high ethanol intake should be considered as an independent risk factor for lobar hematomas in young and middle-aged adults.

Weisberg[78] described six alcoholic patients who developed extensive cerebral hemorrhages with both intraventricular and subarachnoid blood. In all patients there was evidence of liver damage, low platelet counts, and abnormal prothrombin and partial thromboplastin times. All patients were comatose, and one developed delayed neurologic deterioration. In all six patients there were large diffuse cerebral hemispheric hemorrhages, intraventricular blood, and subarachnoid blood on cranial computed tomography. In three, autopsy showed no evidence of aneurysm, vascular malformation, neoplasm, amyloid angiopathy, or arteriolar hypertensive changes.

In summary, the above studies suggest the following about the clinical features of ICH associated with alcohol: (1) hemorrhages tend to be extensive and are associated with liver dysfunction and thrombocytopenia; and (2) hemorrhages may be located in lobar regions of the brain rather than in the basal ganglia and nearby subcortical structures where hypertensive hemorrhages usually occur. These findings will need to be validated by additional well-designed epidemiologic studies.

Treatment

Introduction

The medical and surgical management of ICH is discussed in Chapters 13 and 14. Several aspects of alcohol-related ICH merit special emphasis.

As in stroke of any kind, the general medical condition of the patient greatly influences management decisions.[79] This is especially important in the chronic alcoholic patient with ICH. Liver disease and consequent coagulation factor deficiency may underlie or potentiate hemorrhage and require specific treatment. Malnourishment, gastrointestinal bleeding, anemia and thrombocytopenia, pancreatic dysfunction, and metabolic derangements will further complicate management. Furthermore, neurologic complications of acute alcohol intoxication and chronic alcohol abuse may obscure the acute, hemorrhage-related findings.

For the patient who is an alcohol user, a detailed history of duration and quantity of alcohol use, bleeding complications, liver dysfunction, seizures, and symptoms of withdrawal is important. The general physical examination must carefully assess the cardiovascular and hepatic systems and search for systemic signs of disordered hemostasis. The neurologic examination should focus on cognitive status and determine if there is tremor, ataxia, myopathy, neuropathy, or other evidence of neurologic sequelae of chronic alcohol use, in addition to the manifestations of the ICH.[11] The following section reviews the major systemic complications of alcohol use and serves to alert the clinician to alcohol-related systemic disease that may require standard medical therapy.

The Cardiovascular System

Alcohol use has important effects on the cardiovascular system.[80] Hypertension is associated with chronic alcohol use.[81] Alcohol decreases cardiac contractility, and chronic use is associated with cardiomyopathy.[82,83] Mural thrombus may develop as a consequence of cardiomyopathy and result in thromboembolism to brain, visceral organs, and extremities. Alcohol induces peripheral vasodilatation and, coupled with poor cardiac contractility, may result in postural hypotension. Arrhythmias may develop as a result of cardiomyopathy and the effects of alcohol on the cardiac conduction system.[84] The alcoholic patient with brain hemorrhage requires careful cardiovascular monitoring with attention to blood pressure, heart rhythm, and fluid volume status.

The Gastrointestinal System

Chronic alcohol use induces fatty change, inflammation, and cirrhosis of the liver. Hepatic encephalopathy may complicate management of the patient with stroke and alcohol-related liver failure. Hepatic encephalopathy is a confusional state associated with asterixis, ataxia, and tremor. It may progress to include seizures and coma. In the evaluation of the alcoholic patient with encephalopathy, the possibility of brain hemorrhage may be overlooked. Similarly, the patient with recognized cerebral hemorrhage may subsequently develop hepatic encephalopathy which further complicates examination and treatment.

Drugs such as barbiturates and benzodiazepines may precipitate hepatic encephalopathy. Alcoholic patients may be extremely sensitive to these and other drugs which are metabolized by the liver. Diuretic therapy may result in fluid volume contraction and uremia which may aggravate the encephalopathic state.

Gastrointestinal hemorrhage is common in the alcoholic patient and may be life-threatening. Causes of hemorrhage include esophagitis, esophageal varices, Mallory-Weiss tears, gastritis, and gastric and duodenal ulcers. Blood in the intestinal tract or a diet high in protein increases the serum ammonia level and the likelihood of developing hepatic encephalopathy.

Initial treatment of hepatic encephalopathy is meticulous attention to electrolyte and fluid status as well as treatment of underlying infection. Antibiotics may be used to reduce colonic bacteria and thereby decrease ammonia production. Oral and rectal lactulose decreases bacterial production of ammonia, acidifies the colonic contents, and reduces absorption of ammonia.[85]

Chronic alcohol use predisposes to the development of cancers of the gastrointestinal tract, head and neck, and lungs. Specific mechanisms are not well understood but may relate to local irritation, direct toxic effects, impairment of the immune system, nutritional deficiencies, or concomitant tobacco use.[86] Tumor-associated ICH must be ruled out in the chronic alcohol user.

Coagulation

Among the chief functions of the liver are the production of several of the coagulation factors. Deficiency of coagulation factors, as occurs in patients with alcoholic liver failure, predisposes to cerebral and systemic hemorrhage. Intracerebral hemorrhage from other causes such as hypertension may be potentiated by the coagulopathy of alcoholic liver disease. The liver produces fibrinogen, prothrombin (factor II), and coagulation factors V, VII, IX, and X. In coagulation factor deficiency states, prothrombin and bleeding times are prolonged.

Vitamin K is an essential cofactor in the production of many of the coagulation factors (II, VII, IX, and X). In chronic alcoholism, poor diet and pancreatic or intestinal dysfunction resulting in malabsorption may underlie vitamin K deficiency which exacerbates the coagulation disorder. Antibiotics may act on intestinal bacteria to further interfere with vitamin K production and absorption.

In alcohol-related ICH, vitamin K is used to treat prolonged prothrombin time. However, in alcohol-related hepatocellular disease that is not associated with malnutrition or malabsorption, prolongation of the prothrombin time is not a result of vitamin K deficiency, and thus its replacement will not affect coagulation or the prothrombin time. Transfusion of fresh frozen plasma is required to replace deficient clotting factors.

Alcoholic bone marrow toxicity may result in anemia and thrombocytopenia. In addition to number, platelets may be dysfunctional (altered aggregation) and have shortened survival. Whole blood or platelet transfusions may be required to normalize platelet numbers and function.

Metabolic Derangements

Hypokalemia may result from poor oral intake, vomiting, or diarrhea. Hypokalemia is associated with weakness, hyporeflexia, and cardiac arrhythmias. Hypokalemic metabolic alkalosis may contribute to hepatic encephalopathy.

Hypocalcemia, hypomagnesemia, and hypophosphatemia also result from poor dietary intake, and excess urinary loss of these metabolic factors will often accompany hypokalemia. Hypocalcemia is manifested by paresthesias, tetany, and seizures. Magnesium deficiency is characterized by nausea, weakness, lethargy, paresthesias, muscle cramps, and confusion. Furthermore, athetoid movements, seizures, and tetany may occur. Vitamin D deficiency and hypomagnesemia may be associated with proximal muscle weakness. Magnesium deficiency inhibits parathyroid hormone production and may potentiate hypocalcemia. Hypophosphatemia is associated with generalized weakness and, if severe, obtundation and seizures.

Alcohol may impair hepatic gluconeogenesis and result in symptomatic hypoglycemia. Insulin resistance may result in hyperglycemia. Alcoholic ketoacidosis may follow a period of limited food intake and heavy alcohol consumption and may contribute to stupor and coma in the patient with stroke.[87] Treatment is intravenous administration of glucose and thiamine.

Thiamine Deficiency

Thiamine deficiency in chronic alcoholics is usually due to malnutrition and malabsorption. Wernicke's encephalopathy (confusion, ataxia, and ophthalmoplegia in its classic form) is a major neurologic manifestation of the thiamine deficient state. Wernicke's encephalopathy may be precipitated by administration of intravenous glucose in the absence of concurrent thiamine administration. Treatment consists of daily intravenous thiamine (50 to 100 mg) followed by intramuscular injections. Multivitamin preparations will replace deficiencies in folate, pyridoxine, and niacin which are common in alcoholics.[88]

Alcohol Withdrawal

The management of the chronic alcoholic hospitalized for acute intracranial hemorrhage may be complicated by alcohol withdrawal. In its mild form, withdrawal manifests as anxiety, tremor, and tachycardia. These symptoms usually resolve within 48 hours and usually do not require specific treatment. If withdrawal is severe, agitated confusion, hallucinations, fever, hypertension, and seizures may develop. Delirium tremens usually develop between the third and fifth day of alcohol withdrawal. Severe symptoms should be treated with sedative drugs such as benzodiazepines. Lorazepam has an intermediate half-life and may be safer to use than longer-acting diazepam or chlordiazepoxide. Combination therapy with agents such as propranolol, clonidine, or haloperidol may have usefulness in selected patients.[89]

Alcohol withdrawal seizures are usually generalized, tonic-clonic, and non-recurrent. Anticonvulsant therapy is not normally required. Intracerebral hemorrhage, particularly if lobar, may cause partial and secondarily generalized seizures. Administration of prophylactic anticonvulsant therapy in ICH is controversial, but if a seizure occurs anticonvulsant therapy should be administered promptly. Phenytoin is the drug of choice unless hypersensitivity or severe hepatic dysfunction is present. Phenobarbital or benzodiazepines are alternative anticonvulsants.

References

1. National Institute on Alcohol Abuse and Alcoholism: Sixth special report to the U.S. Congress on alcohol and health. DHHS Publication No. (ADM) 87-1519 U.S. Government Printing Office, Washington, D.C., January 1987.

2. Williams GD, Stinson FS, Parker DA, et al: Demographic trends, alcohol abuse and alcoholism 1985–1995. Alcohol Health and Research World. *Epidemiol Bull* No. 15, NIAAA; 1987.

3. Bullock KD, Reed RJ, Grant I: Reduced mortality risk in alcoholics who achieve long-term abstinence. *JAMA* 1992;267:668.

4. Williams GD, Grant BF, Stinson FS, et al: Trends in alcohol-related morbidity and mortality. *Public Health Rep* 1988;103:592.

5. Burke TR: The economic impact of alcohol abuse and alcoholism. *Public Health Rep* 1988;103:564.

6. Kaplan NM: Bashing booze: the danger of losing the benefits of moderate alcohol consumption. *Am Heart J* 1991;121(6):1854.

7. Eckardt MJ, Harford TC, Kaelber CT, et al: Health hazards associated with alcohol consumption. *JAMA* 1981;246:648.

8. Goedde HW, Agarwal DP: *Alcoholism. Biomedical and Genetic Aspects.* New York: Pergamon Press, 1989.

9. Gorelick PB: The status of alcohol as a risk factor for stroke. *Stroke* 1989; 20:1607.

10. Victor M, Adams RD, Collins GH: *The Wernicke-Korsakoff Syndrome and Related Disorders Due to Alcoholism and Malnutrition.* Philadelphia: FA Davis Company, 1989:1.

11. Charness ME, Simon RP, Greenberg DA: Ethanol and the nervous system. *N Engl J Med* 1989;321:442.
12. Hillbom ME: What supports the role of alcohol as a risk factor for stroke? *Acta Med Scand* 1987;717(suppl):93.
13. Gorelick PB: Alcohol and stroke. *Stroke* 1987;18:268.
14. Sedgwick J: A new treatise on liquors wherein the use and abuse of wine, malt drinks, water, etc are particularly considered in many diseases, institutions and ages with proper manner of using them hot or cold either as physick, diet or both. London:Rivington, 1725.
15. Pakkenberg H: Thrombosis cerebri in young persons: a follow-up examination. *Acta Psychiat Neurol Scand* 1954;29:237.
16. Balow J, Alter M, Resch JA: Cerebral thromboembolism: a clinical appraisal of 100 cases. *Neurology* 1966;16:559.
17. Hillbom M, Kaste M: Does ethanol intoxication promote brain infarction in young adults? *Lancet* 1978;2:1181.
18. Hillbom M, Kaste M: Ethanol intoxication: a risk factor for ischemic brain infarction in adolescents and young adults. *Stroke* 1981;12:422.
19. Hillbom M, Kaste M: Ethanol intoxication a risk factor for ischemic brain infarction. *Stroke* 1983;14:694.
20. Hillbom M, Kaste M: Does alcohol intoxication precipitate aneurysmal subarachnoid hemorrhage? *J Neurol Neurosurg Psychiat* 1981;44:523.
21. Walbran BB, Nelson JS, Taylor JR: Association of cerebral infarction and chronic alcoholism: an autopsy study. *Alcoholism* 1981;5:531.
22. Lee K: Alcoholism and cerebrovascular thrombosis in the young. *Acta Neurol Scand* 1979;59:270.
23. Taylor JR, Coombs-Orme T: Alcohol and strokes in young adults. *Am J Psychiat* 1985;142:116.
24. Kozararevic DJ, Vojvodic N, Dawber T, et al: Frequency of alcohol consumption and morbidity and mortality: the Yugoslavia Cardiovascular Disease Study. *Lancet* 1980;1:613.
25. Kagan A, Yano K, Rhoads GG, et al: Alcohol and cardiovascular disease: the Hawaii experience. *Circulation* 1981;64(suppl III):III-27.
26. Kagan A, Popper JS, Rhoads GG: Factors related to stroke incidence in Hawaii Japanese men. The Honolulu Heart Study. *Stroke* 1980;11:14.
27. Dyken ML, Wolf PA, Barnett HJM, et al: Risk factors in stroke. A statement for physicians by the Subcommittee on Risk Factors and Stroke of the Stroke Council. *Stroke* 1984;15:1105.
28. Report of the WHO Task Force on Stroke and Other Cerebrovascular Disorders: stroke 1989, recommendations on stroke prevention, diagnosis and therapy. *Stroke* 1989;20:1407.
29. Gorelick PB, Rodin MB, Langenberg P, et al: Weekly alcohol consumption, cigarette smoking, and the risk of ischemic stroke: results of a case-control study at three urban medical centers in Chicago, Illinois. *Neurology* 1989;39:339.
30. Tanaka H, Udea Y, Hayashi M, et al: Risk factors for cerebral hemorrhage

and cerebral infarction in a Japanese rural community. *Stroke* 1982;13: 62.

31. Donahue RP, Abbott RD, Reed DM, et al: Alcohol and hemorrhagic stroke: the Honolulu Heart Study. *JAMA* 1986;255:2311.
32. Gill JS, Shipley MJ, Tsementzis SA, et al: Alcohol consumption—a risk factor for hemorrhagic and non-hemorrhagic stroke. *Am J Med* 1991;90: 489.
33. Stampfer MJ, Colditz GA, Willett WC, et al: A prospective study of moderate alcohol consumption and the risk of coronary disease and stroke in women. *N Engl J Med* 1988;319:267.
34. Camargo CA: Moderate alcohol consumption and stroke: the epidemiological evidence. *Stroke* 1989;20:1611.
35. Kurtzke JF: Epidemiology of cerebrovascular disease. In: McDowell FH, Caplan LR, eds: *Cerebrovascular Survey Report*. NINCDS publication, 1985:1.
36. Shimizu Y, Kato H, Lin CH, et al: Relationship between longitudinal changes in blood pressure and stroke incidence. *Stroke* 1984;15:839.
37. Ueda K, Hasuo Y, Kiyohara Y, et al: Intracerebral hemorrhage in a Japanese community, Hisayama: incidence, changing pattern during long-term follow-up, and related factors. *Stroke* 1988;19:48.
38. Brott T, Thalinger K, Hertzberg V: Hypertension as a risk factor for spontaneous intracerebral hemorrhage. *Stroke* 1986;17:1078.
39. Gorelick PB: Stroke from alcohol and drug abuse. A current social peril. *Postgrad Med* 1990;88:171.
40. Reed D: The paradox of high risk of stroke in populations with low risk of coronary heart disease. *Am J Epidemiol* 1990;131:579.
41. Stemmermann GN, Hayashi T, Resch JA, et al: Risk factors related to ischemic and hemorrhagic cerebrovascular disease at autopsy: the Honolulu Heart Study. *Stroke* 1984;15:23.
42. Bozzola FG, Gorelick PB, Jensen J: Epidemiology of intracranial hemorrhage. *Neuroimaging Clin North Am* 1992;2:1.
43. Bonita R, Beaglehole R, North JDK: Subarachnoid hemorrhage in New Zealand: an epidemiological study. *Stroke* 1983;14:342.
44. Bonita R, Thomson S: Subarachnoid hemorrhage: epidemiology, diagnosis, management, and outcome. *Stroke* 1985;16:591.
45. Longstreth WT, Koepsell TD, Yerby MS, et al: Risk factors for subarachnoid hemorrhage. *Stroke* 1985;16:377.
46. Petitti DB, Wingerd J: Use of oral contraceptives, cigarette smoking, and risk of subarachnoid hemorrhage. *Lancet* 1978;2:234.
47. Royal College of General Practitioners' Oral Contraception Study: further analyses of mortality in oral contraceptive users. *Lancet* 1981;1:541.
48. Longstreth WT, Nelson L, Koepsell TD, et al: Risk factors for subarachnoid hemorrhage. *Stroke* 1991;22:149.
49. Sacco RL, Wolf PA, Bharucha NE, et al: Subarachnoid and intracerebral hemorrhage: natural history, prognosis, and precursive factors in the Framingham Study. *Neurology* 1984;34:847.

50. Klatsky AL, Armstrong MA, Friedman GD: Alcohol use and subsequent cerebrovascular disease hospitalizations. *Stroke* 1989;20:741.

51. Stokes GS: Hypertension and alcohol: is there a link? *J Chron Dis* 1982; 35:759.

52. Klatsky AL, Friedman GD, Siegelaub AB, et al: Alcohol consumption and blood pressure. *N Engl J Med* 1977;296:1194.

53. D'Alonzo CA, Pell S: Cardiovascular disease among problem drinkers. *J Occup Med* 1968;10:344.

54. Kannel WB, Sorlie P: Hypertension in Framingham. In: Paul O, ed: *Epidemiology and Control of Hypertension*. New York: Stratton International Medical Book Corp., 1974:553.

55. Caplan LR: Intracerebral hemorrhage revisited. *Neurology* 1988;38:624.

56. Cowan DH: Effects of alcoholism on hemostasis. *Sem Hematol* 1980;17: 137.

57. Lang WE: Ethyl alcohol enhances plasminogen activator secretion by endothelial cells. *JAMA* 1983;250:772.

58. Haselager EM, Vreeken J: Rebound thrombocytosis after alcohol abuse: a possible factor in the pathogenesis of thromboembolic disease. *Lancet* 1977; 1:774.

59. Altura BM, Altura BT, Gebrewold A: Alcohol-induced spasms of cerebral blood vessels: relation to cerebrovascular accidents and sudden death. *Science* 1983, 331.

60. Ettinger PO, Wu CF, De La Cruz C, et al: Arrhythmias and the "holiday heart": alcohol-associated cardiac rhythm disorders. *Am Heart J* 1978;95: 555.

61. Demakis J, Proskey A, Rahimtoola S, et al: The natural course of alcoholic cardiomyopathy. *Ann Intern Med* 1974;80:293.

62. Hutton RA, Fink FR, Wilson DT, et al: Platelet hyperaggregability during alcohol withdrawal. *Clin Lab Haemat* 1981;3:223.

63. Hillbom M, Kaste M, Rasi V: Can ethanol intoxication affect hemocoagulation to increase the risk of brain infarction in young adults? *Neurology* 1983;33:381.

64. Berglund M: Cerebral blood flow in chronic alcoholics. *Alcoholism* 1981;5: 295.

65. Wolf PA: Cigarettes, alcohol and stroke. *N Engl J Med* 1986;315:1087.

66. Landolfi R, Steiner M: Ethanol raises prostacyclin in vivo and in vitro. *Blood* 1984;64:679.

67. Jakubowski JA, Vaillancourt R, Deykin D: Interaction of ethanol, prostacyclin, and aspirin in determining human platelet reactivity in vitro. *Arteriosclerosis* 1988;8:436.

68. Castelli WP, Gordon T, Hjortland MC, et al: Alcohol and blood lipids. The Cooperative Lipoprotein Phenotyping Study. *Lancet* 1977;2:153.

69. Avogaro P, Cazzolato G, Belussi F, et al: Altered apoprotein composition of HDL_2 and HDL_3 in chronic alcoholics. *Artery* 1982;10:317.

70. Reed DM, Resch JA, Hayashi T, et al: A prospective study of cerebral artery atherosclerosis. *Stroke* 1988;19:870.

71. Bogousslavsky J, Van Melle G, Despland PA, et al: Alcohol consumption and carotid atherosclerosis in the Lausanne Stroke Registry. *Stroke* 1990; 21:715.
72. Niizuma H, Suzuki J, Yonemitsu T, et al: Spontaneous intracerebral hemorrhage and liver dysfunction. *Stroke* 1988;19:852.
73. McCormick WF, Rosenfield DB: Massive brain hemorrhage: a review of 144 cases and an examination of their causes. *Stroke* 1973;4:946.
74. Boudouresques G, Hauw JJ, Meninger V, et al: Hepatic cirrhosis and intracranial hemorrhage: significance of the association in 53 pathological cases. *Ann Neurol* 1980;7:204.
75. Cahill DW, Ducker TB: Spontaneous intracerebral hemorrhage. *Clin Neurosurg* 1982;29:722.
76. Niizuma H, Shimizu Y, Nakasato N, et al: Influence of liver dysfunction on volume of putaminal hemorrhage. *Stroke* 1988;19:987.
77. Monforte R, Estruch R, Graus F, et al: High ethanol consumption as risk factor for intracerebral hemorrhage in young and middle-aged people. *Stroke* 1990;21:1529.
78. Weisberg LA: Alcoholic intracerebral hemorrhage. *Stroke* 1988;19:1565.
79. Schuckit MA: *Drug and Alcohol Abuse: A Clinical Guide to Diagnosis and Treatment.* New York: Plenum Medical Book Co., 1989:45.
80. Regan TJ: Alcohol and the cardiovascular system. *J Am Med Soc* 1990; 264:377.
81. Saunders JB: Alcohol: an important cause of hypertension. *Br Med J* 1987; 294:1045.
82. Urbano-Marquez A, Estruch R, Navarro-Lopez F, et al: The effects of alcoholism on skeletal and cardiac muscle. *N Engl J Med* 1989;320:409.
83. Lang RM, Borow MM, Nemann A, et al: Adverse cardiovascular effects of acute alcohol ingestion in young adults. *Ann Intern Med* 1985;102:742.
84. Greenspon AJ, Schaal SF: The "holiday heart": electrophysiological studies of alcohol effects in alcoholics. *Ann Int Med* 1983;98:135.
85. Gammell SH, Jones EA: Hepatic encephalopathy. *Med Clin North Am* 1989;73:793.
86. Lieber CS, Garro A, Leo MA, et al: Alcohol and cancer. *Hepatology* 1986; 6:1005.
87. Fulop M, Ben-Ezra J, Bock J: Alcoholic ketosis. *Alcohol Clin Exp Res* 1986; 10:610.
88. Guthrie SK: The treatment of alcohol withdrawal. *Pharmacotherapy* 1989; 9:131.
89. Rosenbloom A: Emerging treatment options in the alcohol withdrawal syndrome. *J Clin Psych* 1988;49:28.

Chapter 10

Less Common Causes of Intracerebral Hemorrhage

Edward Feldmann, MD

This chapter reviews less common etiologies of intracerebral hemorrhage (ICH). Exploring the mechanisms by which less common disorders lead to hemorrhage may help elucidate the pathophysiology of the more common presentations of ICH. An awareness of unusual causes of ICH will also help diagnose the patient with an atypical presentation, or the patient in whom no obvious cause is present.

Pathophysiology

Several basic pathophysiologic mechanisms likely underly the overwhelming majority of ICHs. However, when considering the uncommon disorders behind ICH, for any one disorder, multiple potential mechanisms exist for producing hemorrhage. For example, the patient with systemic vasculitis may suffer ICH because renal damage has resulted in accelerated hypertension. Despite the presence of systemic vasculitis, the ICH may then merely represent the consequences of hypertension. On the other hand, vasculitis can affect heart valves, leading to embolic brain infarction, or brain infarction can occur secondary to vasculitis of intracerebral vessels. Any of these infarctions may undergo hemorrhagic transformation, thereby producing ICH. The inflammatory process of the vasculitis itself may compromise the integrity of a vessel inside the brain, leading directly to hemorrhage. Many of these patients are prescribed anticoagulants, providing yet another potential source of bleeding. In the following paragraphs, the pathophysiologic events behind the uncommon causes of ICH are discussed, using a handful of specific disorders as examples. The specific disorders themselves are discussed at greater length in the sections that follow.

From Feldmann E (ed). *Intracerebral Hemorrhage*. Armonk, NY: Futura Publishing Company, Inc., © 1994.

Vessel Damage

Damage to the structural integrity of the vessel wall can lead to ICH, as discussed above for vasculitis. The deposition of complement, followed by the release of enzymes from inflammatory cells, is believed to contribute to weakening of the vessel wall in patients with cerebral vasculitis.

Patients with moya-moya disease develop progressive anterior circulation intracranial occlusions, with a compensatory network of small vessel collaterals centered at the base of the brain. While these patients suffer ischemia due to vascular occlusions, damage to and friability of the collateral vessels leads to hemorrhagic events later in life, which are commonly fatal. The collateral vessels are exposed to high volume flow and commonly exhibit weakening of the vessel wall secondary to fibrin deposition, wall thinning, and development of microaneurysms.[1,2]

Bleeding Diathesis

Intracerebral hemorrhage may occur in the setting of hematologic disorders, either hereditary or acquired. Anticoagulant- and thrombolytic-related hemorrhage have been discussed in other chapters. The precise events that initiate hemorrhage and, indeed, the vessel that ruptures are very difficult to identify. Some authorities believe that large hemorrhages represent the consequences of arterial rupture, while smaller, petechial hemorrhages reflect microvascular bleeding. Patients with leukemia in blast crisis are believed to develop ICH when white blood cells plug postcapillary venules.[3] Typically, the location, size, and clinical presentation of ICH in these patients are highly variable.

The relationship between aspirin and ICH is equivocal. No prospective data exist to unequivocally link aspirin use with a higher incidence of ICH. However, aspirin use is becoming increasingly prevalent. An analysis of an aggregate of clinical trials suggests a possible twofold excess risk of hemorrhagic stroke in patients treated with aspirin for stroke prevention.[4] Aspirin irreversibly acetylates and inactivates cyclooxygenase in platelets and endothelium. The mechanism whereby aspirin would lead to ICH and its interaction with other coexistent potential mechanisms of ICH are unknown.[5]

Acute Hemodynamic Changes

Perhaps the most important events underlying ICH in any setting are acute changes in blood pressure and blood volume, leading to autoregulatory failure and vascular rupture. Recent data suggest that the time of onset of ICH parallels the diurnal variation in blood pressure.[6] Moreover, persistent, severe hypertension may be the underlying factor responsible for dramatic expansion of a hematoma after hospital admission.[7] Transient, severe increases in blood pressure or blood volume may overwhelm arteries that are either intrinsically normal or abnormal.[8] The latter situation occurs when blood pressure increases suddenly in a patient whose vessels have been damaged by exposure to chronic hypertension. However, the underlying vessels may be normal when patients who abuse alcohol or sympathomimetics develop ICH (see other chapters). Similar events may occur in patients who develop ICH after exposure to very low temperatures[9] or dental work,[10] and in patients with delayed ICH after head trauma[8] and carotid endarterectomy.[11]

Patients with migraine have been reported to develop ICH after a typical attack. As in ICH associated with sympathomimetic abuse, transient hyperperfusion may follow a period of intense vasoconstriction. Resistance vessels may not adapt rapidly enough to avoid rupture.[12] Another example involves the occurrence of a lobar hematoma in an elderly normotensive patient treated with electroconvulsive therapy. This raises the possibility that even mild blood pressure changes in the elderly, who commonly harbor cerebral amyloid angiopathy, can lead to ICH.[13] In summary, whether ICH is due to chronic hypertension or any of the uncommon causes discussed in this chapter, a combination of pathophysiologic events may form the basis for bleeding. The following sections discuss the less common causes of ICH. Much of the information is presented in tabular form, with references. A detailed discussion of each of these entities is beyond the scope of this volume.

Mechanical

This section discusses ICH occurring in the setting of mechanical invasion of the central nervous system, typically on a therapeutic basis. The major etiologies, their incidence and associated features are summarized in Table 1.

Hematologic

The precise mechanism of ICH in patients with primary or secondary coagulopathies is often unknown. The coagulation disorder is presumed to act in concert with other pathophysiologic events to produce the hemorrhage. The diagnosis of coagulopathy is based upon a careful laboratory evaluation and a high index of suspicion, because the presentation of the hemorrhage is often atypical (unusual site, recurrent bleeding, no risk factors). Anticoagulation-related hemorrhages are discussed in a preceding chapter. Tables 2 and 3 summarize the major etiologies, and clues to their diagnosis and treatment, when a specific therapy is available. Consultation with a hematologist to evaluate and treat these disorders is strongly recommended, especially if surgery is

Table 1

Mechanical Causes of ICH in the Iatrogenic Setting

Clinical Scenario	ICH Incidence	Comment	Reference
Stereotactic biopsy of a mass lesion	< 3% develop ICH	Most survive; may be treated with thrombin administered via the biopsy cannula	14
Endovascular/surgical treatment of an AVM	< 15% develop ICH	Risk increased in posterior fossa and large AVMs with multiple feeders	15
Elective intracranial surgery, not for head trauma, perioperative platelets < 150,000/mm³	40% develop ICH	20% are fatal	16
Removal of chronic subdural hematoma; no underlying brain pathology or hypertension	5% develop ICH	ICH occurs immediately after drainage and may be due to sudden increase in cerebral blood flow	17
Subarachnoid pressure bolt, especially in the setting of coagulopathy	rare	ICH is severe in this setting	18
Postventriculostomy	< 2% develop ICH	Bleeding is intraventricular or parenchymal and usually not severe	19
Caudate implantation of medullary graft for Parkinsonism	5% develop ICH	May require surgical evacuation	20
Dural puncture for myelogram, intrathecal therapy, or analgesia	extremely rare		15
Angioplasty for vasospasm	Uncommon, but data are sparse	Concurrent heparinization is a risk factor	21, 22
Intrathecal thrombolysis for vasospasm	1/65 develop ICH	ICH was pre-existent and merely increased in volume	23–26

contemplated. The therapeutic recommendations detailed in Tables 2 and 3 should serve only as general guidelines.

Vasculitis

Intracerebral hemorrhage is an uncommon complication of vasculitis. The various mechanisms by which cerebral vasculitis can lead to ICH are discussed above. Both brain ischemia and hemorrhage can occur when vasculitis affects

Table 2
Hereditary Hematologic Causes of ICH

Etiology	Clues to Diagnosis	Specific Treatment	Reference
von Willebrand's disease	Usually not spontaneous; complicates surgery or trauma; $\frac{1}{3}$ fatal	Cryo, perhaps epsilon-aminocaproic acid	27
Factor VIII deficiency	Young patient, spontaneous ICH if factor levels < 1%; follows surgery or trauma if levels < 25%	Pure factor VIII or cryo	28, 29
Factor IX deficiency	Similar to factor VIII; deficiency can be acquired in nephrotic syndrome	Factor IX or FFP	30
Deficiency of factor VII, XIII or fibrinogen	ICH occurs spontaneously	For factor VII: FFP or factor concentrates; for XIII: FFP or cryo; for fibrinogen: cryo	31–33

FFP = fresh frozen plasma; cryo = cryoprecipitate.

the brain, and virtually any vessel of any size can be affected. ICH may be the presenting feature of vasculitis, or only one aspect of the complex manifestations of a multisystem disorder causing renal, pulmonary, skin, and perhaps peripheral neuropathic dysfunction. Seizures and cranial neuropathy are important clinical clues suggesting the presence of vasculitis. Diagnosis may be difficult, as cerebrospinal fluid abnormalities are nonspecific or altogether absent, imaging abnormalities are nonspecific, and angiography will be normal if only small arteries are affected. Even when angiography reveals the segmental narrowing and dilatation often associated with vasculitis, the differential diagnosis is still quite broad, including vasospasm from the hemorrhage itself, migraine, multiple emboli, and various other entities.

The neurologist caring for the patient with a systemic vasculitis and ICH will assume that ICH is due to a complication of the systemic disease, if the clinical and radiologic features of the hemorrhage are appropriate and the systemic diagnosis is firmly established. If the systemic diagnosis is not established, serologic studies or a biopsy of peripheral tissues may establish the nature of the systemic illness. Biopsy of the brain is a less commonly chosen option. In a significant number of patients, the brain biopsy may fail to reveal vasculitic changes. In such instances, the physician institutes treatment presumptively, based on the systemic features of the illness and any supportive serologic studies. However, it is important to attempt to obtain diagnostic tissue, even from the brain, especially when considering the serious toxicity associated with treatment of these disorders. Obviously, the patient with disease

Table 3
Acquired Hematologic Causes of ICH

Etiology	Clues to Diagnosis	Specific Treatment	Reference
Disseminated intravascular coagulation	Severe neoplastic, inflammatory, or infectious illness; low platelets, hemolysis, anemia; any CNS hemorrhage type and infarction may occur together	Treat primary problem, replace factors and blood components; transfuse platelets to > 150,000/μl; cryo to keep fibrinogen >150 mg/dl; FFP if PT/PTT increased	5, 34–36
Uremia	Increased bleeding time	DDAVP and cryo	37–39
Immune thrombocytopenic purpura	Platelets < 10,000/μl; usually serious ICH; may occur with lymphoproliferative disorder	Platelet transfusion, ± i.v. steroids, gamma globulin, pheresis, or splenectomy	40–43
Thrombotic thrombocytopenic purpura	Fever, low platelets, renal failure, hemolysis, focal neurologic findings; infarction more common than ICH	Plasma exchange with FFP	35
Multiple myeloma	Low platelets and amyloid deposition are risk factors	Treat primary disease; pheresis for platelet abnormalities	5, 44
Acute promyelocytic leukemia	Low platelets and procoagulant released by tumor cells are risk factors; DIC occurs, especially in type Fab M3	Treat primary disease; heparin ± cryo, FFP, platelet transfusions	45–49
Acute myelogenous leukemia	Platelets < 10,000/μl or consumptive coagulopathy, which are usually due to treatment	Treat primary disease; platelet transfusion to > 50,000/μl	49, 50
Chronic myelogenous leukemia	Platelets < 10,000/μl, due to primary disease or due to treatment	Treat primary disease; platelet transfusion to > 50,000/μl	5
Essential thrombocythemia	Abnormal platelet function and microinfarction common	Treat primary disease + thrombocytopheresis or platelet transfusion	51
L-Asparaginase	Used in treatment of acute lymphoblastic leukemia; ICH occurs especially in setting of coagulopathy	Stop drug; cryo for low fibrinogen ± FFP, platelet transfusion	52
Deficiency of vitamin K	Seriously ill hospitalized adult, especially on antibiotics	FFP; vitamin K	53

FFP = fresh frozen plasma; cryo = cryoprecipitate.

confined to the brain represents the most difficult diagnostic challenge in this setting.

Therapy is typically immunosuppressive and tailored to the nature of the primary, systemic vasculitis. The hemorrhage itself is treated supportively. Table 4 lists the vasculitic diseases more commonly associated with ICH.

Table 4
Vasculitic Causes of ICH and Clues to Their Diagnosis

Disease	Systemic Clues	Neurologic Clues	Diagnostic Approach	Treatment	Reference
Primary CNS angiitis	No systemic manifestations, by definition	Headache, encephalopathy, infarction, seizures, and subarachnoid hemorrhage also common	Biopsy of meninges and underlying brain	Prednisone and cyclophosphamide	54–56
Polyarteritis nodosa	Systemic disease common, especially fever, hypertension, skin, joint, gastrointestinal, and cardiac disease	Neuropathy, headache, seizures, and cerebral infarction also common	Biopsy of systemic tissue, muscle or nerve	Prednisone and cyclophosphamide	57–60
Wegener's granulomatosus	Renal and pulmonary involvement; joints, eyes, and cardiac abnormalities less common; **anticytoplasmatic antineutrophil antibody**	Peripheral and cranial neuropathy common; brain can also be involved by granuloma or contiguous extension from sinuses, as well as vasculitis	Pulmonary biopsy preferable to renal biopsy	Prednisone and cyclophosphamide	61–66
Systemic lupus erythematosus	Any organ may be involved; **antinuclear antibodies specific for double-stranded DNA**	Brain involvement common, but CNS vasculitis rare; encephalopathy, seizures, headache, infarction, and subarachnoid hemorrhage more common than ICH	Systemic serologies or biopsy of peripheral tissues	Prednisone	67, 68
Rheumatoid arthritis	Nodules and rheumatoid factor typically present in patients with ICH; **IgM rheumatoid factor**	None	Systemic serologies	Prednisone + other immune suppressants	69, 70
Sjögren's syndrome	Salivary gland inflammation; dry eyes; dry mouth; may have concomitant rheumatoid arthritis; **SSA and SSB**	Seizures, encephalopathy, and subarachnoid hemorrhage more common than ICH	Systemic serologies and salivary gland biopsy	Little data to support the use of steroids	71

Serologic tests in **bold** typeface.

Table 5
Infectious Causes of ICH

Disease/ Organism	Mechanism of ICH	Reference
Purulent meningitis	Venous occlusion	72
Tuberculosis	Damage to vessels by tuberculoma	73
Aspergillosis/other fungal infection	Arterial/venous thromboses with secondary hemorrhage or mycotic aneurysm	74, 75
Varicella zoster virus	Granulomatous angiitis secondary to viral infection	76
HIV	Either granulomatous angiitis, thrombocytopenia, toxoplasmosis, CMV, nonbacterial thrombotic endocarditis with embolism, metastatic Kaposi's sarcoma, or lymphoma	77, 78
HTLV-1	Cerebral vasculitis of the isolated angiitis type	79

Infectious

Infectious disorders may be associated with ICH, most often via the blood borne dissemination of organisms to cerebral vessels, with secondary vessel wall weakening, aneurysmal dilatation, and hemorrhage. Treatment involves antimicrobial therapy specific for the organism in question, with surgery to repair intracranial aneurysms in selected patients. Bacterial endocarditis was specifically discussed in the chapter on vascular malformations. Other infectious disorders and the mechanisms by which they produce ICH are listed in Table 5.

References

1. Suzuki J, Kodama N: Moyamoya disease: a review. *Stroke* 1983;14:104.
2. Taveras JM: Multiple progressive intracranial arterial occlusion: a syndrome of young adults. *Am J Roentgenol* 1969;106:235.
3. Fritz RD, Forkner CD, Freireich EJ: The association of fatal intracranial hemorrhage and "blastic crisis" in patients with acute leukemia. *N Engl J Med* 1959;261:59.
4. Mayo NE, Levy AR, Goldberg MS: Aspirin and hemorrhagic stroke. *Stroke* 1991;22:1213.
5. del Zoppo GJ, Mori E: Hematological causes of intracerebral hemorrhage and their treatment. *Neurosurg Clin North Am* 1992;3:637.
6. Sloan MA, Price TR, Foulkes MA, et al: Circadian rhythmicity of stroke onset. Intracerebral and subarachnoid hemorrhage. *Stroke* 1992;23:1420.

7. Bae HG, Lee KS, Yun IG, et al: Rapid expansion of hypertensive intracerebral hemorrhage. *Neurosurgery* 1992;31:35.
8. Caplan L: Intracerebral hemorrhage revisited. *Neurology* 1988;38:624.
9. Caplan LR, Neely S, Gorelick P: Cold-related intracerebral hemorrhage. *Arch Neurol* 1984;41:227.
10. Barbas N, Caplan L, Baquis G, et al: Dental chair intracerebral hemorrhage. *Neurology* 1987;37:511.
11. Caplan LR, Skillman JJ, Ojemann R, et al: Intracerebral hemorrhage following carotid endarterectomy. *Stroke* 1978;9:457.
12. Cole AJ, Aube M: Migraine with vasospasm and delayed intracerebral hemorrhage. *Arch Neurol* 1990;47:53.
13. Weisberg LA, Elliott D, Mielke D: Intracerebral hemorrhage following electroconvulsive therapy. *Neurology* 1991;41:1849.
14. Chimowitz MI, Barnett GH, Palmer J: Treatment of intractable arterial hemorrhage during stereotactic brain biopsy with thrombin. Report of three patients. *J Neurosurg* 1991;74:301.
15. Gibbons KJ, Guterman LR, Hopkins LN: Iatrogenic intracerebral hemorrhage. *Neurosurg Clin North Am* 1992;3:667.
16. Chan KH, Mann KS, Chan TK: The significance of thrombocytopenia in the development of postoperative intracranial hematoma. *J Neurosurg* 1989;71:38.
17. Modesti LM, Hodge CJ, Barnwell ML: Intracerebral hematoma after evacuation of chronic extracerebral fluid collections. *Neurosurgery* 1982;10:689.
18. Bobo H, Miller JD, Evans OB, et al: Delayed intracerebral hematoma at the site of a subarachnoid bolt pressure monitor. Case report. *J Neurosurg* 1986;64:673.
19. Narayan RK, Kishore PR, Becker DP, et al: Intracranial pressure: to monitor or not to monitor? A review of our experience with severe head injury. *J Neurosurg* 1982;56:650.
20. Lopez-Lozano JJ, Bravo G, Abascal J, et al: Grafting of perfused adrenal tissue into the caudate nucleus of patient's with Parkinson's disease. *J Neurosurg* 1991;75:234.
21. Linskey ME, Horton JA, Rao GR, et al: Fatal rupture of the intracranial carotid artery during transluminal angioplasty for vasospasm induced by subarachnoid hemorrhage. *J Neurosurg* 1991;74:985.
22. Higashida RT, Halbach VV, L.D. C, et al: Transluminal angioplasty for treatment of intracranial arterial vasospasm. *J Neurosurg* 1989;71:648.
23. Findlay JM, Weir BKA, Kassell NF, et al: Intracisternal recombinant tissue plasminogen activator after aneurysmal subarachnoid hemorrhage. *J Neurosurg* 1991;75:181.
24. Mizoi K, Yoshimoto T, Fujiwara S, et al: Prevention of vasospasm by clot removal and intrathecal bolus injection of tissue-type plasminogen activator: preliminary report. *Neurosurgery* 1991;28:807.
25. Ohman J, Servo A, Heiskanen O: Effect of intrathecal fibrinolytic therapy on clot lysis and vasospasm in patients with aneurysmal subarachnoid hemorrhage. *J Neurosurg* 1991;75:197.

26. Zabramski JM, Spetzler RF, Lee KS, et al: Phase I trial of tissue plasminogen activator for the prevention of vasospasm in patients with aneurysmal subarachnoid hemorrhage. *J Neurosurg* 1991;75:189.

27. Rapaport SI: Preoperative hemostatic evaluation. Which tests, if any? *Blood* 1983;61:229.

28. Kerr CB: Intracranial hemorrhage in hemophilia. *J Neurol Neurosurg Psychiat* 1964;27:166.

29. Vioconti EB, Hilgartener MW: Recognition and management of central nervous system hemorrhage in hemophilia. *Paediatrician* 1980;9:127.

30. Hendley DA, Lawrence JR: Factor IX deficiency in the nephrotic syndrome. *Lancet* 1967;1:1079.

31. Petri M, Ellman L, Carey R: Acquired factor XIII deficiency with chronic myelomonocytic leukemia. *Ann Intern Med* 1983;99:638.

32. Ragni MV, Lewis JH, Spero JH, et al: Factor VII deficiency. *Am J Hematol* 1981;10:79.

33. Ratnoff OD, Forman WB: Criteria for the differentiation of dysfibrinogenemic states. *Semin Hematol* 1976;13:141.

34. Mant MJ, King EG: Severe, acute disseminated intravascular coagulation. *Am J Med* 1979;67:557.

35. Silverstein A: Intracranial hemorrhage in patients with bleeding tendencies. *Neurology* 1991;36:310.

36. Schwartzman RJ, Hull JB: Neurologic complications of disseminated intravascular coagulation. *Neurology* 1982;32:791.

37. Janson P, Jubelirer SJ, Weinstein MJ, et al: Treatment of the bleeding tendency of uremia with cryoprecipitate. *N Engl J Med* 1980;303:1318.

38. Steiner RW, Coggins C, Carvalho ACA: Bleeding time in uremia. *Am J Hematol* 1979;7:107.

39. Mannucci P, Remuzzi G, Pusineri F, et al: Deamino-8-delta-arginine vasopressin shortens the bleeding time in uremia. *N Engl J Med* 1983;308:8.

40. Berchtold P, McMillan R: Therapy of chronic idiopathic thrombocytopenic purpura in adults. *Blood* 1989;74:2309.

41. Kelton JG, Gibbons S: Autoimmune platelet destruction: idiopathic thrombocytopenic purpura. *Semin Thromb Hemost* 1982;8:83.

42. McMillan R: Chronic idiopathic thrombocytopenic purpura. *N Engl J Med* 1981;304:135.

43. Novak R, Wilimas J: Plasmapheresis in catastrophic complications of idiopathic thrombocytopenic purpura. *J Pediatr* 1978;92:434.

44. Nilehn N, Nilsson IM: Coagulation studies in different types of myeloma. *Acta Medica Scand* 1966;179:194.

45. Andoh K, Kubota T, Takada M, et al: Tissue factor activity in leukemia cells. Special reference to disseminated intravascular coagulation. *Cancer* 1987;59:748.

46. Pollack A: Acute promyelocytic leukemia with disseminated intravascular coagulation. *Am J Clin Pathol* 1971;56:155.

47. Gralnick HR, Bagley J, Abrell E: Heparin treatment for the hemorrhagic diathesis of acute promyelocytic leukemia. *Am J Med* 1972;52:167.

48. Hoyle CF, Swirsky DM, Freedman L, et al: Beneficial effect of heparin in the management of patients with APL. *Br J Haematol* 1988;68:283.

49. Olson JD: Hemostasis and hematological conditions in intracerebral hemorrhage. In: Kaufman HH, ed: *Intracerebral Hematomas*. New York: Raven Press, 1992:151.

50. Leavy RA, Kahn SB, Brodsky I: Disseminated intravascular coagulation: a complication of therapy in acute myelomonocytic leukemia. *Cancer* 1970; 26:142.

51. Singh AK, Wetherley-Mein G: Microvascular occlusive lesions in primary thrombocythemia. *Br J Haematol* 1977;36:553.

52. Urban C, Sager WD: Intracranial bleeding during therapy with L-asparaginase in childhood acute lymphocytic leukemia. *Eur J Pediatr* 1981;137: 323.

53. Payne NR, Hasegawa DK: Vitamin K deficiency in newborns: a case report in alpha-1-antitrypsin deficiency and a review of factors predisposing to hemorrhage. *Pediatrics* 1984;73:712.

54. Biller J, Loftus CM, Moore SA, et al: Isolated central nervous system angiitis first presenting as spontaneous intracranial hemorrhage. *Neurosurgery* 1987;20:310.

55. Calabrese LH, Malleck JA: Primary angiitis of the central nervous system. Report of 8 new cases, review of the literature and proposal for diagnostic criteria. *Medicine* 1987;67:20.

56. Clifford-Jones RE, Love S, Gurusinghe N: Granulomatous angiitis of the central nervous system: a case with recurrent intracerebral hemorrhage. *J Neurol Neurosurg Psychiat* 1985;48:1054.

57. Moore PM, Cupps TR: Neurological complications of vasculitis. *Ann Neurol* 1983;14:155.

58. Conn DL: Update on systemic necrotizing vasculitis. *Mayo Clin Proc* 1989; 64:535.

59. Ford RG, Siekert RG: Central nervous system manifestations of periarteritis nodosa. *Neurology* 1965;15:114.

60. Moore PM, Fauci AS: Neurologic manifestations of systemic vasculitis: a retrospective and prospective study of the clinicopathological features and responses to therapy in 25 patients. *Am J Med* 1981;71:517.

61. Drachman DA: Neurologic complications of Wegener's granulomatosis. *Arch Neurol* 1963;8:45.

62. Fauci AS, Haynes BF, Katz P, et al: Wegener's granulomatosis: prospective clinical and therapeutic experience with 85 patients for 21 years. *Ann Intern Med* 1983;98:76.

63. Hoffman GS, Leavitt RW, Fleisher TA, et al: Treatment of Wegener's granulomatosis with intermittent high-dose intravenous cyclophosphamide. *Am J Med* 1990;89:403.

64. Nishino H, Rubino RA, Parisi JE: The spectrum of neurologic involvement in Wegener's granulomatosis. *Neurology* 1993;43:1334.

65. Nishino H, Rubino FA, DeRemee RA, et al: Neurologic involvement in Weg-

ener's granulomatosis: an analysis of 324 consecutive patients at the Mayo Clinic. *Ann Neurol* 1993;33:4.

66. Berlit P, Moore PM, Bluestein HG: Vasculitis, rheumatic disease and the neurologist: the pathophysiology and diagnosis of neurologic problems in systemic disease. *Cerebrovasc Dis* 1993;3:139.

67. Ellis SG, Verity MA: Central nervous system involvement in systemic lupus erythematosus: a review of neuropathologic findings in 57 cases, 1955–1977. *Semin Arthritis Rheum* 1979;8:212.

68. Johnson RT, Richardson EP: The neurologic manifestations of systemic lupus erythematosus. *Medicine* 1968;47:337.

69. Ramos S, Mandybur T: Cerebral vasculitis in rheumatoid arthritis. *Arch Neurol* 1975;32:271.

70. Watson P, Fekete J, Deck J: Central nervous system vasculitis in rheumatoid arthritis. *Can J Neurol Sci* 1977;4:269.

71. Alexander GE, Provost TT, Stevens MB, et al: Sjogren syndrome: central nervous system manifestations. *Neurology* 1981;31:1391.

72. Schochet SS, Nelson J: Vasculitis and vasculopathies. In: Kaufman HH, ed: *Intracerebral Hematomas.* New York: Raven Press, 1992:127.

73. Talamas O, Del Brutto OH, Garcia-Ramos G: Brain-stem tuberculoma. An analysis of 11 patients. *Arch Neurol* 1989;46:529.

74. Horton B, Abbott G, Porro R: Fungal aneurysms of intracranial vessels. *Arch Neurol* 1976;33:577.

75. Hadley MN, Martin NA, Spetzler RF, et al: Multiple intracranial aneurysms due to *Coccidioides immitis* infection. Case report. *J Neurosurg* 1987;66:453.

76. Fukumoto S, Kinjo M, Hokamura K, et al: Subarachnoid hemorrhage and granulomatous angiitis of the basilar artery: demonstration of the varicella zoster virus in the basilar artery lesions. *Stroke* 1986;17:1024.

77. Mizusawa H, Hirano H, Llena JF, et al: Cerebrovascular lesions in acquired immune deficiency syndrome (AIDS). *Acta Neuropathol* 1988;76:451.

78. Trenkwalder P, Trenkwalder C, Feiden W, et al: Toxoplasmosis with early intracerebral hemorrhage in a patient with the acquired immunodeficiency syndrome. *Neurology* 1992;42:436.

79. Smith D, Lucas S, Jacewicz M: Multiple cerebral hemorrhages in HTLV-I-associated myelopathy. *Neurology* 1993;43:412.

Part III

Diagnosis of Intracerebral Hemorrhage

Chapter 11

Clinical Syndromes of Intracerebral Hemorrhage

Lawrence M. Brass, MD

Intracerebral hemorrhage (ICH) accounts for about 10% to 15% of all strokes. The syndrome of the chronically hypertensive patient who presents with sudden onset of severe headache, vomiting, depressed consciousness, and focal neurologic signs has been associated with ICH since the autopsy studies of Aring and Merritt reported in 1935.[1] The classic teaching that nearly all cases of spontaneous ICH occur in older people with chronic hypertension may not be correct.

Although stroke is predominantly a disease of the elderly, many young people get stroke. The incidence of stroke in young adults is twice that of multiple sclerosis, and hemorrhage accounts for about half of all strokes in young and middle-aged people.[2] Although much attention has been focused on subarachnoid hemorrhage (SAH) in this age group, recent community-based studies using computed tomography (CT) suggest that ICH is at least as common as SAH and just as deadly.[3]

In the past, most ICHs were attributed to hypertension, even if the hypertension was first noted following the hemorrhage. The role of acute hypertension in ICH is speculative.[4] For chronic hypertension to be convincingly implicated as the etiology for a hemorrhage, it should have been present prior to the ictus with other evidence of hypertensive vasculopathy in the eyes, heart, brain, or kidney. As few as half of the cases of ICH may be caused by hypertension.[5,6]

Improved neurodiagnostic techniques have expanded the list of known causes of ICH (Table 1), and several large retrospective surveys over the past decade have helped clarify the relative importance of these factors. Commonly cited nonhypertensive etiologies include amyloid angiopathy, small vascular malformations, brain tumors, drug abuse (cocaine, amphetamines), and the use of anticoagulants. Intracerebral hemorrhage has also been reported in a wide variety of atypical situations such as exposure to cold weather, drug use

From Feldmann E (ed). *Intracerebral Hemorrhage.* Armonk, NY: Futura Publishing Company, Inc., © 1994.

Table 1
Causes of ICH and Clinical Clues

Etiology	Clinical Clues
Hypertension (HTN)	
Chronic Effects	History of HTN, myocardial infarction, stroke; signs of retinal, cardiac, or renal evidence of hypertensive changes; usually a single hemorrhage
Malignant	
Hypertension	Most common in second to fourth decades in those with a history of renal disease; sudden onset of headache, nausea, vomiting, visual symptoms, anxiety, and agitation; seizures may occur; optic disc swelling and "cotton-wool" spots seen on funduscopic examination
Drugs	Most reported cases are in chronic uses with hemorrhage occurring in association with recent use
Cocaine	Increased cardiac contraction, increased blood pressure, tachycardia, peripheral vasoconstriction, dilated pupils, and fever. May be sleeplessness, irritability, agitation, dysphoria, paranoia, hallucinations, or frank psychosis
Pseudoephedrine	Tachycardia, hypertension, and a history of recent use of decongestants or bronchodilators
Amphetamines	Excitement, agitation, tremor, talkativeness, insomnia, increased tendon reflexes. Other sympathetic effects include tachycardia, hypertension, peripheral vasoconstriction, and fever; in high dose, coma and vascular collapse may occur
Methamphetamine	(Amphetamine derivative, speed) see amphetamines above
Talwin-pyribenzamine	Analgesia, sedation along with dysphoric and psychotomimetic symptoms including hallucinations
Phenylpropanolamine	Young women with no history of hypertension. Eating disorders, with excessive doses, are commonly seen for diet preparations. History of recent cold/flu may suggest use of cough suppressants or decongestants
Phencyclidine	Euphoria, emotional liability, symptoms of diffuse numbness; intermediate doses—confusion, excitation, body disorientation, decreased sensory perception; higher doses—psychosis, myoclonus, nystagmus, seizures, coma
Vascular abnormalities	Younger patients without a history of hypertension
Cavernous angiomas	Tend to be multiple with a family history; there may be a preceding history of headache or seizure
Saccular aneurysms	Similar preceding symptoms (sentinel bleed), focal syndrome corresponding to common location for aneurysms
Arteriovenous malformations	Often history of seizures, headache, or progressive neurologic deficits. Larger and dural AVMs may produce cranial bruit or tinnitus. In more severe cases, signs of hydrocephalus or cardiac failure
Mycotic aneurysms	Associated endocarditis often with cardiac murmur, fever, and sytstemic embolization
Abnormal Arteries	
Arteritis	Often preceding headache, prior focal neurologic symptoms (including infarction), seizures, and progressive cognitive decline
Amyloid angiopathy	Older patients, especially normotensive or with preceding dementia, recurrent bleeds (simultaneous hematomas); parietal and occipital syndromes most common

(continued)

Table 1 *(continued)*

Etiology	*Clinical Clues*
Bleeding Diatheses	
Fibrinolytic agents	The use of fibrinolytic agents is usually obvious, but should always be considered in the setting of myocardial infarction or arterial thrombosis
Anticoagulants	More prolonged bleeding, may occur in the setting of an acute ischemic stroke, high prothrombin time
Blood dyscrasias/ coagulopathy	Presence of prior bleeding tendency (mucosal or easy bruising) or family history of bleeding disorder
Head Trauma	
Brain contusion	Usually multiple, especially involving syndromes of inferior frontal and anterior temporal lobe
Delayed hemorrhage	Worsening of original deficit, especially in patients with coagulopathy secondary to trauma. May also present as "Spät" hemorrhage, ie, apoplectic appearance of a deficit after an asymptomatic period (may be up to weeks, but usually less than 48 hours) following head trauma
Pre-existing Lesions	New neurologic deficit, or worsening of a previous subtle deficit, in the setting of nonspecific neurologic symptoms such as headache, decreased mental performance
Tumors—primary	Atypical ICH syndromes because of the hemispheric white matter location of primary tumors associated with bleeding (glioblastoma multiform)
Tumors—secondary	Lobar syndromes (superficial) most commonly seen (corticosubcortical location most common site for metastatic tumors). Pre-existing symptoms associated with the most common primary tumors are in the lung (bronchogenic carcinoma), skin (melanoma), pelvis (choriocarcinoma), or kidney (renal cell cancer). Most of these tumors are malignant and signs and symptoms related to the primary tumor are present.
Granulomas	Associated with chronic inflammatory process, most commonly tuberculosis or syphilis. May be history of seizures, focal deficit, or underlying infection; often silent
Meningitis	Recent fever, headache, seizures, impaired consciousness, and stiff neck
Ischemic stroke	Sudden onset of focal deficit with later worsening; recent use of anticoagulants, antiplatelet agents, or thrombolytic therapy
Abscess	Recent history of headache, drowsiness, seizures, and focal deficits. May have prior infection in ear, sinus, or lung
Genetic	
Familial ICH	Younger age, autosomal dominant pattern, ancestry in Iceland or the Netherlands
Spontaneous	No prior neurologic syndrome; no history of vascular risk factors

(phenylpropanolamine), severe dental pain, surgery for trigeminal neuralgia, embolic cerebral infarction, carotid endarterectomy, following cardiac surgery, and as a late consequence of head trauma.

Intracerebral hemorrhages more commonly occur during the day, with a peak in the morning after awakening. The onset of hemorrhage is often associated with activity. One third are associated with moderate or strenuous activity at onset.[7] It is very uncommon for a patient to awaken with an ICH. The clinical syndrome of transient ischemic attacks (TIAs) usually does not occur, although prodromal symptoms may be reported. They are usually nonspecific, such as headache, syncope, and confusion, and do not suggest a focal process.

The initial symptoms of ICH are usually focal and vary with the size and location of the hematoma. The onset is often abrupt. In larger hemorrhages, there may be bilateral signs from the onset, reflecting that the process of hemorrhage does not respect a single vascular territory. Tendon reflexes may be abnormal bilaterally. As with ischemic stroke, there may be a period of several hours of hyporeflexia before the development of hyperreflexia.

More than half of patients show progression over hours or days, especially those taking anticoagulants.[6] One third have maximal symptoms at onset.[8,9] In some instances, the syndrome may evolve slowly over days, simulating a brain tumor. Fewer than 5% have stepwise progression or fluctuation, profiles suggesting an ischemic etiology for the stroke syndrome.

The reasons for a progressive, deteriorating course are still being investigated. Initial deficits and worsening may be associated with tissue disruption, mass effect, edema, diaschisis, and progressive bleeding. The role of rebleeding, especially within the first 6 hours, is also being reevaluated. Early work by Herbstein and Schaumburg suggested that bleeding does not occur after presentation.[10] They labeled red blood cells with ^{51}Cr and injected them into patients shortly after presentation of ICH. Those who came to autopsy were examined for the presence of ^{51}Cr in the intracerebral hematoma, which would indicate that bleeding had occurred after injection of the labeled red blood cells. This was not found. More recently, however, reports have appeared with serial CT scans, performed within hours of the onset of the hemorrhage, demonstrating enlargement of the hematoma.[11,12]

The clinical syndromes associated with ICH have also been revised during the past 2 decades since the introduction of CT scanning. Prior to this, the syndromes associated with ICH were affected by a severe selection bias. Before the introduction of CT scanning, the diagnosis of hemorrhage was often made only at autopsy. Many hematomas do not become large enough to be fatal. In the past, small hemorrhages were diagnosed as ischemic infarctions and many clinical syndromes of ICH went unrecognized in clinical reports.

The clinical syndrome associated with an ICH is determined primarily by the location and size of the hematoma. In addition, dissection along white matter tracts or rupture into the ventricular system or subarachnoid space can also profoundly affect the clinical presentation. Secondary signs are usually related to herniation or increased intracranial pressure. These signs reflect compression of neural tissue from the hematoma or edema, infarction from entrapment of vascular structures, and hydrocephalus from occlusion of cerebrospinal fluid (CSF) pathways.

The incorporation of CT scanning into the management of patients with stroke has had a great impact on brain hemorrhage. The diagnosis can now be reliably made. The improved detection of minor cases of brain hemorrhage has led to an increased incidence, decreased mortality, and improved outcome, as well as expansion of the clinical syndromes of ICH.[13]

Symptoms Associated with ICH

In this chapter, we will consider two broad categories of clinical manifestations of ICH. First, there are signs and symptoms related to the specific location of hemorrhage in the brain. These are outlined in Table 2 and are reviewed in detail later in this chapter. Second, there are core features common to all ICHs. This includes abrupt onset, features of intracranial hypertension (headache, vomiting, impaired consciousness), and signs of meningeal irritation or stretching. The frequency and severity of these symptoms varies with the size, location,

Table 2
Brain Hemorrhages: Common and Clinical Syndromes

Location	Syndrome
Putaminal	Hemiparesis (smooth and steady onset); may progress to involve hemisensory loss, hemianopia, and aphasia (dominant hemisphere) or neglect (nondominant hemisphere); often associated with gaze deviation. Syndrome may progress to coma and death
Lobar	
Occipital	Pain around eye and dense hemianopsia
Temporal	Mild pain anterior to ear, aphasia (posterior), partial field defect
Frontal	Begins with severe arm weakness, minimal leg and face weakness, and frontal headache. Behavior changes, including abulia, are often seen
Parietal	Anterior temporal headache, hemisensory deficit; may also see cognitive and behavioral abnormalities along with visual neglect
Thalamic	Initial deficit of hemisensory loss, later hemiparesis. With enlarging size, there may be vertical gaze palsy, retraction nystagmus, skew deviation, loss of convergence, ptosis and miosis, anisocoria, or unreactive pupils. If the hematoma is large, coma may be present from the onset. Compression of CSF pathways may lead to hydrocephalus
Cerebellar	Sudden onset of nausea, vomiting, and inability to walk. Also present may be headache, dizziness, impaired consciousness, appendicular ataxia, facial palsy, and ipsilateral gaze palsy
Pontine	Rapid onset of quadriplegia, decerebrate posturing, pinpoint pupils, oculomotor disturbances (bilateral horizontal gaze palsy), fever, and coma
Caudate	Headache, vomiting, decreased alertness, and stiff neck, because of their common association with intraventricular extension

and mechanism of the hemorrhage. These nonfocal symptoms are seen in about half of all cases. These are covered below.

Headache

Although headache is an important symptom suggestive of ICH, severe headache is present at onset in only 30% to 40% of cases. One third of patients do not report any headache. Headache is most commonly seen with superficial and larger hemorrhages and those more likely to stretch the meninges. Lobar, cerebellar, and caudate hemorrhages are the locations most commonly associated with headache. The combination of headache with vomiting, especially if present at onset of the syndrome, suggests a cerebellar hemorrhage.[14]

Seizures

Seizures are associated with nontraumatic ICH in about 15% of cases.[15,16] This most often occurs at the onset of the hemorrhage, while 20% are delayed. Seizures rarely have onset beyond 4 months after bleeding.[16] About two thirds of seizures are generalized, and the remainder are focal. Focal seizures involve the body contralateral to the hemorrhage.

The incidence of seizures varies with the location of the hemorrhage. Hematomas involving the cerebrum are likely to be associated with seizures, which are most common with lobar hemorrhages, less so far basal ganglia, and rarely seen with bleeding in the thalamus, brainstem, or cerebellum. Also, extension of blood into the cerebral cortex is eight times more likely to be associated with seizures.[15] There is no association with the size of the bleed, hydrocephalus, shift of intracranial structures, or extension into the subarachnoid space or ventricular system. Seizures at onset and recurrent seizures are more commonly associated with an underlying neoplastic or vascular etiology for the hemorrhage.[16]

The occurrence of seizures is unrelated to level of consciousness on admission, the Glasgow coma score, or clinical features such as headache, vomiting, acute hypertension, respiratory changes, focal motor or sensory deficits, or cranial nerve abnormalities.[15] There may be an increased incidence of seizures in blacks. Patient with a bleeding diathesis (anticoagulation or thrombocytopenia) were also more likely to have seizures.

Impaired Consciousness

Alterations in consciousness can occur in a variety of settings in brain hemorrhage. Increased intracranial pressure can lead to depressed consciousness and coma. Increased intracranial pressure can be seen with SAH or obstructive hydrocephalus. Locally, hematomas can lead to impaired consciousness by interruption of the reticular activating system and ascending projections. At least half of patients have some alteration in consciousness. About 20% of patients present in coma.[8] Coma at onset is suggestive of pontine hemorrhage.[14] Coma is associated with a very poor prognosis. An exception is thalamic and intraventricular hemorrhage, where good recovery can be seen even with initially impaired consciousness. In lobar hemorrhage, impaired consciousness is associated with lateral shifts greater than 8 mm) of the pineal gland.[17,18] Other mechanisms for stupor and coma include diencephalic or upper brainstem destruction or distortion by the hematoma, with interruption of reticular activating system and projections, or hydrocephalus.[18]

Nausea and Vomiting

Nausea and vomiting are common in ICH. Vomiting is more common with posterior fossa (69%) versus hemispheric (39%) hemorrhage.[8] It is especially common in cerebellar hemorrhage.

Differential Diagnosis of the Clinical Syndrome

The differential diagnosis of the clinical syndromes associated with ICH include SAH, ischemic stroke, hypertensive encephalopathy, meningitis, brain abscess, and a variety of other pathologies (Table 1).

A key factor in the initial management of patients with an acute stroke syndrome is the differentiation of ischemic infarction from brain hemorrhage. Although there is overlap, the clinical syndromes of ICH differ from those of ischemia. In ischemic stroke, the infarction follows the course of a vascular territory. In ICH, the hematoma usually dissects along white matter fiber tracts and may affect several vascular territories.

The history and physical examination do not reliably distinguish between hemorrhage and ischemia. Brain imaging will remain the standard where the technology is available. There are, however, clinical features which suggest a hemorrhagic mechanism in a patient presenting with an acute stroke syndrome (Table 3).[19]

In many parts of the world, cost concerns limit the use of brain imaging in acute stroke. In these settings, clinicians must rely on simple clinical findings to help distinguish between hemorrhage and infarction. The Siriraj Stroke Score[20] uses five clinical variables to differentiate cerebral hemorrhages from infarctions: dulled consciousness, vomiting, headache, and higher diastolic blood pressure were predictors of hemorrhage. The presence of vascular risk factors such as diabetes, claudication, or angina was associated with infarction.

Table 3
Differentiation Between Brain Infarction and Hemorrhage

Factors Associated with Hemorrhage	Factors Associated with Infarction
• Sudden onset of headache, vomiting, and stiff neck • Drowsiness or loss of consciousness (within 24 hours) • High diastolic blood pressure after 24 hours • Bilateral extensor plantar responses	• History of hypertension, diabetes, angina, or claudication • TIA, stroke, or myocardial infarction within 6 months • Aortic or mitral murmur • Atrial fibrillation, cardiomyopathy or cardiac failure, or cardiomegaly on chest x-ray

In applying their rules, about 20% had equivocal scores. For those with suggestive scores, the instrument correctly predicted 89% of hemorrhages and 93% of infarctions.[20] The incidence of cerebral hemorrhage is higher among Asian peoples, and the results may not directly apply to Western populations. The Siriraj Stroke Score[20] was devised in Thailand, where up to half of all strokes are hemorrhagic. This may be due to genetic differences and poorer control of hypertension.

Stroke scoring systems such as the Siriraj Stroke Score may be useful in nations with very limited access to imaging technology, but may not perform as well in industrialized nations. It is unlikely that this type of information will be useful for the hospital evaluation of stroke patients; however, this type of scoring system could prove useful in the field. As thrombolytic agents are introduced into the clinical management of stroke, it is highly likely that the earlier thrombolysis can be achieved, the better. If clinical criteria applied by emergency personnel in the field could reasonably differentiate between ischemia and hemorrhage, it may be possible to identify a subgroup with a very high likelihood of an ischemic syndrome. In this group, there may be a high enough risk-benefit ratio to justify the use of a thrombolytic agent, especially if the therapy is highly effective and the effect is strongly time dependent.[21]

Syndromes by Location

The most common sites for ICH are shown in Table 4.[22,23] The clinical syndromes for all forms of parenchymal brain hemorrhage have been dramatically revised since the application of CT scanning. Many syndromes attributed to ischemia are now recognized to be caused by hemorrhage. Parenchymal hemorrhages are now recognized to cause nearly all the syndromes also associated with large and small ischemic strokes.

Putaminal Hemorrhage

This is the most common site for ICH, accounting for 30% to 50% of ICHs. The medial putamen is the most common site of bleeding, followed by the poste-

Table 4
Location of Primary ICH

Location	Frequency
Putamen	30% to 50%
Lobe	20% to 30%
Thalamus	10% to 15%
Cerebellum	8% to 10%
Pons	7% to 10%
Caudate	4%
Other	5%

rior and anterior regions.[24] The internal capsule, thalamocortical radiations, the thalamus itself, and optic radiations are all in this region. The classic syndrome for putaminal hemorrhage is an abrupt onset with smooth, steady progression of hemiplegia, hemisensory deficits, and visual field defects.[25]

A motor deficit is nearly always present because of the proximity to the internal capsule. Sensory deficits are seen in 65% of cases.[25] Other signs commonly seen include conjugate eye deviation toward the side of the hemorrhage. If the dominant hemisphere is involved, an aphasia may be present. With nondominant hemisphere putaminal hemorrhage, neglect for the clinical deficit can be seen.

Putaminal hemorrhages may be large enough to interrupt or compress the arcuate fasciculus. This large white matter bundle was believed to be associated with conduction aphasia; however, this is rarely seen with putaminal hemorrhage.[26] Because most aphasia syndromes were originally described in patients with ischemic stroke involving the cerebral cortex, it is not surprising that the classic aphasias are usually not seen with these deep hemorrhages.[27]

Because these hemorrhages are deep and often do not distort the meninges, headache is usually not a prominent feature. It is seen only in one quarter of patients. Of those with headache, only half reported the headache at the onset of hemorrhage.[22] The clinical deficit may evolve over several hours. Just over half of cases are associated with a smooth and progressive onset, while one third present with a deficit maximal at onset. The size of the hemorrhage determines both the clinical syndrome and the prognosis. Small hemorrhages usually result in moderate weakness and sensory loss. Larger hemorrhages are associated with greater amounts of weakness and, additionally, hemianopia, lateral gaze preference, and aphasia. Those hemorrhages extending into the brainstem may be associated with third nerve palsies or vertical gaze abnormalities from midbrain involvement. Compression of the reticular activating system or its cortical projections results in impaired consciousness or coma. In the largest hemorrhages, coma may be present early. This is a very poor prognostic sign.

Small putaminal hemorrhages may mimic lacunar syndromes such as pure motor weakness[28] or dysarthria clumsy hand syndrome.[29] For the smaller hemorrhages, the clinical syndrome may provide information about where in the putamen the hemorrhage is located.[30] The anterior putamen, supplied by the recurrent artery of Heubner, is associated with contralateral gaze paresis (eyes deviated toward hemorrhage). This may also be seen with midputaminal hemorrhages, and much less commonly with small posteriorly located hematomas. Although they may differ from the classic aphasia syndromes described in patients with ischemic syndromes, more anteriorly located putaminal hemorrhages are associated with poorly articulated, sparse speech resembling a Broca's aphasia.

The medial putamen is adjacent to the internal capsule, globus pallidus, caudate nucleus, and near the lateral ventricles. Weakness is the cardinal symptom for hematomas in this location.[8,24,31] Very small hemorrhages here may mimic a lacunar stroke with a pure motor syndrome.[28] Hemichorea has also been reported with small hemorrhages in this region.[32] Those extending more posteriorly, affecting the internal capsule, may have sensory abnormalities including impaired joint position sense and contralateral ataxisa.[30] Another lacunar syndrome, ataxic hemiparesis, may be mimicked by hemorrhage in this area or in the internal capsule.[33] Those extending even further posteriorly into the posterior white matter can cause visual field defects.[31]

The lateral putamen is beneath the insula. Autonomic changes and aphasia may be present. From this location, the hematoma may dissect into the Sylvian fissure and subarachnoid space with a resultant syndrome of SAH.

Posterior putaminal hematomas can cause a fluent aphasia resembling a Wernicke's aphasia. A posterior putaminal hematoma with aphasia, hemisensory changes, and a visual field defect may be difficult to distinguish clinically from an inferior division middle cerebral artery infarction.[34] In the nondominant hemisphere, anterior putaminal hemorrhages may be associated with abulia and motor impersistence. The more posterior hematomas can present with parietal symptoms including contralateral neglect, anosognosia, constructional apraxia, and dysprosody of speech.[30,31]

Lobar Hemorrhage

Lobar hemorrhages arise in the hemispheric white matter. This type of hemorrhage is important to identify because there is a better prognosis. Also important is identification of candidates for surgical evacuation of the hematoma, which may improve the outcome.

The syndrome will vary with location of the hematoma, which is most commonly parietal-occipital. The onset of the clinical syndrome, though rapid, typically evolves over minutes to an hour.[23,35]

Seizures are most common with this type of intracranial hemorrhage because the blood is adjacent to or directly involves the cortex. Similarly, severe headache is relatively more common (70% to 80%)[23,35] in this type of hemorrhage because of proximity to the superficial vessels and meninges. The location of the headache is related to the innervation of the meninges than the location of the hematoma.

Small hemorrhages can occur in nearly any location within the brain. Non-hypertensive etiologies such as a vascular malformation should be strongly considered when the hemorrhage occurs in an atypical area, for example a small frontal hemorrhage deep in the white matter.

Frontal Lobe

Contralateral weakness and severe bifrontal headache, worse on the side of hemorrhage, are the classic signs of a frontal lobe hemorrhage.[35] Seizures, frontal release signs (sucking, grasping), lethargy, and apathy are also seen. With larger hemorrhages, gaze preference or supranuclear gaze palsy, with eyes deviated toward the side of the lesion, may be seen. The presence of frontal lobe signs out of proportion to hemiparesis suggests a hemorrhage in the frontal lobe.[30,35] Pure motor monoparesis and hemiparesis have been described with ICH confined to the primary motor area.[36]

Parietal Lobe

In parietal hemorrhages, contralateral sensory changes and parietal or temporal headache[35] are associated with mild weakness, as 40% of the corticospinal tract arises from neurons posterior to the Rolandic fissure.[37] Gerstmann's Syndrome (finger agnosia, confusion of laterality, agraphia, and acalculia) was originally described with ICH in the dominant hemisphere.[38] Constructional and dressing apraxias are commonly seen with hemorrhages in the nondominant parietal hemisphere.

Temporal Lobe

Interruption of the optic radiations in the temporal lobes results in a hemianopia or quadrantanopia. Headache may be referred to the ear.[35] Hemorrhage in the posterior region of the dominant hemisphere may result in a Wernicke's aphasia or related syndrome, such as impaired comprehension with good repetition. Hematoma in this location may also present with only agitation, delirium, and minimal motor or sensory loss. Larger hemorrhages are associated with uncal herniation syndromes.

Occipital Lobe

The headaches associated with occipital hemorrhage are often referred to the area around the ipsilateral eye.[35] This is because the majority of the supratentorial meninges are supplied by the ophthalmic division of the trigeminal nerve. Visual field defects are the most common neurologic sign. Weakness and sensory loss are uncommon, but have been reported, possibly due to diaschisis or secondary to compression from upper midbrain shifts.

Thalamic Hemorrhage

The thalamus is deep within the cerebral hemispheres. In addition to serving as a major relay center for ascending fiber pathways, with widespread reciprocal connections with the cerebral cortex, the thalamus lies adjacent to major white matter tracts such as the optic radiations and the internal capsule. The classic syndrome of thalamic hemorrhage begins with widespread hemisensory loss. Depending on the size of the lesion, the adjacent internal capsule is usually involved, resulting in weakness. The weakness is less severe than the sensory loss. Headache is uncommon.[25]

Many of the signs associated with thalamic hemorrhage can be seen in a variety of stroke syndromes. The ocular motility disturbances, however, strongly suggest the diagnosis of thalamic hemorrhage.[39] The most frequent abnormalities are vertical gaze palsies, often with downward eye deviation, and convergence spasm. Miotic pupils are seen in over half the patients, usually bilaterally.[40] When anisocoria is present, the smaller pupil is usually ipsilateral to the lesion. When pupillary dilatation is seen, transtentorial herniation may be present.

In dominant hemisphere thalamic lesions, aphasia, disorientation, and memory disturbances may be seen.[41] The aphasia is often fluent, with paraphasic errors and neologisms. Although similar to Wernicke's aphasia, repetition is usually not significantly impaired.[27] The aphasic syndrome may also begin with a brief period, lasting hours or days, of mutism. Also described are aphasic syndromes characterized by brief periods of drowsiness with logorrhea and neologistic paraphasias with decreasing vocal volume eventually leading to silence, alternating with alert periods with little or no deficits in speech or language.[42] Although uncommon, this fluctuating language deficit is characteristic of thalamic lesions.

With nondominant lesions, there may be constructional apraxia and impaired visuospatial performance.[41] Contralateral hemineglect is also seen in thalamic hemorrhage with either dominant or nondominant lesions.[43]

Extension of the hemorrhage caudally into the upper brainstem is common, resulting in ocular abnormalities. Vertical gaze palsy, downward eye deviation and paresis of upward gaze, retraction nystagmus, skew deviation, loss of convergence or hyperconvergence (pseudo-VIth palsy), ptosis and miosis, anisocoria, or unreactive pupils may be seen.[22] Conjugate gaze palsy may also be seen. The deviation may be toward the lesion, as is seen in more superficial cerebral lesions, or the "wrong way," with the eyes looking away from the side of the hemorrhage.[44]

Stupor or coma at onset is more common in patients with intraventricular extension of a thalamic hemorrhage. Alteration in consciousness is also seen in the larger hemorrhages and with obstructive hydrocephalus secondary to compression of the ventricles or Aqueduct of Sylvius.

As with putaminal hemorrhages, the use of CT scans has expanded the early, classic syndrome of thalamic hemorrhage derived from larger, fatal hemorrhages. The syndromes associated with small thalamic hemorrhages (less than 3 cm) have recently been correlated with their intrathalamic location. Kawahara and colleagues described four types based on topographic location.[45]

Posterolateral hematomas are the most common small thalamic hemorrhage. They arise from the posterolateral inferior thalamic arteries and cause severe sensory and motor deficits. The lateral part of the thalamus abuts the posterior limb of the internal capsule. Small hemorrhages in this area may cause syndromes similar to those seen with internal capsule lesions, but there is an important difference in the clinical presentation. Simultaneous sensory and motor involvement is rarely seen with ischemic lesions of the internal capsule, because the perforating arteries supplying the sensory and motor fibers typically originate in different circulations. Although sensory-motor strokes do occur from ischemia, they are relatively uncommon.

Dysesthesias are a sign of lateral thalamic injury. Ataxia and choreiform movements have been reported for thalamic hemorrhages.[46] Ataxic hemiparesis has also been described in association with small hemorrhages. In these cases, hypesthesia was also present.[47]

The prognosis for hematomas in this region varies with the extent of the hemorrhage. Those confined to the anterior two thirds of the thalamus usually show significant improvement. If the hematoma extends laterally through the internal capsule, there is usually little recovery.

Medial hematomas are associated with alterations in the level of consciousness during the acute stage, followed by behavioral, prefrontal, signs.[48] These signs include loss of spontaneity, speaking to oneself, change in character, memory disturbance, and impaired learning, possibly due to injury of the dorsomedial nucleus and its connections to prefrontal cortex.

The alterations in consciousness associated with medial thalamic lesions can occur because of extension into the ventricular system. About half of thalamic hemorrhages extend medially into the ventricular system. Ventricular extension is associated with more severe deficits and higher mortality. Vomiting, nuchal rigidity, severe headache, and impaired consciousness are more common in those patients with intraventricular extension of a thalamic hemorrhage.[43] Impaired consciousness can also follow injury to the intralaminar nuclei. The intralaminar nuclei help maintain consciousness through connections with the midbrain reticular formation and cortical projections.[37]

Anterolateral hematomas result in mild prefrontal signs, with only mild sensory changes or weakness. The prefrontal signs are similar to those reported in medial thalamic hematomas and occur because of compression of tracts from the thalamus to the prefrontal cortex in the anterior limb of the internal capsule.

Dorsal hematomas are associated with ipsilateral parieto-occipital signs. In the dominant hemisphere there is often an aphasia. In the nondominant hemisphere there are constructional apraxia and topographic memory changes. These patients usually have mild deficits and make an excellent recovery.

Cerebellar Hemorrhage

The syndrome of cerebellar hemorrhage is among the most important to recognize. The morbidity and mortality associated with cerebellar hemorrhage is strongly dependent on prompt and accurate diagnosis.

Classically, the patient presents with sudden onset of dizziness or vertigo, nausea, vomiting, and midline ataxia, nearly always impairing walking.[25] The clinical syndrome has been divided into three stages (Table 5).[49] The first stage corresponds to an early or small hemorrhage localized to the cerebellum, usually located near the dentate nucleus. The second stage involves mild compression or shift in the region of the fourth ventricle and underlying medullary

Table 5
Features of Cerebellar Hemorrhage

Symptoms	*Signs*
A. Early Stage	
Headache	Truncal ataxia
Dizziness	Nystagmus
Nausea	Appendicular ataxia
Vomiting	Stiff neck
Lack of balance	Dysarthria
B. Intermediate Stage	
Irritability	Pseudo-VI nerve palsy
Confusion	VI nerve palsy
Drowsiness	Gaze paresis
	Forced gaze deviation
	Babinski signs
	Peripheral facial palsy
	Homer's syndrome
	Mild hemiparesis
	Small pupils reactive to bright light
C. Late Stage	
	Stupor
	Coma
	Posturing
	Cardiovascular instability
	Pinpoint pupils
	Ataxic respirations
	Apnea

tegmentum. The final stage involves frank brainstem compression and tonsillar herniation.

A classic triad of ataxia, ipsilateral gaze palsy, and ipsilateral facial nerve palsy has been described for cerebellar hemorrhage. Two of these three signs were present in 73% of cases in reports compiled shortly after the introduction of CT scanning. With more widespread use of brain imaging in acute stroke, the number of cerebellar hemorrhages presenting with this triad is likely to decrease, because smaller hemorrhages are now routinely diagnosed.

Although it is convenient to classify the syndrome into stages, it must be noted that progression can be rapid and unpredictable, and may occur many days after the initial hemorrhage.[50] The decision for surgery is based on the size of the hemorrhage and secondary compression, as well as the clinical features, especially level of consciousness and progression of signs and symptoms.[49,50] The management of this neurologic emergency should be familiar to all clinicians.

Pontine Hemorrhage

Early reports of pontine hemorrhage predominantly described larger hemorrhages, usually centered in the midpons at the junction of the basis pontis and the pontine tegmentum. The classic syndrome was dramatic, with sudden onset of coma, respiratory abnormalities, small but reactive pupils, loss of horizontal eye movements, including caloric stimulation and oculocephalic maneuvers, hyperthermia, and quadriparesis.[51,52] The weakness often begins asymmetrically and usually progresses rapidly. Initially there may also be stiffness and abnormal movements including tremors or twitching. Extensor posturing may be seen later.[30]

The pontine gaze center, medial longitudinal fasciculus (MLF), and VI nerve nucleus are often involved. There may be eye deviation away from the side of the lesion. Fisher[53] described the "one and a half" syndrome with hemorrhages in this area. The only intact ocular movement is abduction of the eye opposite the hemorrhage. Ipsilateral gaze is interrupted because of involvement of the pontine gaze center and the VI nerve/nucleus. Adduction of the eye is impaired because of involvement of the MLF.[53] Fisher also described ocular bobbing, quick downward jerks with a slow upward drift back to the primary position.[54] This eye movement has been described in both pontine hemorrhage and basilar artery thrombosis.

The pupils are small because of interruption of the sympathetic tracts in the dorsal medial brainstem, but they do react. Magnification and a bright light may be needed to detect this. Other autonomic signs include fever, more common in larger hemorrhages, neurogenic bladder, respiratory problems, and abnormal sweating, more common in smaller hemorrhages.[55]

Over the past 2 decades, the syndrome of partial pontine hemorrhage has been recognized and associated with small bleeds, less than 20 mm in diameter. These partial syndromes are also associated with a favorable prognosis.[56,57]

Caplan and Goodwin described three locations for pontine hemorrhages: lateral basis pons, paramedian, and lateral tegmental.[58] Other classifications have also been devised.[59,60] There appears to be considerable overlap in the clinical syndromes from the hemorrhage in these locations. The prognosis for most of these smaller pontine hemorrhages is good.

The small lateral basal hematomas, limited to the basis pontis, may present with a pontine lacunar syndrome: pure motor hemiparesis,[61] or ataxic hemiparesis.[62] The syndrome associated with paramedian pontine hemorrhage consists of ipsilateral miosis, horizontal gaze paresis, lower motor neuron facial paresis, contralateral hemisensory loss, mild and often transient hemiparesis or asymmetric bilateral weakness, dysarthria, and normal or mildly impaired consciousness.[56] Lateral tegmental pontine hemorrhages are less common, but these hematomas have a good prognosis. Full recovery is the usual outcome.[59] They may present as crossed (ipsilateral face/contralateral body) sensory loss, ataxia, ocular motor nerve palsies, including horizontal gaze paresis or the "one and a half" syndrome, and ipsilateral cranial nerve signs (facial weakness, deafness, dysarthria). The medial lemniscus and spinothalamic tracts merge in the upper pons. Hemorrhage affecting this area is more likely to involve both pain/temperature and touch/joint position sense.[37]

Complex hallucinations, both auditory and visual, have been reported in up to half of mild cases of pontine hemorrhage. The visual hallucinations are more common. The images are recognizable objects, and the scenes tend to be complex and colorful. The patients usually recognize the images as unrealistic, which disappear within days to a couple of weeks.[55]

Caudate Hemorrhage

The clinical syndrome of primary caudate hemorrhage can easily be mistaken for SAH. Hemorrhage in the caudate nucleus often extends medially and ruptures into the ventricular system. The presenting symptoms are related more to the intraventricular blood, and patients present with headache, nausea and vomiting, stiff neck, and decreased consciousness or confusion. Mild weakness may be present.

Until recently, localized caudate hemorrhages were most often classified along with putaminal hemorrhages, yet different vessels and structures are involved. The blood supply to the medial caudate nucleus comes from the recurrent artery of Heubner, a branch off the anterior communicating artery.[37] Changes in cognition and behavior are often seen including apathy and abulia, restless agitation, and impaired memory.

The hematoma may also extend posterolaterally into or through the anterior limb of the internal capsule. Weakness and conjugate eye deviation are usually seen. Sensory loss, if present, is minor. Less commonly, the hematoma may extend inferiorly into the hypothalamus, causing a Horner's syndrome, or into the thalamus and upper midbrain.

Hemorrhage in Other Locations

Other locations for hemorrhage are very rare. Midbrain hemorrhage can present with ipsilateral ocular motor paralysis and contralateral weakness for small hemorrhages, with coma and hydrocephalus seen with larger hematomas. Medullary hemorrhages have rapid onset of coma and death. A few cases of very small medullary hematomas have been reported in patients who present with vertigo and lower cranial nerve dysfunction.[63]

Syndromes by Pathology

The most common etiology for ICH is hypertension, but nearly half of brain hemorrhages may be associated with nonhypertensive mechanisms including tumor, aneurysms, vascular malformations, inflammatory and degenerative vasculopathies, and hematologic and iatrogenic disorders of coagulation.[22] Clinical clues may suggest one of these mechanisms and alter the diagnostic and therapeutic plans. These are outlined in Table 1. Several etiologies are reviewed here in greater detail.

Hemorrhage into a Brain Tumor

Hemorrhage into a tumor accounts for 5% to 10% of ICH, and intracranial bleeding occurs in about 5% of all intracranial tumors. Bleeding is most commonly intratumor, but subarachnoid, subdural, and epidural hemorrhages also may occur.

Bleeding occurs most often with malignant tumors which invade the blood vessels. The most common metastatic brain tumors associated with hemorrhage are bronchogenic carcinoma, melanoma, choriocarcinoma, and renal cell carcinoma. Of the primary brain tumors, glioblastomas are the most likely to bleed, followed by oligodendrogliomas. In children, medulloblastomas are associated with bleeding, usually in the cerebellum.

Of the benign brain tumors, meningioma and pituitary adenomas are the most likely to bleed. Hemorrhage into a pituitary tumor, typically an adenoma, can cause a sudden increase in the size of the pituitary. The associated clinical syndrome is referred to as pituitary apoplexy. It is characterized by headache, often referred to a localized area in the midline between the eyes, visual impairment, especially bitemporal field defects, and ophthalmoplegia.[64] Autopsy studies have documented that many pituitary adenomas contain small hemorrhages but remain asymptomatic.[65]

Hemorrhage into a tumor has also been associated, although uncommonly, with therapeutic interventions in tumor patients including placement of a ventricular catheter and intracranial pressure monitoring, anticoagulation, and embolization for vascular tumors.[66]

Although a stroke syndrome may be the reason a patient with an ICH first seeks medical care, there are often clues from the history or examination to suggest a pre-existing mass lesion. This includes a prior history of headache or subtle neurologic deficits, such as mildly impaired cognition. During the initial evaluation, bleeding into a tumor is suggested by early papilledema on examination. On a CT scan, there may be multiple or ring-shaped hemorrhages, and more edema and shift than expected for the size of the hemorrhage.

The location of the tumor influences the syndrome associated with bleeding. Gliomas occur within the white matter. Metastatic tumors tend to grow in the superficial white matter. Bleeding most common occurs at the margin of the tumor.[67]

The prognosis is worse when ICH is associated with tumor. Over the first month, mortality may exceed 90%. This is attributed to the decreased volume available for the intracranial hematoma caused by the pre-existing tumor, and the progression of underlying tumor, with those bleeding tending to be more malignant.

Aneurysmal Intracerebral Hemorrhage

About 20% of large ICHs are caused by a ruptured aneurysm.[68] For patients with a ruptured aneurysm, up to 40% will have some bleeding into the brain parenchyma.[69] These syndromes are important to recognize because of the need to consider surgery and antispasm therapies. The prognosis in this form of intracranial hemorrhage is also poor, both for rebleeding and mortality.

Clinical clues to this form of intracranial hemorrhage include the presence of recent, similar neurologic events. In many instances, aneurysmal rupture is preceded by a "sentinel bleed." The symptoms may be minor or unrecognized at the time by patient or physician. A warning bleed is rare with hypertensive ICH.

The clinical presentation for a ruptured intracranial aneurysm depends heavily on the location and degree of bleeding. Headache at onset remains the major symptom for most patients. In SAH, the symptoms are usually nonfocal and include confusion, neck stiffness, photophobia, nausea, vomiting, and blurred vision. The presence of focal signs other than sixth nerve palsies in the setting of an SAH suggests an intracranial hematoma. The location of the ICH and the associated clinical syndrome correspond to the site of the intracranial aneurysm.

ICA Aneurysms

About 20% of ICA aneurysms produce ICH. Most frequently, bleeding occurs into the temporal and frontal lobes. Bleeding into the medial aspect of the temporal lobe can occur when a posterior communicating aneurysm has its dome above the tentorium and directed laterally. The more common anatomy is for the dome to be directed posteriorly and downward. Hematomas into the putamen, with hemiplegia, are commonly seen.

MCA Aneurysms

Aneurysms at the MCA bifurcation and within the Sylvian fissure are bounded by the frontal and temporal lobes. The dome of the aneurysm commonly points laterally and slightly downward. Intracerebral hemorrhage from these lesions is associated with hemiparesis, aphasia, and anosognosia. Larger lesions may be associated with uncal herniation. Bleeding also occurs less commonly into the basal ganglia.

Other common syndromes include: leg weakness, confusion, and bilateral Babinski signs in anterior communicating artery aneurysms, and homonymous hemianopsia in posterior cerebral artery aneurysms.

Vascular Malformations

Approximately 10% of ICHs are due to small vascular malformations.[70] This includes arteriovenous malformations, cavernous angiomas, and venous angiomas. These most commonly present in the third or fourth decade. There may be a higher incidence in women.[71]

There is a tendency for these vascular malformations to occur in the superficial or deep white matter, especially in the cerebral convexities. The syndromes associated with these hemorrhages are not specific, and merely reflect the location of the bleeding. The prodrome is very similar to tumor except that the mean age of the patients with vascular malformations and hemorrhage is younger than tumor. The stroke is often preceded by headaches and seizures. The occurrence of ICH in a young nonhypertensive women should especially raise the suspicion for a vascular malformation. In addition, there is often a family history of ICH.

Cavernous malformations have received a great deal of attention in recent years because of increased detection with improved imaging technology (MRI). The cavernous malformations are blood-filled sinusoidal channels lined by endothelium, but without smooth muscle or elastin. This type of malformation also presents with seizures in 40% to 70% of cases. Focal findings are present in 35% to 50% of related hemorrhages and reflect the location of the malformation. Headache is a major symptom in 25% to 30% of cases.[72] With heightened clinical awareness and improved diagnostic techniques, the proportion of strokes attributed to small vascular malformations, and specifically cavernous malformations, is likely to increase.

Inflammatory and Degenerative Vasculopathy

Cerebral Amyloid Angiopathy

In this condition, amyloid is deposited in the media and adventitia vessels of small and medium arteries of the brain. The involved arteries are usually located in the superficial layers of the cerebral cortex.[73] Because of this, the syndromes associated with basal ganglia hemorrhages nearly never occur. Amyloid-affected vessels tend to be in the parietal and occipital cortices, and lobar hemorrhage most commonly occurs in this location.[70] The acute syndromes reflect bleeding in these locations. There are also reports of associated subarachnoid or subdural bleeding, possibly because of the superficial location of the diseased vessels.

Bleeding associated with cerebral amyloid angiopathy typically affects older people and accounts for up to one third of intracerebral hematomas in this age group. In autopsy studies, amyloid vascular changes are seen in 8% of those in their sixties, but nearly 60% of those over age 90.[73] Pathologically, neuritic plaques are often seen. Clinically, an associated dementia has been reported in 10% to 30% of cases of hemorrhage attributed to amyloid angiopathy.[70,74] In addition, there is a tendency for bleeding to recur over years or to have bleeding in two locations simultaneously. The presence of either dementia or prior ICH should suggest the diagnosis.

The clinical presentation of patients with biopsy-proven amyloid angiopathy includes headache, nausea and vomiting, loss of consciousness, and focal neurologic deficits such as hemiplegia and blindness.[75] There may also be a history of seizures or focal neurologic signs, without hemorrhage, although it is unclear if this represents prior injury by infarction, small hemorrhagic foci, or some other lesion.[76] Bleeding in patients with amyloid angiopathy has also been reported in association with minor head trauma, anticoagulation, and antiplatelet therapy.[76]

Hematologic and Iatrogenic Vasculopathy

Oral Anticoagulants

Anticoagulant use increases the risk of primary ICH. The risk seems highest in the first year of treatment, but may occur after many years of treatment.[77] Overtreatment is more common in those who develop intracranial bleeding, and for those who develop bleeding, the mortality is higher and the outcome worse than for other ICHs.[78]

Warfarin use is associated with bleeding in about 5% of patients receiving the drug, but only 1% of bleeding complications are intracranial. The most common site for intracranial bleeding is the subdural space, followed by intracerebral and subarachnoid bleeding. Anticoagulation increases the risk of ICH 10-fold. There are clinical features which may contribute to the risk of ICH for those taking warfarin. These include age greater than 65 to 70 years,[79] hypertension,[80] prior ischemic stroke,[81] development of malignant disease,[77] and excessive prolongation of the prothrombin time and duration of treatment.[70] In some series, up to one third of patients reported mild trauma within 48 hours preceding the hemorrhage.[77]

In about half the cases, the initial symptoms of anticoagulant-related hemorrhage are headache associated with nausea and vomiting.[77] The focal syndromes are similar to those from ICH of other etiologies except that gradual or slow progression is seen in about half of these cases. The progression may continue for 48 to 72 hours.[6] There is usually an absence of bleeding elsewhere in the body.

Heparin Therapy

Heparin, like oral anticoagulation, is commonly used in many patients with thromboembolic stroke, especially cardiogenic embolism. Intracerebral hemorrhage has been associated with heparin therapy. Defining the clinical syndrome has been difficult because both hemorrhagic conversion and ICH occur in the setting of cerebral infarction not treated with heparin. The syndromes usually involve worsening of the original stroke because of bleeding into the area of infarction. The most often cited clinical predictors are age, sex, hypertension, and degree of anticoagulation.

The clinical syndromes of heparin-associated ICH are difficult to define because of the difficulty in linking the use of heparin with the bleeding. Heparin may not induce ICH, but rather worsen the hemorrhages which occur spontaneously.[82] Heparin is commonly used in combination with antiplatelet agents, other anticoagulants, and, more recently, thrombolytic agents. In addition, hemorrhagic transformation is common in ischemic stroke, even in the absence of any anticoagulant therapy. Hemorrhagic conversion appears to be most common in cardioembolic stroke, the stroke subtype most likely to be treated with heparin therapy.[83]

There has been no consistent location reported for anticoagulant-related hemorrhage. The bleeding usually occurs in the area of infarction. Low platelet count, recent head trauma, underlying coagulopathies, and excessive anticoagulation are all probably risk factors, but these do not define a distinct clinical syndrome for heparin- (and coumadin-) associated ICH.

Hemorrhagic transformation usually occurs within the first 48 hours following a stroke. Clinical deterioration within the first days following a large, cardioembolic stroke, especially when heparin was started within the first 12 hours in the presence of one of the risk factors mentioned above, should raise suspicion of the diagnosis.[82]

Fibrinolytic Therapy in Myocardial Infarction

The use of fibrinolytic agents is associated with stroke in several ways. These agents have procoagulant effects and may cause ischemic stroke or reocclusion of the symptomatic coronary artery.[84] Ischemic stroke increases the risk for hemorrhagic transformation with consequent ICH. Because of the risk of subsequent ischemia in this setting, the use of anticoagulation may increase the risk for ICH. Fibrinolytic agents may directly increase the risk of intracranial hemorrhage.[85] The effect appears to be dose dependent, with higher rates of hemorrhage noted with total tPA doses of over 150 mg.[86] The difference in the rate of ICH between fibrin selective agents (such as tPA) and nonselective agents (streptokinase) has not been resolved.[87]

Most of the hemorrhages from fibrinolytic therapy are associated with clinical deterioration within the first 24 hours. The hemorrhages are most often lobar, and cortical syndromes predominate. Putaminal hemorrhages are rare. Higher doses (greater than 100 mg of tPA) have been associated with an increased risk of bleeding complications,[88] as have prolonged and excessive use of heparin.[89]

Multiple hemorrhages may be seen. Fluid levels have been noted within hematomas, suggesting that continuing bleeding commonly occurs. Amyloid angiopathy may play a significant role in these bleeds.[90]

Intracerebral hemorrhage is a severe, but infrequent, complication of myocardial infarction.[88] Intracerebral hemorrhage has been associated with myocardial infarction even in the absence of thrombolytic therapy.

Fibrinolytic Therapy in Ischemic Stroke

There is much less experience with ICH after fibrinolytic therapy for ischemic stroke. Part of the problem arises from changes in imaging technology and an evolving understanding of the natural history of spontaneous bleeding in different subtypes of ischemic stroke.

In pilot studies of ischemic stroke, 85 to 95 mg/kg doses of tPA started 90 to 180 minutes after the onset were associated with a 17% risk of bleeding.[91] The rate of bleeding with these doses was not statistically significantly higher than with lower doses or historical controls. Unfortunately, a therapeutic effect has not been demonstrated for these regimens either.

An aggregate analysis of 379 patients treated with thrombolytic therapy in the setting of an acute stroke showed that hemorrhagic transformation occurred in 8% to 53% of cases, with an average of only 7% of patients experiencing clinical worsening due to intracranial bleeding.[92]

In a large, prospective study which enrolled patients up to 8 hours following stroke onset, the rate of hemorrhagic infarction was 20%, and parenchymal hematoma occurred in 11%.[93] Overall, neurologic worsening associated with hemorrhage was seen in 10% of patients treated with tPA. Most deteriorations were associated with parenchymal hemorrhage. This was a dose escalation study. At no dose up to 0.75 MI U/kg was there a significant increase in the risk of bleeding or therapeutic benefit.

Larger infarcts and those with early changes on CT scan are also associated with a higher rate of hemorrhagic complications following fibrinolytic therapy. Also at higher risk are patients with surface infarcts and those with a time-to-treatment greater than 6 hours.[94] Most bleeding occurred in the ischemic territory.

Ongoing trials have not yet identified a dose associated with an increased risk of bleeding. Similarly, no maximally effective dose has been determined. The clinical variables such as age, gender, or degree or type of clinical impairment associated with an increased risk of bleeding have not been clearly defined.

Disease Associated with Clotting Disorders

Intracerebral hemorrhage has been reported in a variety of clotting disorders. The initial symptom of bleeding in these patients is headache followed by deterioration of consciousness. The onset may be slow and the syndrome may evolve over several days.[25] Intracerebral hemorrhages may be associated with mild trauma.

Carotid Endarterectomy

Intracerebral hemorrhage has been associated with carotid endarterectomy in two settings. Intracerebral hemorrhage is seen as a result of hemorrhagic transformation, usually seen when the procedure is performed in the setting of a large ischemic stroke. If the hemorrhage is large, there may be clinical deterioration. This complication usually occurs when surgery is performed within the first days following infarction. The situation may be more common in the setting of anticoagulation or embolic stroke.

Second, hemorrhage may occur after repair of a high-grade stenosis of the internal carotid artery where there is postoperative dysautoregulation of the cerebral circulation and secondary hyperperfusion.[95] The hemorrhage usually occurs within a week of surgery. The onset of weakness, headache, or seizures suggests the diagnosis.[96]

Miscellaneous

Hemorrhagic Conversion

Hemorrhagic conversion occurs commonly after cerebral infarction, especially with cerebral embolism. It is usually asymptomatic. More than one third of autopsied cases of CT-documented cerebral infarction demonstrate a hemorrhagic component.[97] With MRI and a cardioembolic source, up to 70% of patients will show hemorrhagic transformation at 3 weeks after ischemic stroke.[98]

Two types of hemorrhagic conversion have been described. The first and most common are small petechial hemorrhages within the area of infarction. The occurrence of bleeding is usually asymptomatic. These changes develop hours or days following an infarction. Only 5% of patients will have blood within an area of ischemia at the time of presentation,[99] but this rises to about 40% by the first month.[100]

The second type of hemorrhage is a single frank hematoma. It originates within the infarct, but may extend beyond its boarders. This type of hemorrhage usually occurs within the first days following infarction and may be associated with neurologic worsening. Bleeding into an area of ischemia may also occur so early that the initial CT scan may be interpreted as a primary cerebral hemorrhage.[101] This early spontaneous hematoma associated with cerebral infarct occurs more commonly with prior TIAs, silent infarction on CT, and a cardioembolic mechanism.

The clinical syndrome associated with hemorrhagic conversion usually mimics progression of a branch occlusion of the middle cerebral artery. This is because the middle cerebral artery territory is the most common location for embolic infarction.[99] Typical signs include hemiparesis, hemisensory deficit, hemianopia, somnolence, aphasia, and hemineglect. Another common area for hemorrhagic conversion is the cerebellar hemisphere.[99]

When worsening occurs in the setting of acute cerebral ischemia, especially worsening hemiparesis with disturbance of consciousness, and especially in older people with larger areas of ischemia and a history of hypertension or anticoagulant therapy, the possibility of an intrainfarction hematoma must be considered.

The implications of hemorrhagic conversion are unclear. In the setting of early stroke, reperfusion into an ischemic area with hemorrhagic transformation in an area of nonviable tissue may be of little concern if the patient enjoys simultaneous clinical improvement.[102]

Drug Use

Intracerebral hemorrhage has been associated with the use of many agents including cocaine, amphetamines, and other sympathomimetic drugs.[103] Many of the reported bleeds occur shortly after use of the drug and, for illicit drugs, signs of intoxication may still be present.[104] This may create a bias in screening and reporting of cases, especially as nonhypertensive mechanisms have been proposed.

Transient hypertension has been proposed as a mechanism, as has vasculitis.[105,106] Most reported cases are in chronic users, and signs of chronic substance abuse may suggest drugs as the etiology for hemorrhage. The most common location is the subcortical white matter with a lobar syndrome.[107]

Phenylpropanolamine use has been reported in association with ICH in young people.[108,109] It is, however, one of the most common over-the-counter medications and is found in diet preparations and cough and cold remedies. Given the frequency of use, it is not surprising that cases have been reported. A causal link remains to be established. Many of the reported cases were in young women with eating disorders who took excessive doses.

Drug use should be included in the clinical evaluation of all patients with ICH, especially those with signs of illicit drug use or the potential for abuse of diet or other over-the-counter medications.

Head Trauma

The most common symptoms associated with traumatic intracranial hemorrhage are focal neurologic deficits and seizures. The most common location for the bleeding is the inferior frontal lobe and anterior pole of the temporal lobe. It may be difficult to separate the signs and symptoms due to the ICH from those of the traumatic brain injury. The trauma in patients with traumatic ICH is often severe, diffuse, and may affect consciousness. This decreases the ability to reliably identify subtle frontal lobe signs or the behavioral signs associated with small traumatic ICH.

Although intracranial bleeding may occur at the time of the head trauma, many cases of ICH associated with trauma occur after a delay. Spät hemorrhage (delayed traumatic ICH) refers to the sudden appearance of signs or symptoms of serious ICH related to recent head trauma in a previously asymptomatic individual. CT scanning has demonstrated that this syndrome may be related to different mechanisms, including delayed bleeding, early bleeding with loss of compensatory mechanisms for maintaining normal intracranial pressure, or rebleeding. Since the advent of CT scanning, it has become clear that there are many patients with late bleeding who do not show any evidence of clinical deterioration.[110]

The reported incidence of delayed bleeding or rebleeding with worsening of the original signs range from 7.5% to 50%.[110-112] The highest rates are reported in those trauma cases that develop secondary coagulopathies. These hematomas often develop in the area of the original injury and are often associated with clinical deterioration, beginning with worsening of the original deficit. This mechanism is difficult to differentiate from the natural history of brain injury, but should always be considered, especially when the brain injury is associated with multisystem trauma.

Clinical Deterioration

The early course of ICH is unpredictable. The smooth onset over minutes is usually attributed to a period of active bleeding. The active bleeding is believed rarely to persist beyond 1 hour.[10]

Changes in the clinical status of a patient with ICH are important to recognize, especially deterioration. This may signal new bleeding or a secondary medical complication that is potentially amenable to treatment. Clinical deterioration is most often manifested as a worsening of the original syndrome. Changes in consciousness are the best guide to prognosis.

Recently, several studies have begun to evaluate patients with ICH early, and to reevaluate them early, often with repeat CT scans.[11,113,114] These studies have shown that bleeding does occur beyond the first hour, but it is uncommon. About 3% of patients will have a clinical deterioration associated with rapid expansion of an ICH.[114] This has been reported most commonly for thalamic and putaminal hemorrhages. For those patients who have expansion of their hematoma, there is neurologic deterioration.

Clinical series have documented that once the clinical deficit associated with an ICH stabilizes, worsening and rebleeding are uncommon.[115] When it does occur, the usual syndrome is worsening of the original deficit, decreased consciousness, and anisocoria. Rebleeding has been reported up to 4 to 5 days after the onset of the hemorrhage, with a mean time of 40 hours. In these reports, repeat CT scanning was prompted by clinical deterioration. This introduces a selection bias to identify rebleeding for those cases with a worsening clinical course. It is likely rebleeding also occurs with only minor fluctuations in the clinical course. This has been more difficult to document in clinical studies.

The clinical course of ICH beyond the first hours or day is strongly influenced by secondary injury caused by the mass of the hematoma, edema, or hydrocephalus. With the initial bleeding and expansion of the hematoma, there can be tearing of previously uninvolved vessels, with additional bleeding. The hematoma may be large enough to deform the intracranial anatomy, impairing the normal flow of cerebrospinal fluid, leading to an obstructive hydrocephalus. Hydrocephalus can also occur with intraventricular extension of the blood. As

Table 6
Medical Complications of ICH

Complications	Frequency
Pneumonia	16%
Urinary tract infection	15%
Arrhythmia	8%
Seizure	8%
Septicemia	7%
Hypotension	7%
Other infection	5%
Gastrointestinal bleeding	4%
Hydrocephalus	4%
Respiratory arrest	4%
Renal failure	2%
Thrombophlebitis	2%
Congestive heart failure	1%

injured tissue becomes edematous, additional brain shifts may occur. The shifts in the intracranial contents can lead to mechanical disruption of the brain, compression of cranial nerves, obstruction of the ventricular system, stretching and tearing of small vessels with additional bleeding, or compression of blood vessels with secondary infarction.

When late worsening occurs, it may also be associated with medical complications. These should be considered in the differential diagnosis of the patient who experiences worsening (Table 6).[14]

Conclusions

The use of imaging technology has profoundly influenced the diagnosis and management of patients with ICH, especially at the time of initial presentation or clinical deterioration. The accuracy of CT and MRI in detecting ICH has often overshadowed the clinical examination. This is unfortunate because the neurologic examination and brain imaging complement each other. For patients with ischemic stroke, CT scanning did not eliminate the need for clinical skill, but allowed for refinement of the clinical assessment.

The clinical examination of the patient with a neurologic syndrome is underdeveloped in modern medical practice. This is unfortunate. The clinical status and outcome are central to diagnostic and therapeutic decisions for patients with ICH. Although imaging technology will remain an essential part of patient management, it is best viewed as an extension of the process that begins at the bedside with the clinical evaluation of a patient with a stroke syndrome. No longer does the physician have to labor over whether the cause of the stroke syndrome is hemorrhagic or ischemic. This can free the physician to place more emphasis on getting a better picture of what is going on with the individual patient by integrating the clinical, laboratory, and imaging data. This approach will not only be more rewarding for patient and physician, it will also result in better care for the patient with ICH.[116]

References

1. Aring CD, Merritt HH: Differential diagnosis between cerebral hemorrhage and cerebral thrombosis. *Arch Intern Med* 1935;56:435.
2. Bamford J, Sandercock P, Dennis M, et al: A prospective study of acute cerebrovascular disease in the community: Oxfordshire community stroke project: 1981–1986. 2-Incidence, case fatality rates, and overall outcome at one year of cerebral infarction, primary intracerebral and subarachnoid hemorrhage. *J Neurol Neurosurg Psychiat* 1990;53:16.
3. Broderick JP, Brott T, Tomsick T, et al: Intracerebral hemorrhage more

than twice as common as subarachnoid hemorrhage. *J Neurosurg* 1993; 78:188.

4. Caplan LR: Intracerebral hemorrhage revisited. *Neurology* 1988;38:624.

5. Brott T, Thalinger K, Hertzberg V: Hypertension as a risk factor for spontaneous intracerebral hemorrhage. *Stroke* 1986;17:1078.

6. Kase CS, Robinson RK, Stein RW, et al: Anticoagulant-related intracerebral hemorrhage. *Neurology* 1985;35:943.

7. Wroe SJ, Sandercock P, Bamford J, et al: Diurnal variation in incidence of stroke: Oxfordshire community stroke project. *Br Med J* 1992;304:155.

8. Mohr JP, Caplan LR, Melski JW, et al: The Harvard Cooperative Stroke Registry. *Neurology* 1978;26:754.

9. Foulkes MA, Wolf PA, Price TR, et al: The Stroke Data Bank. *Stroke* 1988; 19:547.

10. Herbstein DJ, Schaumburg HH: Hypertensive intracerebral hemorrhage. *Arch Neurol* 1974;30:412.

11. Chen ST, Chen SD, Hsu CY, et al: Progression of hypertensive intracerebral hemorrhage. *Neurology* 1989;39:1509.

12. Fujitsu K, Muramoto M, Ikeda Y, et al: Indications for surgical treatment of putaminal hemorrhage. *J Neurosurg* 1990;73:518.

13. Schuetz H, Dommer T, Boedeker RH, et al: Changing pattern of brain hemorrhage during 12 years of computed axial tomography. *Stroke* 1992; 23:653.

14. Hier DB, Babcock DJ, Foulkes MA, et al: Influence of site on course of intracerebral hemorrhage. *J Stroke Cerebrovasc Dis* 1993;3:65.

15. Berger AR, Lipton RB, Lesser ML, et al: Early seizures following intracerebral hemorrhage: implications for therapy. *Neurology* 1990;38:1363.

16. Weisberg LA, Shamsnia M, Elliott D: Seizures caused by nontraumatic parenchymal brain hemorrhages. *Neurology* 1991;41:1197.

17. Ropper AH, Gress DR: Anatomic causes of coma in large cerebral hemorrhage. *Ann Neurol* 1989;26:161.

18. Ropper AH, Gress DR: Computerized tomography and clinical features of large cerebral hemorrhages. *Cerebrovasc Dis* 1991;1:38.

19. Allen C: Clinical diagnosis of the acute stroke syndrome. *Q J Med* 1983; 208 (new series LII):515.

20. Poungvarin N, Viriyavejakul A, Komontri C, et al: Siriraj stroke score and validation study to distinguish supratentorial intracerebral hemorrhage from infection. *Br Med J* 1991;302:1565.

21. Marshall RS, Mohr JP: Current management of ischaemic stroke. *J Neurol Neurosurg Psychiat* 1993;56:6.

22. Ojemann RG, Heros RC: Spontaneous brain hemorrhage. *Stroke* 1983;14: 468.

23. Kase CS, Williams JP, Wyatt DA, et al: Lobar intracerebral hematomas: clinical and CT analysis of 22 cases. *Neurology* 1982;32:1146.

24. Koba T, Yokoyama T, Kaneko M: Correlation between the location of hematoma and its symptoms in the lateral type of hypertensive intracerebral hemorrhage. *Stroke* 1977;8:676.

25. Ojemann RG, Mohr JP: Hypertensive brain hemorrhage. *Clin Neurosurg* 1975;23:220.
26. Tuhrim S, Berndt R, Joslyn JN: Transient conduction aphasia following putaminal hemorrhage. *Cerebrovasc Dis* 1991;1:113.
27. Alexander MP, Loverme SR: Aphasia after left hemispheric intracerebral hemorrhage. *Neurology* 1980;30:1193.
28. Tapia JF, Kase CS, Mohr JP: Hypertensive putaminal hemorrhage presenting as pure motor hemiparesis. *Stroke* 1983;14:505.
29. Minemsatsu K, Tagawa K, Yamaguchi T: A case of putaminal hemorrhage presenting with dysarthria-clumsy hand syndrome. *Neurol Med* 1981;14: 291.
30. Wityk RJ, Caplan LR: Hypertensive intracerebral hemorrhage: epidemiology and clinical pathology. *Neurosurg Clin North Am* 1992;3:521.
31. Kier DB, Davis KR, Richardson EP, et al: Hypertensive putaminal hemorrhage. *Ann Neurol* 1977;1:152.
32. Jones HR, Baker RA, Kott HS: Hypertensive putaminal hemorrhage presenting with hemichorea. *Stroke* 1985;16:130.
33. Mori E, Yamadori A, Kudo Y, et al: Ataxic hemiparesis from small capsular hemorrhage. *Arch Neurol* 1984;41:1050.
34. Caplan LR: *Stroke: A Clinical Approach,* 2nd Ed. Boston: Butterworth-Heinemann, 1993.
35. Ropper AH, Davis KR: Lobar cerebral hemorrhages: acute clinical syndromes in 26 cases. *Neurology* 1980;8:141.
36. Yoneda Y, Mori E, Tabuschi M, et al: Pure motor monoparesis due to intracranial hemorrhage. *Stroke* 1993;24:142.
37. Carpenter MB, Sutin J: *Human Neuroanatomy.* 8th Ed. Baltimore: Williams & Wilkins, 1983.
38. Gerstmann J: Some notes on the Gertsmann syndrome. *Neurology* 1957; 7:866.
39. Barraquer-Bordas L, Illa I, Escartin A, et al: Thalamic hemorrhage: a study of 23 patients with diagnosis by computed tomography. *Stroke* 1981; 12:524.
40. Walshe TM, Davis KR, Fisher CM: Thalamic hemorrhage: a computed tomographic-clinical correlation. *Neurology* 1977;27:217.
41. Graff-Radford NR, Damasio H, Yamada T, et al: Nonhemorrhagic thalamic infarction. *Brain* 1985;108:485.
42. Mohr JP, Watters WC, Duncan GW: Thalamic hemorrhage and aphasia. *Brain & Lang* 1975;2:3.
43. Steinke W, Sacco RS, Mohr JP, et al: Thalamic stroke: presentation and prognosis of infarcts and hemorrhages. *Arch Neurol* 1992;49:703.
44. Pessin MS, Adelman LS, Prager RJ, et al: "Wrong-way eyes" in supratentorial hemorrhage. *Ann Neurol* 1981;9:79.
45. Kawahara N, Sato K, Muraki M, et al: CT classification of small thalamic hemorrhages and their clinical implications. *Neurology* 1986;36:165.
46. Dobato JL, Villaneuva VA, Giménez-Roldan S: Sensory ataxic hemiparesis in thalamic hemorrhage. *Stroke* 1990;21:1749.

47. Pu-An Y, Qiu-Yue W, Jing-Chang F: Hypesthetic ataxia hemiparesis and thalamic-capsular hemorrhage. *Cerebrovasc Dis* 1991;1:357.
48. Caplan LR: Intracerebral hemorrhage. *Lancet* 1992;339:656.
49. Heros RC: Cerebellar hemorrhage and infarction. *Stroke* 1982;13:106.
50. Ott KH, Kase CS, Ojemann RG, et al: Cerebellar hemorrhage: diagnosis and treatment. A review of 56 cases. *Arch Neurol* 1974;31:150.
51. Fisher CM: Pathological observations in hypertensive cerebral hemorrhage. *J Neuropathol Exp Neurol* 1971;30:536.
52. Goto N, Kaneko M, Hosaka Y, et al: Primary pontine hemorrhage: clinicopathological correlations. *Stroke* 1980;11:84.
53. Fisher CM: Some neuro-ophthalmological observations. *J Neurol Neurosurg Psychiat* 1967;30:383.
54. Fisher CM: Ocular bobbing. *Arch Neurol* 1964;11:543.
55. Nakajima K: Clinicopathological study of pontine hemorrhage. *Stroke* 1983;14:485.
56. Lancman M, Norscini J, Mesropian H, et al: Tegmental pontine hemorrhages: clinical features and prognostic factors. *Can J Neurol Sci* 1992;19:236.
57. Kase C, Maulsby G, Mohr JP: Partial pontine hematomas. *Neurology* 1981;30:652.
58. Caplan LR, Goodwin JA: Lateral tegmental brainstem hemorrhages. *Neurology* 1982;32:252.
59. Chung CS, Park CH: Primary pontine hemorrhage. *Neurology* 1992;42:830.
60. Tanaka Y, Nishiya M, Ogasawara S, et al: Clinical study of hypertensive pontine hemorrhage. *Brain Nerve* 1982;34:601.
61. Gobernado JM, Fernandez de Molina AR, Gimeno A: Pure motor hemiplegia due to hemorrhage in the lower pons. *Arch Neurol* 1980;37:393.
62. Schnapper RA: Pontine hemorrhage presenting as ataxic hemiparesis. *Stroke* 1982;13:518.
63. Shuaib A: Benign brainstem hemorrhage. *Can J Neurol Sci* 1991;18:356.
64. Oliver RM, Craft TM, Shaw KM: Bleeding intracranial aneurysm? Pituitary apoplexy! *Br J Clin Pract* 1991;45:150.
65. Fraioli B, Esposito V, Palma L, et al: Hemorrhagic pituitary adenomas: clinicopathological features and surgical treatment. *Neurosurgery* 1990;27:741.
66. Gibbons KJ, Guterman LR, Hopkins LN: Iatrogenic intracerebral hemorrhage. *Neurosurg Clin North Am* 1992;3:667.
67. Little JR, Dial B, Bellanger G, et al: Brain hemorrhage from intracranial tumor. *Stroke* 1979;10:238.
68. Mutlu N, Berry RG, Alpers BJ: Massive cerebral hemorrhage: clinical and pathological correlations. *Arch Neurol* 1963;8:644.
69. Pasqualin A, Bazzan A, Cavazzani P, et al: Intracranial hematomas following aneurysmal rupture: experience with 309 cases. *Surg Neurol* 1986;25:6.

70. Kase CS: Intracerebral hemorrhage: non-hypertensive causes. *Stroke* 1986;17:590.

71. Steiger HJ, Tew JM: Hemorrhage and epilepsy in cryptic cerebrovascular malformations. *Arch Neurol* 1984;41:722.

72. Robinson JR, Awad IA: Clinical spectrum and natural course. In: Awad IA, Barrow DL, ed: *Cavernous Malformations*. Park Ridge: American Association of Neurological Surgeons, 1993;25–36.

73. Vinters HV, Gilbert JJ: Cerebral amyloid angiopathy: incidence and complications in the aging brain II. The distribution of amyloid vascular changes. *Stroke* 1983;14:915.

74. Kalyan-Raman UP, Kalyan-Raman K: Cerebral amyloid angiopathy causing intracerebral hemorrhage. *Ann Neurol* 1984;16:321.

75. Yong WH, Robert ME, Secor DL, et al: Cerebral hemorrhage with biopsy-proven amyloid angiopathy. *Arch Neurol* 1992;49:51.

76. Feldman E, Tornabene J: Diagnosis and treatment of cerebral amyloid angiopathy. *Clin Geriat Med* 1991;7:617.

77. Forsting M, Mattle HP, Huber P: Anticoagulant-related intracerebral hemorrhage. *Cerebrovasc Dis* 1991;1:97.

78. Fogelholm R, Eskola K, Kiminkinen T, et al: Anticoagulant treatment as a risk factor for primary intracerebral hemorrhage. *J Neurol Neurosurg Psychiat* 1992;55:1121.

79. Furlan AJ, Whisnant JP, Elveback LR: The decreasing incidence of primary intracerebral hemorrhage: a population study. *Ann Neurol* 1979;5:367.

80. Wintzen AR, de Jonge H, Loeliger EA, et al: The risk of intracerebral hemorrhage during oral anticoagulant treatment: a population study. *Ann Neurol* 1984;16:553.

81. Lieberman A, Hass WK, Pinto R, et al: Intracerebral hemorrhage and infarction in anticoagulated patients with prosthetic heart valves. *Stroke* 1978;9:18.

82. Cerebral Embolism Task Force: Cardiogenic stroke, early anticoagulation, and brain hemorrhage. *Arch Intern Med* 1987;147:636.

83. Cerebral Embolism Task Force: Cardiogenic brain embolism: the second report of the cerebral embolism task force. *Arch Neurol* 1989;46:727.

84. Owen J, Friedman KD, Grossman BA, et al: Thrombolytic therapy with tissue plasminogen activator or streptokinase induces transient thrombin activity. *Blood* 1988;72:616.

85. ISIS-3 (Third International Study of Infarct Survival) Collaborative Group: ISIS-3: a randomized comparison of streptokinase vs tissue plasminogen activator vs antistreplase and of aspirin plus heparin vs aspirin alone among 41,299 cases of suspected acute myocardial infarction. *Lancet* 1992;239:753.

86. Braunwald E, Knatterud GL, Passamani E: Announcement of protocol change in Thrombolysis in Myocardial Infarction trial. *J Am Coll Cardiol* 1987;9:467.

87. Sobel BE, Collen D: Strokes, statistics and sophistry in trials of thrombolysis for acute myocardial infarction. *Am J Cardiol* 1993;71:424.

88. Gore JM, Sloan M, Price TR, et al: Intracerebral hemorrhage, cerebral infarction, and subdural hematoma after acute myocardial infarction and thrombolytic therapy in the Thrombolysis in Myocardial Infarction Study. *Circulation* 1991;83:448.

89. Kase CS, O'Neal AM, Fisher M, et al: Intracranial hemorrhage after use of tissue plasminogen activator for coronary thrombolysis. *Ann Intern Med* 1990;112:17.

90. Wijdicks EFM, Jack CR: Intracerebral hemorrhage after thrombolytic therapy for acute myocardial infarction. *Stroke* 1993;24:554.

91. Haley EC, Levy DE, Brott TG, et al: Urgent therapy for stroke: part II. Pilot study of tissue plasminogen activator administered 91-180 minutes from onset. *Stroke* 1992;23:641.

92. Teal PA, Pessin MS: Hemorrhagic transformation: the spectrum of ischemia-related brain hemorrhage. *Neurosurg Clin North Am* 1992;3:601.

93. del Zoppo GJ, Poeck K, Pessin MS, et al: Recombinant tissue plasminogen activator in acute thrombotic and embolic stroke. *Ann Neurol* 1992;32:78.

94. Wolpert SM, Bruckmann H, Greenlee R, et al: Neuroradiological evaluation of patients with acute stroke treated with recombinant tissue plasminogen activator. *AJNR* 1993;14:3.

95. Bernstein M, Fleming JF, Deck JH: Cerebral hyperperfusion after carotid endarterectomy: a cause of cerebral hemorrhage. *Neurosurgery* 1984;15:50.

96. Pomposelli FB, Lamparello PJ, Riles TS, et al: Intracranial hemorrhage after carotid endarterectomy. *J Vasc Surg* 1988;7:248.

97. Hart RG, Easton JD: Hemorrhagic infarcts. *Stroke* 1986;17:586.

98. Hornig CR, Bauer T, Simon C, et al: Hemorrhagic transformation in cardioembolic cerebral infarction. *Stroke* 1993;24:465.

99. Bogousslavsky J, Van Melle G, Regli F, for the Lausanne Stroke Registry Group: The Lausanne Stroke Registry: analysis of 1000 consecutive patients with first stroke. *Stroke* 1989;10:1083.

100. Hornig CR, Dorndorf W, Agnoli AL: Hemorrhagic cerebral infarction: a prospective study. *Stroke* 1986;17:179.

101. Bogousslavsky J, Regli F, Uské A, et al: Early spontaneous hematoma in cerebral infarct: is primary cerebral hemorrhage overdiagnosed? *Neurology* 1991;41:837.

102. Lyden PD, Zivin JA: Hemorrhagic transformation after cerebral ischemia: mechanisms and incidence. *Cerebrovasc Brain Metab Rev* 1993;5:1.

103. Delaney P, Estes M: Intracranial hemorrhage with amphetamine use. *Neurology* 1980;30:1125.

104. Harrington H, Heller HA, Dawson D, et al: Intracerebral hemorrhage and oral amphetamine. *Arch Neurol* 1983;40:503.

105. Citron BP, Halpern M, McCarron M, et al: Necrotizing angiitis associated with drug abuse. *N Engl J Med* 1970;283:1003.

106. Stoessl AJ, Young GB, Feasby TE: Intracerebral haemorrhage and angiographic beading following ingestion of catecholaminergics. *Stroke* 1985; 16:734.

107. Salanova V, Taubner R: Intracerebral haemorrhage and vasculitis secondary to amphetamine use. *Postgrad Med J* 1984;60:429.

108. Fallis RJ, Fisher M: Cerebral vasculitis and hemorrhage associated with phenylpropanolamine. *Neurology* 1985;35:405.

109. Kikta DG, Devereaux MW, Chander K: Intracranial hemorrhages due to phenylpropanolamine. *Stroke* 1985;16:510.

110. Gudeman SK, Kishore PRS, Miller JD, et al: The genesis and significance of delayed traumatic intracerebral hematoma. *Neurosurgery* 1979;5:309.

111. Touho H, Hirakawa K, Hino A, et al: Relationship between abnormalities of coagulation and fibrinolysis and postoperative intracranial hemorrhage in head injury. *Neurosurgery* 1986;19:523.

112. Soloniuk D, Pitts LH, Lovely M, et al: Traumatic intracerebral hematomas: timing of appearance and indications for operative removal. *J Trauma* 1986;26:787.

113. Broderick JP, Brott TG, Tomsick T, et al: Ultra-early evaluation of intracerebral hemorrhage. *J Neurosurg* 1990;72:195.

114. Bae HG, Lee KS, Yun IG, et al: Rapid expansion of hypertensive intracerebral hemorrhage. *Neurosurgery* 1992;31:35.

115. Fisher CM: Clinical syndrome in cerebral hemorrhage. In: Fields WS, ed: *Pathogenesis and Treatment of Cerebrovascular Disease*. Springfield: Charles C. Thomas, 1961:1.

116. Prichard JW, Brass LM: New anatomical and functional imaging methods. *Ann Neurol* 1992;32:395.

Chapter 12

Laboratory Evaluation of Intracerebral Hemorrhage

Jeffrey I. Frank, MD, José Biller, MD

The preceding chapters addressed the various etiologies and clinical presentations of nontraumatic intracerebral hemorrhage (ICH). Laboratory studies are central to the diagnosis and treatment of patients with ICH, and an understanding of the available diagnostic armamentarium is paramount for all physicians involved in the acute care of these patients.

This chapter focuses on the most useful laboratory tests for patients with ICH, balancing comprehensiveness with practical clinical applicability. The first section discusses each test separately, emphasizing its utility and limitations in the diagnosis of ICH. The second section suggests a rational approach to the laboratory evaluation of patients with ICH by brain region.

The Main Diagnostic Armamentarium for ICH

There are many laboratory tests helpful in the diagnosis and management of patients with ICH, each with its own advantages and limitations. An understanding of these issues maximizes their utility in the evaluation of patients with ICH.

Computed Tomography (CT) Scanning

The development and application of CT scanning in the 1970s had a profound impact on our ability to diagnose ICH by allowing direct imaging of the blood collection.[1-3] Previously, angiography could only provide indirect evidence of a hematoma when it was large enough to exert mass effect and disrupt the

From Feldmann E (ed). *Intracerebral Hemorrhage*. Armonk, NY: Futura Publishing Company, Inc., © 1994.

normal vascular architecture,[4] or acute enough to allow seepage of contrast material.[5]

The contemporary availability of CT allows for prompt diagnosis of ICH. Although magnetic resonance imaging (MRI) has enhanced our understanding of the sequential changes in hematoma composition over time, it has not replaced CT. Brain CT is more accessible and rapidly performed than MRI, and it is more sensitive for the detection of intracranial calcification, intrinsic bone lesions and acute hemorrhage.

Brain CT scanning involves a narrow beam of x-rays which scan the head at various angles, usually between 180 to 360 degrees, confined to a section of tissue of designated thickness, usually 5 to 10 mm. Photon detectors measure beam attenuation, and the absorption values of tissues are processed by computer. The x-ray absorption coefficients are calculated for blocks of tissue, and the density values are displayed on an adjustable gray scale as a matrix pattern of small squares, approximately 1 mm on transverse section. Each small square represents the mean calculated attenuation for a volume of tissue portrayed by the cross-sectional area of the matrix cell and the thickness of the scanned tissue. Most CT equipment arbitrarily defines the attenuation of water as zero and the attenuation of other substances to be proportionately above (e.g., most tissue, calcification, bone, blood) or below (e.g., air, lipids) that of water.

The technique used for CT scanning can be tailored to the physician's specific questions. Most CT scanners can adjust the background window to accentuate intracranial blood (e.g., "blood" windows). In addition, thinner sections can be scanned to detect more subtle lesions (e.g., 3 mm posterior fossa cuts). This can be particularly advantageous in patients with suspected posterior fossa hemorrhage. In certain circumstances, adjustment of patient position and scanning orientation, albeit cumbersome, can alter the plane of study (e.g., temporal lobe cuts). This is often useful in patients with suspected temporal lobe pathology when conventional CT images are complicated by extensive bony artifact.

Cerebrospinal fluid is dark (black) on CT, and blood appears white. However, it is important to note that the attenuation of circulating whole blood varies linearly with the hematocrit and hemoglobin values. Severe anemia may therefore challenge CT detection of hemorrhage in certain locations, since extravasated blood with a hematocrit of 20% has a similar attenuation as cerebral hemispheric gray matter.[6] Intracranial calcification appears as an area of increased attenuation (white) on CT and must be differentiated from a hematoma. Fortunately, benign intracranial calcifications occur in certain regions or are bilaterally symmetric. The pineal gland is calcified in most adults. Calcification can also involve the choroid plexus, basal ganglia, and dentate nuclei, usually in a bilaterally symmetric manner. Dural calcification is also common, most visibly involving the falx cerebri and the tentorium cerebelli, and calcification frequently occurs within neoplasms (e.g., meningioma, oligodendroglioma) and vascular malformations. Occasionally, analysis of the attenuation values (Hounsfield units) directly on the CT scanner can assist in differentiating hemorrhage from calcification when that determination is in question. Notably,

ICH often has associated edema which increases over the first week (Figure 1A, 1B).

The residual CT abnormalities after ICH are highly variable. One prospective follow-up study evaluated CT scans of 42 patients with spontaneous ICH 2 to 24 months after the ictus.[7] These investigators found 17% without any residual CT abnormalities, 12% with only focal atrophy, 5% with only focal calcification, 14% with slit-like lesions (after deep hemorrhages), and 50% with rounded hypodense areas frequently connected to the ventricular system. These diverse, often nonspecific post-ICH CT changes illustrate the difficulty in retrospectively making the diagnosis, except for the characteristic slit-like lesions which occasionally occur after basal ganglia hematomas.

When CT is performed after the administration of intravenous radiographic contrast material, vascular structures are outlined as radiodense (white). In addition, a loss of integrity of the blood-brain-barrier may allow seepage of the radiodense contrast material leading to regional "enhancement." This technique can be helpful for identifying ICH due to cerebral aneurysm,[8] vascular malformation,[9] other vasculopathies,[10] neoplasm,[11,12] and sagittal

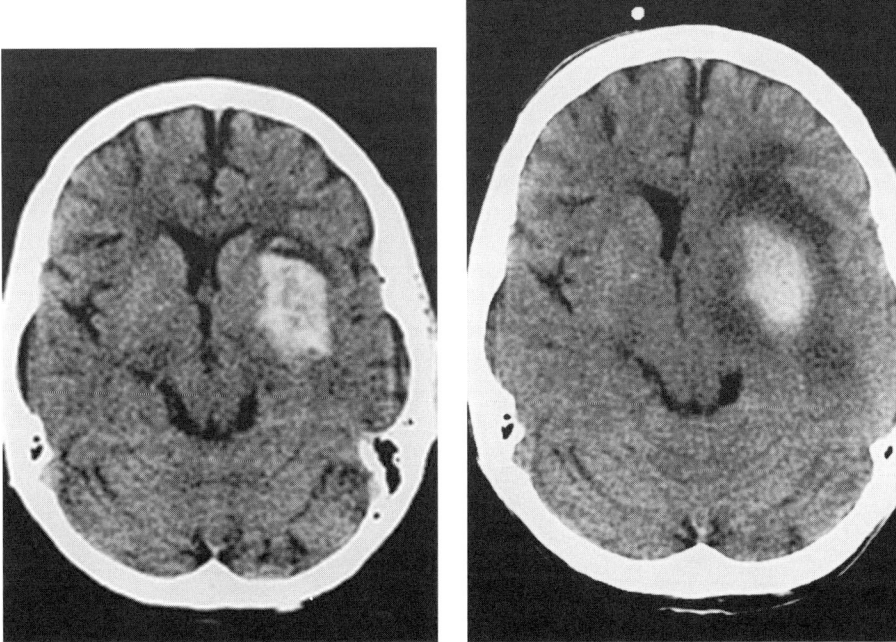

Figure 1A   **Figure 1B**

Figure 1: Noncontrast axial CT sections in a 57-year-old woman with acute right hemiparesis and a nonfluent aphasia. **A.** Scan several hours after onset of her symptoms reveals a left basal ganglia hematoma. **B.** Scan from day #11 reveals the same hematoma. The more extensive peripheral area of low attenuation represents cerebral edema.

sinus thrombosis. Regional "ring"-like enhancement is common with ICH, but it can also occur with vascular-rich neoplasms and abscesses. Differentiating neoplastic and infectious enhancement from the characteristic enhancement pattern observed with ICH is challenging and imperfect. Notably, corticosteroids attenuate the enhancement of ICH,[13] as they do with neoplasms.

Computed tomography is the diagnostic test of choice for acute ICH and should be performed in any patient with this diagnostic consideration. Special instructions should be provided to the CT technician to tailor the study to the patient's syndrome (e.g., blood windows, thin posterior fossa cuts).

Primary ICH is usually homogeneous and well demarcated. A heterogeneous appearance to the hemorrhage is highly suspicious of an underlying structural lesion such as a neoplasm, vascular malformation, or hemorrhagically converted infarction (Figure 2). As already mentioned, CT can miss very small hemorrhages and ICH in severely anemic patients, particularly those localized to gray matter.[6,14] A strong clinical suspicion should lead to further diagnostic testing in these situations, such as MRI. CT is also valuable for the diagnosis of ICH in the posterior fossa,[15-19] but CT scans of this region are often encum-

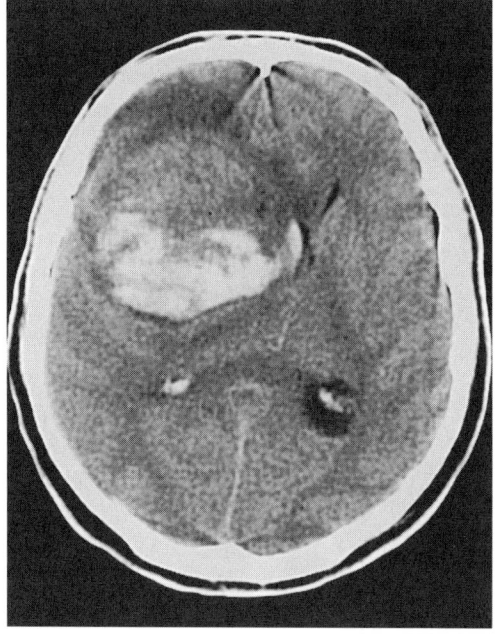

Figure 2: Noncontrast axial CT section in a 55-year-old man after the sudden onset of left body weakness. He had a 2-week history of recurrent, transient confusion prior to his presenting with acute and persistent left hemiplegia, left homonymous hemianopsia, and left hemineglect. Note the large area of mixed high and low attenuation in the deep right frontal region obliterating the right lateral ventricle causing subfalcian herniation. This represents an acute right frontal hemorrhage into a glioblastoma. The outermost rim of lower attenuation is edema.

bered by excessive bony artifact compromising the ability to diagnose small hemorrhages or clarify their extent.[20]

Computed tomography has expanded our understanding of the spectrum of ICH severity, often by identifying hemorrhage in patients suspected to have cerebral infarction.[21] It has also demonstrated interesting and important phenomena such as hyperacute clot retraction,[22] progression of hypertensive ICH,[23–25] and early hemorrhagic infarction appearing as primary ICH.[26]

Some characteristic CT abnormalities can provide clues about the pathophysiology of the hemorrhage. Dilated tortuous blood vessels in the posterior fossa, often with calcification of the vessel wall or intraluminal thrombus, in a patient with brainstem hemorrhage is highly suggestive of a dolichoectactic vertebrobasilar arterial system (Figure 3A, 3B).[10] The "empty delta sign," seen with sagittal sinus thrombosis, is characterized by a triangular extra-axial region of nonenhancement at the level of the confluence of the sinuses. The "nidus sparing sign" is a region spared of extravasated blood in a patient with ICH suggestive of an underlying arteriovenous malformation (AVM),[27] but this is rarely present.

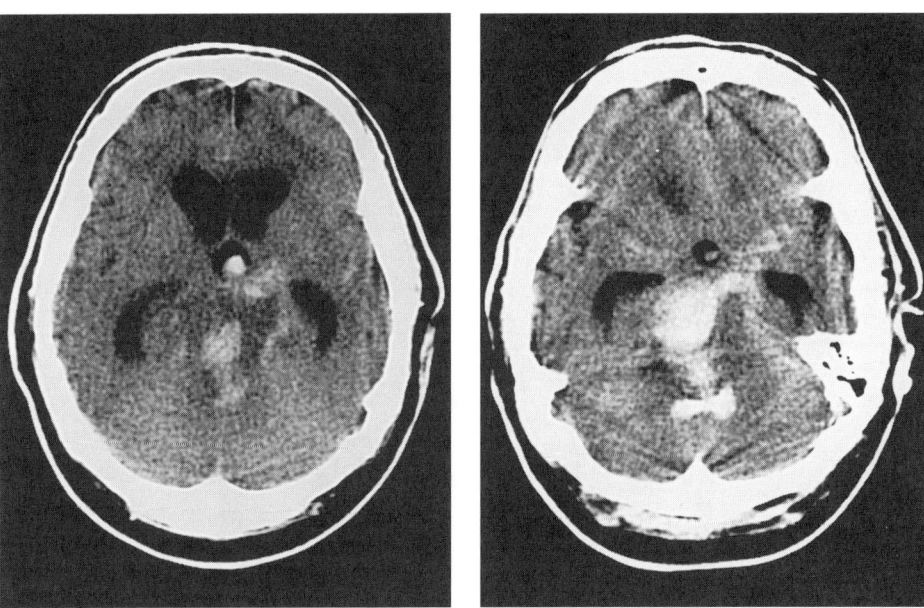

Figure 3A   **Figure 3B**

Figure 3: Noncontrast axial CT sections in a 75-year-old man after acute onset of headache, depression of consciousness, diplopia, dysarthria and quadriparesis. **A.** Note the right midbrain tectal hematoma with associated perimesencephalic and intraventricular hemorrhage. The lateral and third ventricles are dilated (hydrocephalus). **B.** A more inferior section of the same CT demonstrates a well-circumscribed high attenuation extra-axial mass compressing the brainstem. Angiography revealed a partially thrombosed, large dolichoectatic basilar artery aneurysm.

Table 1
Common Sites of ICH By Etiology

ICH Etiologies	Lobar	Basal Ganglia/ Thalamus	Brainstem	Cerebellar	Comment
Hypertension	+	+	+	+	
Arteriovenous malformation	+	+	+	+	
Venous angioma	+				
Cavernous angioma	+		+		
Aneurysm	+				Temporal, frontal
Primary neoplasm	+				
Metastatic neoplasm(s)	+				Gray-white junction
Cerebral amyloid	+				
Coagulopathy	+			+	Occasionally multiple
Sinovenous occlusive	+				Occasionally bilateral, high convexities

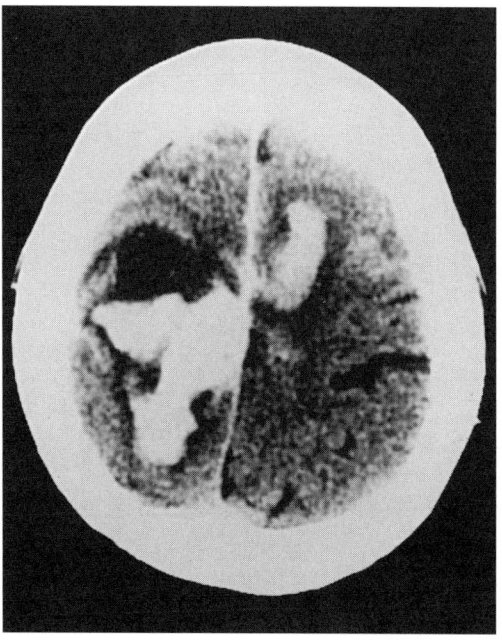

Figure 4: High convexity noncontrast axial CT section in a 58-year-old woman with a several week history of headaches followed by acute quadriparesis and confusion. Note the bilateral parenchymal hematomas with surrounding areas of low attenuation likely representing venous infarction. MRI revealed a superior sagittal sinus thrombosis.

Other features of the CT scan can be helpful in prioritizing potential etiologies of ICH. The location of the ICH, coupled with the clinical history, allows estimation of the most reasonable diagnostic possibilities (Table 1). Also, the presence of multiple separate areas of ICH can raise important diagnostic considerations including trauma, coagulopathy, vasculitis, metastatic neoplasms, sinovenous occlusive disease, and cerebral amyloid angiopathy (Figures 4 and 5A, 5B). Multiple intracranial hemorrhages with fluid-blood levels may be more characteristic of patients on anticoagulant therapy.[28-29]

Computed tomography has become incorporated into other aspects of managing patients with ICH. Stereotactic hematoma evacuation is becoming increasingly popular and depends on CT or MRI for planning intervention.[30-34] In addition, many authors have used CT to determine if surgical evacuation is indicated and to predict clinical status and prognosis based on hemorrhage volume, location, presence of intraventricular blood, and horizontal tissue

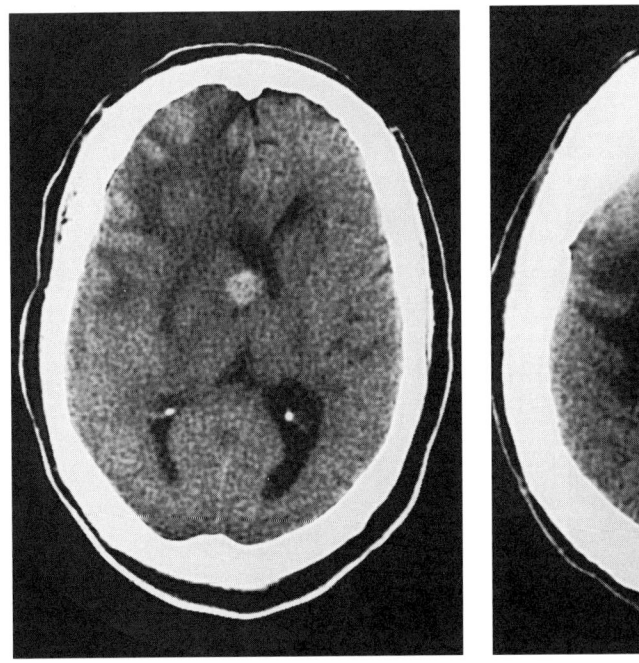
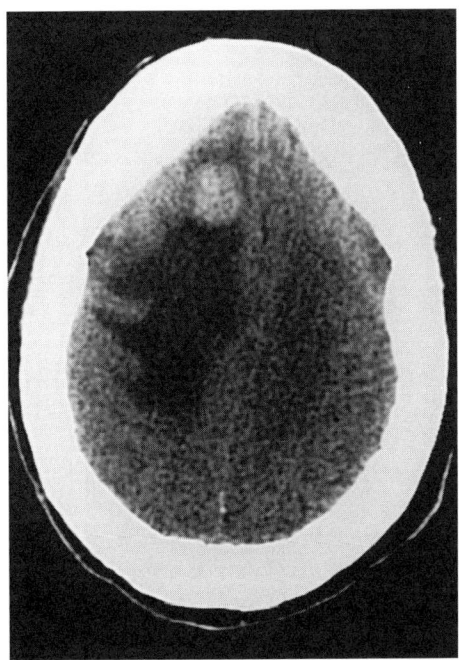

Figure 5A   **Figure 5B**

Figure 5: Noncontrast axial CT sections of a 65-year-old woman with known renal cell carcinoma with acute worsening of left-sided weakness and confusion which had been progressive for several weeks. **A.** Note the focal area of hemorrhage in the region of the head of the right caudate nucleus. There is extensive edema extending within the right frontal white matter. **B.** A more superior axial section in the same patient shows an additional area of hemorrhage in the right frontal region with edema in the adjacent white matter. Both hemorrhagic areas (scans **A** and **B**) represent hemorrhagic brain metastases from renal cell carcinoma diagnosed by biopsy of the right frontal lesion.

shifts.[35-42] Since the details of these applications are beyond the scope of this chapter, the reader is referred to the listed references for more information.

Magnetic Resonance Imaging

Magnetic resonance imaging utilizes a powerful magnetic field and selected pulsations of electromagnetic radiofrequency waves to obtain multiplanar images of the body. The images reflect the distribution of hydrogen nuclei and the tissue environment affecting them.

When patients are exposed to the MRI magnet, the protons within the studied body region align with the magnetic field. Then, pulsations of electromagnetic radiofrequency waves are introduced to excite these protons out of their alignment. Since protons within diverse tissue environments respond variably to each radiofrequency pulsation sequence and have different relaxation rates, focusing on these distinct relaxation rates highlights tissue differences. The shorter pulsation sequences (T_1) reveal exquisite anatomic detail. The longer T_2 sequences demonstrate subtle changes in tissue water content and, therefore, are more sensitive to pathologic processes. Although the detailed physical principles of MRI imaging are beyond the scope of this text, reference is made to many useful reviews on the subject.[43-49] A contrast agent (gadolinium-DTPA) can be administered to enhance vasculature, vascular-rich structures, and regions with a loss of integrity of the blood-brain-barrier.

Magnetic resonance imaging has many advantages over CT, including multiplanar imaging capabilities, increased sensitivity to subtle tissue pathology, the ability to image rapidly flowing blood, less bony artifact, use of nonionizing radiation, and contrast material with a higher safety margin than that used for CT. Some disadvantages of MRI include the high cost, longer study time which can be prohibitive with agitated or confused patients, and limited access for obese patients (more than 300 lbs) or those with pacemakers or metallic implants. In addition, the long scanning duration and flat positioning of patients for MRI can be cumbersome, if not dangerous, for some unstable patients. However, MRI can be performed successfully in patients even on ventilators at some medical centers with the proper scanner and MRI compatible ventilators. Of course, the MRI physical plant must be able to accommodate the ventilator and other equipment (e.g., suctioning apparatus) in case of respiratory decompensation.

Perhaps the most important disadvantage of MRI in patients with ICH is its limitation in the hyperacute period. Since hemorrhage has no characteristic MRI signal intensity within the first 24 hours of bleeding, it may be difficult to differentiate ICH from soft tissue abnormalities. As a result, CT remains the diagnostic test of choice for hyperacute ICH.

The dynamic composition of intracerebral hematomas can be documented by the evolution in their appearance on MRI (Table 2). Many studies have focused on the MRI features of ICH.[43-45,48-52] Hyperacute hematoma contains

Table 2
ICH Characteristics on MRI

Timing Issues	Changing Blood Component	Signal Intensity on T_1 Weighted Images	Signal Intensity on T_2 Weighted Images
Hyperacute (0 to 24 hours)	Intracellular oxyhemoglobin	Decreased	Increased
Acute (24 hours to 1 week); Begins centrally	Intracellular deoxyhemoglobin	Isointense or decreased	Decreased
Subacute (1 to 4 weeks); Begins peripherally	Intracellular methemoglobin	Increased	Decreased
Subacute—Chronic	Extracellular methemoglobin	Increased	Increased
Chronic (> 2 to 4 weeks)	Hemosiderin	No Change	Decreased
Hyperacute—Subacute (0 to 4 weeks)	Edema	Decreased	Increased

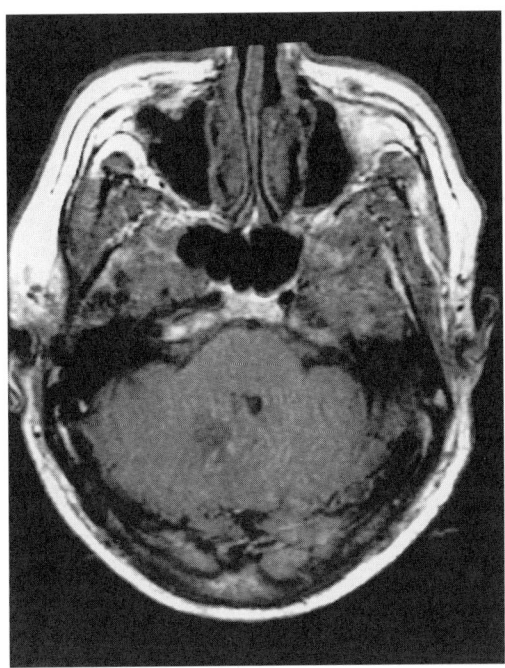

Figure 6: Axial T_1 weighted MRI (SE 516/19) performed 36 hours after an acute right cerebellar hemorrhage. There is an area of ill-defined decreased signal intensity in the right cerebellar hemisphere. The finding is vague and nonspecific.

intracellular oxyhemoglobin and plasma and, therefore, projects on MRI as a protein-rich fluid with a hypointense signal on T_1 weighted images and a hyperintense signal on T_2 weighted images (Figure 6).

Acute hematomas (24 hours to 1 week) change from the hyperacute period as the plasma fraction significantly resorbs and the intracellular oxyhemoglobin converts to intracellular deoxyhemoglobin. The process begins in the central portion of the hematoma. A hematoma in this stage is isointense or slightly hypointense relative to gray matter on T_1 weighted images and hypointense on T_2 weighted images. Surrounding edema may cause a hyperintense signal around the periphery on T_2 weighted images (Figure 7).

The subacute stage (1 to 4 weeks) involves the conversion of intracellular deoxyhemoglobin (T_1 isointense/hypointense) to intracellular methemoglobin (T_1 hyperintense), beginning around the hematoma periphery. Thus, the hematoma gradually becomes hyperintense on T_1 weighted images from the outside inward. With red blood cell lysis and resorption leading to free methemoglobin, the hematoma becomes hyperintense on all image sequences (Figure 8A, 8B).

In the chronic stage (more than 1 month), all of the red blood cells have lysed and the hematoma appears hyperintense on all image sequences due to

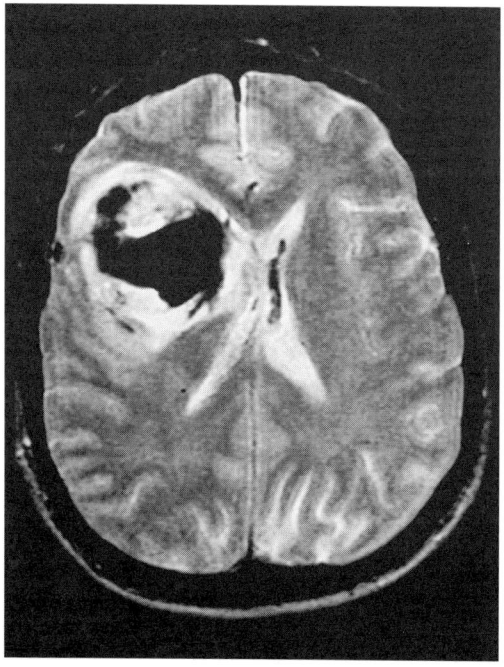

Figure 7: Axial T_2 weighted MRI (SE 2400/70) in a man 4 days after a right frontal hemorrhage. The area of markedly decreased signal centrally demonstrates the evolution of appearance of blood products on MRI in the acute period after ICH. The hypointense core is predominantly intracellular deoxyhemoglobin and the surrounding area of high signal represents associated edema.

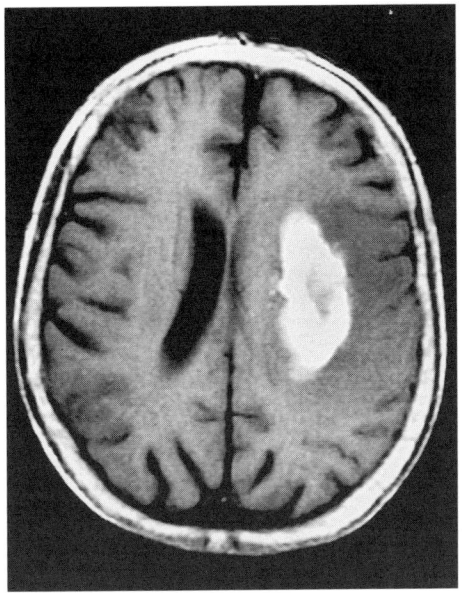
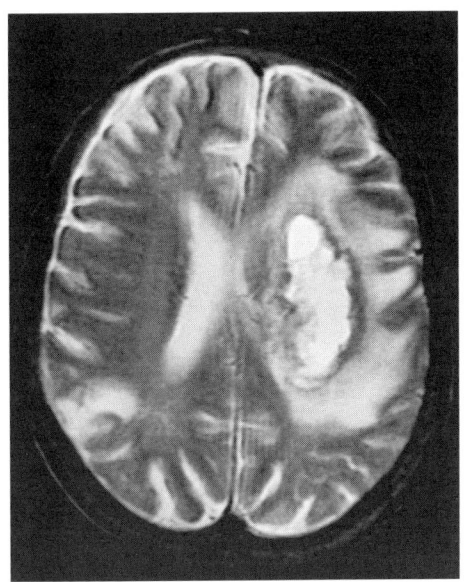

Figure 8A **Figure 8B**

Figure 8: A. Axial T_1 weighted MRI (SE 616/19) reveals a well-circumscribed area of hemorrhage in the left basal ganglia 15 days after the ictus. The main area of hyperintensity is due to intracellular methemoglobin and contrasts to the central region of lower attenuation from residual intracellular deoxyhemoglobin. **B.** Axial T_2 weighted MRI (SE 2416/80) in the same patient demonstrates subacute hematoma (mainly extracellular methemoglobin) and a surrounding area of high (but lesser) signal intensity due to surrounding edema.

free dilute methemoglobin. A thin rim of hypointensity due to hemosiderin deposition may persist indefinitely (Figure 9).

Magnetic resonance imaging is helpful for the evaluation of ICH in several ways. Its sensitivity and specificity for post-hyperacute ICH makes it valuable for the detection of previous, perhaps asymptomatic, hemorrhage.[53,54] In addition, MRI's ability to clearly image posterior fossa structures makes it very useful in cases of brainstem hemorrhage (Figure 10).

Magnetic resonance imaging has also demonstrated vascular malformations undetectable by cerebral angiography.[45,55–57] An underlying neoplasm may be detected by MRI,[11,58] while evasive to other diagnostic modalities, but MRI is also imperfect for this diagnosis.[59] Clinicians should avoid false comfort from the "normal" MRI or the one revealing "only the ICH already detected by CT." Patients with clinically suspected neoplastic hemorrhage should have serial contrast studies or, if appropriate, biopsy.

As with CT, MRI has nondiagnostic roles in the management of patients with ICH. It can be used to plan stereotactic hematoma aspiration.[28] In addition, its multiplanar imaging abilities can clarify the mass effect and brain tissue shifts due to the hematoma.

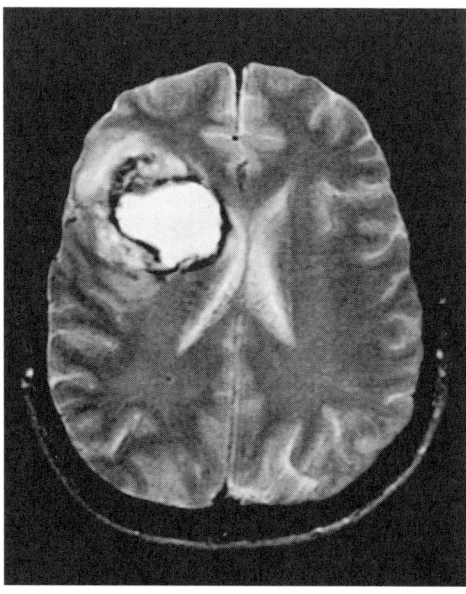

Figure 9: Axial T_2 weighted MRI (SE 2400/80) demonstrates a right frontal hematoma 26 days after the ictus. Note the predominant high signal intensity centrally with a peripheral rim of low intensity due to extracellular methemoglobin surrounded by hemosiderin, respectively.

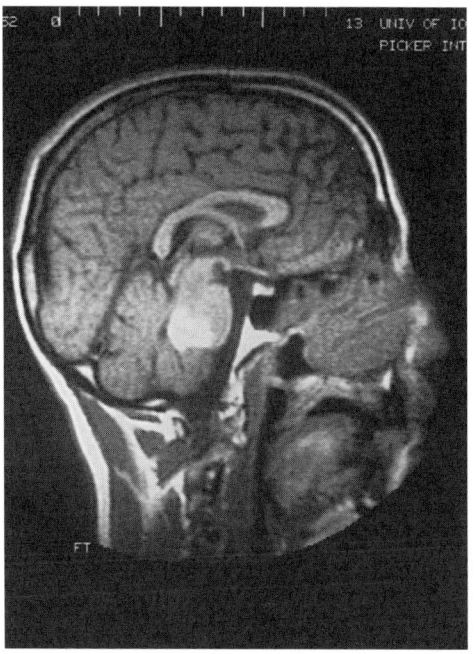

Figure 10: Sagittal T_1 weighted MRI (SE 616/19) reveals an inferior pontine hematoma 8 days after presentation.

Ultrasound/Magnetic Resonance Angiography

The anterior fontanelle allows effective ultrasound identification of intraparenchymal hemorrhage and intraventricular hemorrhage in infants, particularly neonates.[60] In adults, noninvasive diagnostic alternatives for evaluating cerebral vasculature include transcranial Doppler sonography and magnetic resonance angiography (MRA). However, neither of these studies has an established role in the evaluation of patients with ICH. Magnetic resonance angiography provides very attractive images of the intracranial circulation, but its efficacy and accuracy are only now being investigated and established.

Cerebral Angiography

Cerebral angiography involves the intravascular administration of a radiopaque contrast material to outline the cerebral vasculature. This typically requires selective intra-arterial injection of contrast through long, flexible, plastic, disposable catheters inserted through a femoral artery approach. The various filming (projecting in several planes) and computerized image processing alternatives provide a wide spectrum of sophistication for identifying intracranial cerebrovascular pathology. Selection of the particular vessels to be studied should be established in cooperation with the neuroradiologist performing the procedure. Although intravenous digital subtraction angiography (IV-DSA) does not involve intra-arterial catheter manipulations, it requires a higher contrast load than "conventional" angiography, the image quality is highly variable, and it is ineffective for confident evaluation of the intracranial vasculature.[61] In general, IV-DSA has no role in the evaluation of patients with ICH.

Complications from conventional cerebral angiography in the hands of an experienced neuroradiologist are uncommon,[62–65] but may include regional hematoma or infection at the site of arterial puncture, distal lower extremity emboli, arterial dissections, embolic stroke, cardiac arrhythmia, allergic reaction, renal failure, and death.

In general, angiography is indicated when cerebral aneurysm, AVM, vasculitis, and moya-moya disease are important diagnostic considerations and determining their presence will affect patient management. Although angiography is also valuable for the detection of sinovenous occlusive disease, MRI is similarly impressive for establishing this diagnosis (Figure 11).

One angiography-based review of 97 patients with ICH found angiography to be diagnostic in 12.8% of hypertensive patients and 44% of nonhypertensive patients. The angiograms identified aneurysms, arteriovenous malformations, moya-moya disease, and superior sagittal sinus thrombosis. The highest yield of arteriographic abnormalities was found in lobar hemorrhages in the nonhypertensive group and intraventricular hemorrhages in the hypertensive group. Angiography was not useful in hypertensives with putaminal hemorrhage.[66]

Angiography is also helpful in the diagnosis of carotid cavernous fistulae[67,68]

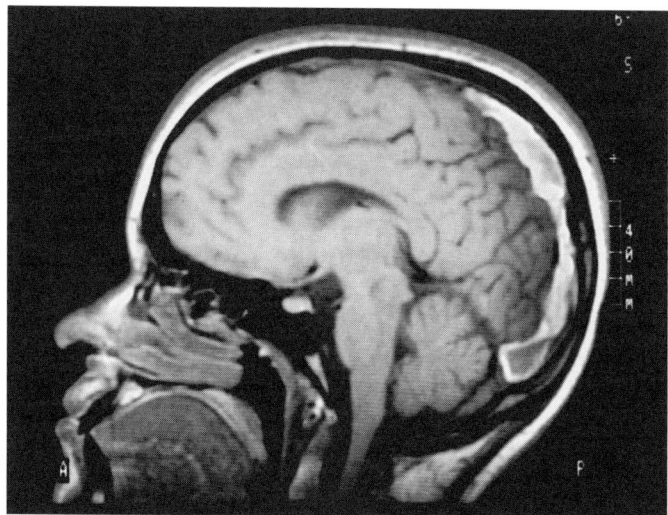

Figure 11: Sagittal T_1 weighted MRI (SE 766/19) in a 25-year-old pregnant woman with subacute onset headaches, nausea, vomiting, and diplopia. Note the abnormal increased signal within the posterior aspect of the superior sagittal sinus representing thrombosis.

and vasculitis,[69-72] but the occurrence of angiographically-negative vascular malformations[55,73] and vasculitis[74] emphasize the limited diagnostic significance of a "normal" angiogram in the individual patient with ICH. Nonetheless, negative angiograms may have prognostic significance, since angiographically occult vascular malformations may have a better prognosis than those demonstrable by angiography.[75]

In addition to the diagnostic indications for angiography in patients with ICH, angiography can assist in the planning and performance of endovascular embolization of vascular neoplasms[76] and arteriovenous malformations[77,78] and balloon[79] or thrombotic electrolytic detachable coil[80] obliteration of cerebral aneurysms.

Nonradiologic Studies

Laboratory Studies

Some studies should be performed in all patients with ICH, whereas others can be performed depending on the specific details of the case (Table 3). Prothrombin time (PT), partial thromboplastin time (PTT), and platelet count should be performed in all patients, since patients with known structural intra-

Table 3
Nonradiologic Laboratory Studies Indicated in Patients With ICH

All Patients:
—CBC, platelet count
—PT, PTT
—Alkaline phosphatase, serum glutamic oxalacetic transaminase
—Erythrocyte sedimentation rate
—BUN, creatinine
—Urinalysis
—Toxicology screen
Selected Patients:
—Examination of peripheral blood smear
—Blood cultures
—Fibrinogen, fibrinogen degradation products
—Bleeding time
—Platelet aggregation studies
—Hemoglobin electrophoresis
—Plasminogen assay, plasminogen activation studies
—Human immunodeficiency virus-type I antibody studies
—In patients with sinovenous occlusive disease:
   Protein C, protein S, antithrombin III assays
   Antiphospholipid and anticardiolipin antibody titers
   Urinary and serum homocysteine levels

cranial lesions prone to hemorrhage could have precipitation of their bleeding episode from a concomitant bleeding disorder. Elevated liver enzymes or malnutrition should raise suspicion of acquired coagulation factor deficiencies. Bleeding time, platelet aggregation studies, and fibrinogen assay can also be revealing in this setting, as disorders of platelet function and certain forms of dysfibrinogenemia have been associated with early rehemorrhage.[81]

A toxicology screen should be sent from the emergency room, particularly in younger patients without known risk factors for ICH. In patients with a family history of bleeding, a search for inherited bleeding disorders such as factor VIII deficiency or factor IX deficiency should ensue. Blood cultures, fibrin degradation products, and analysis of the peripheral blood smear for fragmented erythrocytes should be performed when disseminated intravascular coagulation is suspected. Erythrocyte sedimentation rate, C-reactive protein, complement levels, and various rheumatologically-associated antibody assays have limited value for detecting vasculitis. Hemoglobin electrophoresis is indicated in patients at risk for sickle cell disease. Acquired immune deficiency syndrome and its multitude of related complications should always be considered as a potential etiology of ICH.

Patients with ICH from sinovenous occlusive disease should have a thorough investigation for a hypercoagulable state including assays for protein-C, protein-S, antithrombin III, lupus anticoagulant, anticardiolipin antibodies, cold agglutinins, serum protein electrophoresis, and immunoelectrophoresis.

Analysis of plasminogen can rarely demonstrate defects in the intrinsic fibrinolytic pathway. Patients with proteinuria on screening urinalysis should be investigated for nephrotic syndrome since it can be associated with a "hypercoagulable" state. Older patients without other identifiable causes of sinovenous occlusive disease should be evaluated for an underlying malignancy.

Biopsy

Histologic evaluation of brain tissue can be diagnostic of cerebral amyloid angiopathy,[82-86] cerebral vasculitis,[74,87] and neoplasm.[88] Any patient undergoing surgical evacuation of an ICH should have the margins of the hematoma explored and biopsied unless a confident diagnosis of its etiology has already been established.

In patients who would not otherwise be considered candidates for hematoma evacuation, the role of biopsy in the diagnosis of cryptogenic ICH is controversial. Stable patients with a homogeneous ICH on CT and no unusual areas of enhancement on MRI should be afforded an interval of close observation. If the clinical history suggests focal neurologic dysfunction or seizure disorder antedating the ICH, or if the imaging characteristics are suggestive of an underlying neoplasm or vasculitis, then the alternative of biopsy should at least be considered. However, the risk of biopsy (anesthesia-related complications, hemorrhage, infection, seizures) must be carefully weighed against the potential contribution of the gathered information on patient management and outcome. In most circumstances, serial MRI with gadolinium is the most prudent approach to these patients.

Multiple ICHs, particularly lobar hematomas in older patients, are suggestive of cerebral amyloid angiopathy when other causes of bleeding have been properly excluded. A more detailed discussion of cerebral amyloid angiopathy is contained in another chapter. When the clinical features and temporal profile of the patient's illness is suggestive of vasculitis and the angiogram is not diagnostic, leptomeningeal and brain biopsy may be efficacious[74,87] in order to confidently proceed with immunosuppressive therapy.

Cerebrospinal Fluid Examination

The advent of CT and MRI scanning has had a significant negative impact on the frequency and utility of cerebrospinal fluid (CSF) examination in patients with ICH. The most important studies analyzing CSF in patients with ICH were performed in the pre-CT era.[88-92] Increased CSF pressure is common (>50% of patients). Red blood cells (RBC) are variably present with ICH, depending on subarachnoid or intraventricular extension, and interpreting their significance requires distinguishing true hemorrhage from traumatic puncture.[93]

The CSF white blood cell count (WBC) may be elevated in a proportion reflecting the serum WBC/RBC ratio, or in excess if there is significant tissue necrosis. Initially, the CSF protein levels vary after ICH and may be proportional to the quantity of RBCs in the CSF. Eventually protein levels may elevate out of proportion to the cell count, ranging from 40 to 2,200 mg/dl.[89] The CSF glucose is most often normal in the patients with ICH, as opposed to the occasional decrease in patients with subarachnoid hemorrhage.[89-92]

The examination of CSF in patients with ICH is so nonspecific that it is rarely of significant diagnostic utility. In addition, the potential risk of promoting life-threatening brain tissue shifts by withdrawal of CSF from the spinal subarachnoid space in a patient with a known intracranial space occupying lesion further emphasizes the low utility of lumbar puncture in this setting.

An Approach To Laboratory Evaluation of ICH by Brain Region

The predilection of various ICH etiologies for certain brain regions is discussed in the preceding chapters, and much of the subsequent narrative is based on that information. The premise for the remainder of the chapter is that any patient with an acute neurologic deficit even remotely suspicious for ICH should have a CT scan of the brain without contrast. Figure 12A through 12E summarizes our usual investigational strategy for patients with ICH, although we readily adjust this approach to each patient's individual situation. Our approach is based on a combination of scientific information, experience, and the compulsiveness which defines our approach to medical management. We advocate this strategy as a sound way to avoid missing the opportunity to diagnose a treatable problem or prevent recurrent hemorrhage.

The best time to perform these tests depends on each specific clinical situation, and is beyond the scope of this chapter. In general, the diagnostic tests should be done at a time when the information obtained will affect patient management decisions. It is never appropriate to perform diagnostic studies on unstable patients, particularly those who require transport or are invasive, if the information will not lead to a temporally proximate alteration in patient management. Obviously, an aggressive diagnostic and therapeutic approach may not be justified in patients who are neurologically devastated by the hemorrhage or too medically frail to undergo the diagnostic studies safely.

All patients with ICH should have initial blood and urine evaluations as listed in Table 3, tailored to the individual patient's history and potential risk factors for hemorrhage. Patients strongly suspected of having ICH but without CT evidence of hemorrhage should have an MRI scan. This is particularly important in patients with significant anemia or brainstem localization by examination.

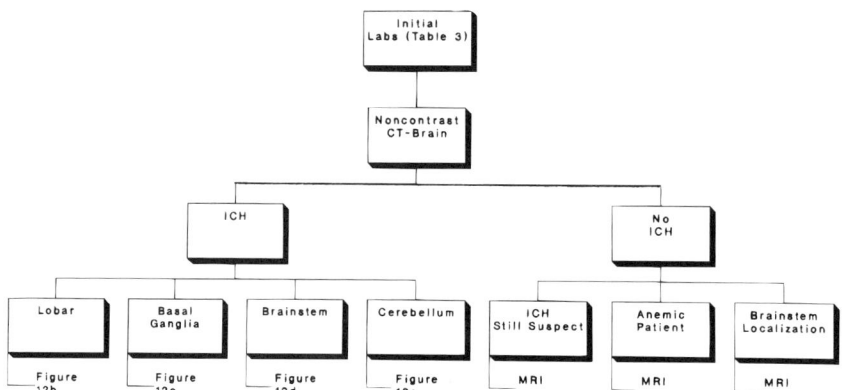

Figure 12A

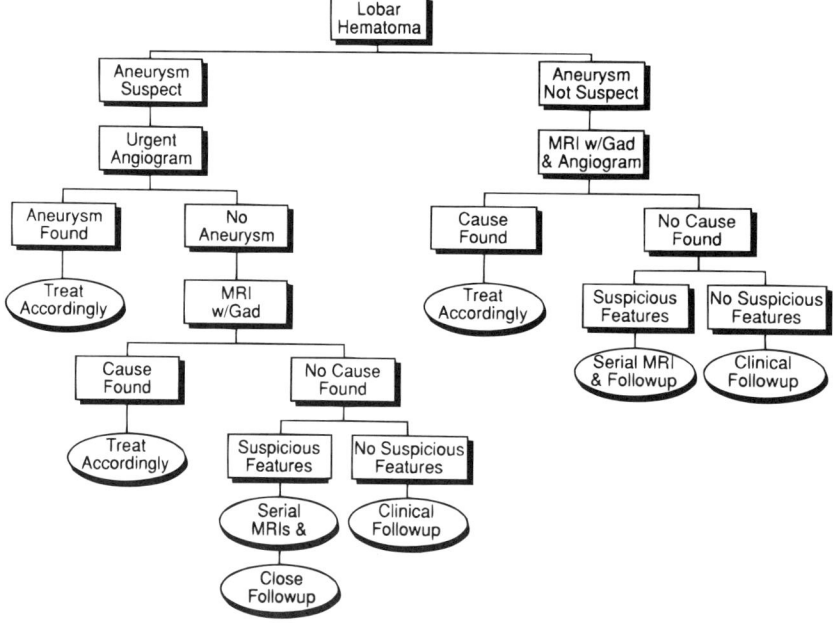

Figure 12B

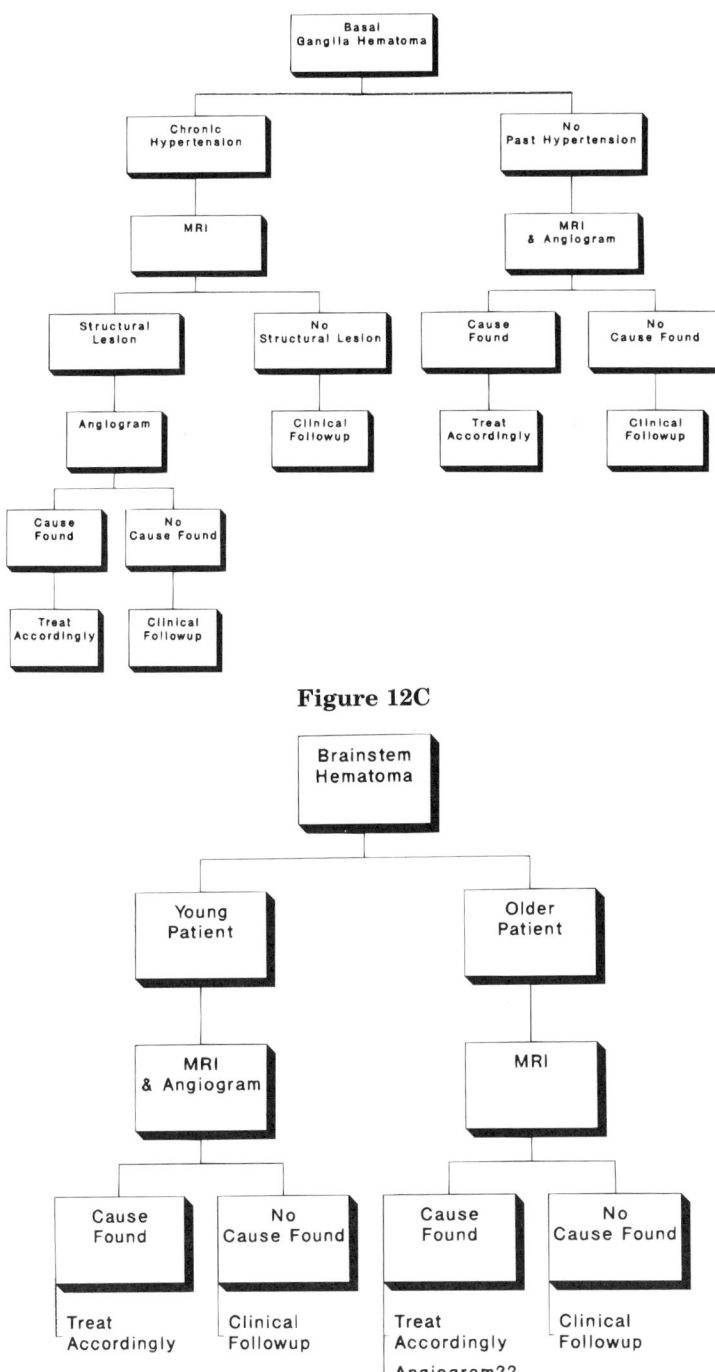

Figure 12C

Figure 12D

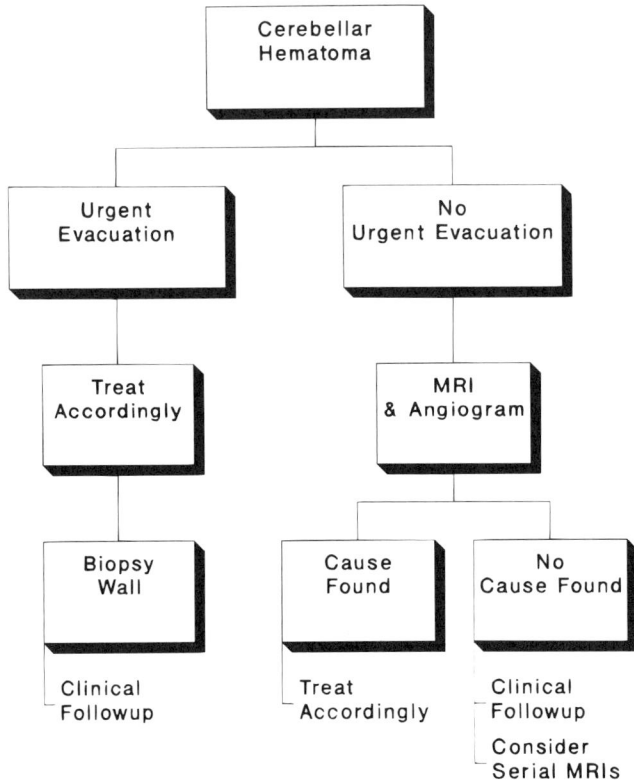

Figure 12E

Figure 12: A. Suggested diagnostic strategy for patients presenting with nontraumatic ICH. **B.** Approach to patients with lobar hematoma after initial CT and laboratory evaluations. **C.** Approach to patients with basal ganglia hematoma after initial CT and laboratory evaluations. **D.** Approach to patients with brainstem hematoma after initial CT and laboratory evaluations. **E.** Approach to patients with cerebellar hematoma after initial CT and laboratory evaluations.

Lobar Hematomas

The high incidence of structural brain pathology responsible for lobar hematomas warrants a thorough diagnostic evaluation even in patients with a long history of hypertension. This aggressive diagnostic approach to lobar hematomas is supported by a CT/angiography correlative study of 67 consecutive patients with nontraumatic lobar hematoma. Angiography was diagnostic in 43% of the cases. Notably, the diagnostic yield of angiography increased from 27% without subarachnoid hemorrhage (SAH) to 77% with SAH.[94] MRI is also incorporated into the evaluation of patients with lobar ICH, providing potentially useful noninvasive diagnostic information.

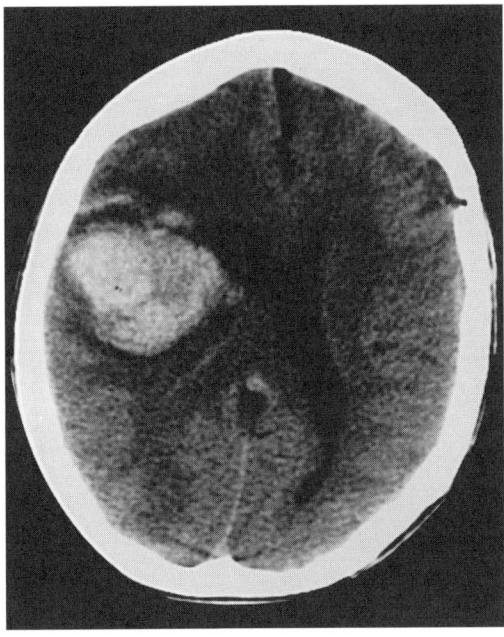

Figure 13: Axial noncontrast CT section reveals a well-defined area of acute hemorrhage in the right frontoparietal region with surrounding edema and mass effect.

When CT demonstrates a lobar hematoma (Figure 13), an angiogram should be performed acutely if the pattern of hemorrhage is consistent with a ruptured aneurysm (e.g., perisylvian hematoma, deep inferior frontal hematoma, or subarachnoid or intraventricular blood) (Figure 14). If aneurysm is not highly suspect, MRI with Gd-DTPA should be performed to determine if there are findings suspicious for an underlying structural lesion. If a primary or metastatic neoplasm is confidently identified by MRI, then angiography is not necessarily indicated. Biopsy may be appropriate in certain situations, especially if these patients undergo surgical evacuation of the hematoma.

When the MRI does not demonstrate an underlying neoplasm or is logistically prohibited, angiography should be performed in most patients to identify an underlying AVM, unsuspected aneurysm, or inflammatory vascular disorder (Figure 15). Although MRI is very useful in detecting AVMs (Figure 16) and any area of prior hemorrhage, the hematoma and associated mass effect may compromise its sensitivity. Even if a vascular malformation is detected by MRI, angiography is indicated to determine the type of vascular malformation (e.g., AVM, cavernous angioma, venous angioma) and to plan either surgical or endovascular therapy.[95]

Due to the high incidence of structural lesions causing lobar hematoma, particularly frontal and temporal,[94] any patient with a history suspicious for previous focal neurologic deficit or seizure disorder or any subtle, albeit nondi-

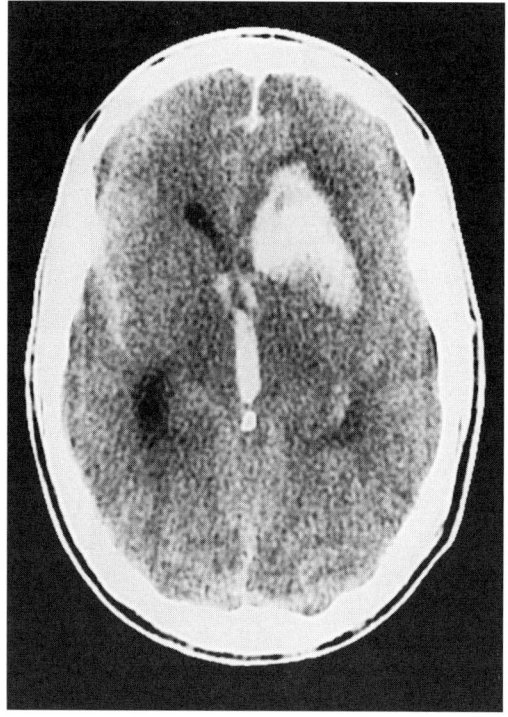

Figure 14: Axial noncontrast CT section in a 28-year-old man with acute onset coma and right motor changes, demonstrates a deep left frontal acute hematoma with associated subarachnoid and intraventricular blood due to a ruptured left anterior communicating artery aneurysm.

agnostic, abnormalities by CT, MRI, or angiography should have serial MRI scans with gadolinium and close clinical follow-up.

Putaminal, Thalamic, and Caudate Hematomas

Recognizing that hypertensive patients can have structural brain pathology which causes ICH independent of their hypertension, skepticism is recommended when approaching a chronically hypertensive patient with ICH in the putamen, thalamus, or caudate nucleus. "Hypertensive" ICH is a diagnosis of exclusion, always deserving careful analysis of all clinical details and intense scrutiny of available laboratory and radiographic information. Patients with a known history of chronic hypertension and putaminal, (Figure 17) thalamic, (Figure 18) or caudate hematoma should have an MRI with Gd-DTPA to determine if there is an underlying vascular malformation, neoplasm, or inflammatory vascular disorder. However, if nothing suspicious is found, only clinical

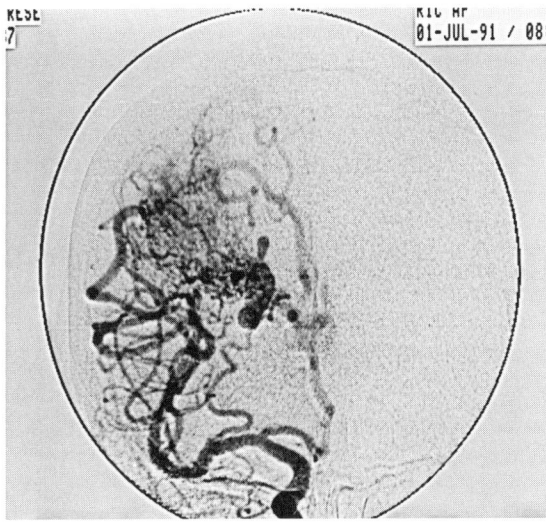

Figure 15: AP angiographic projection of the early arterial phase of a selective right internal carotid artery injection demonstrates early venous drainage of an arteriovenous malformation.

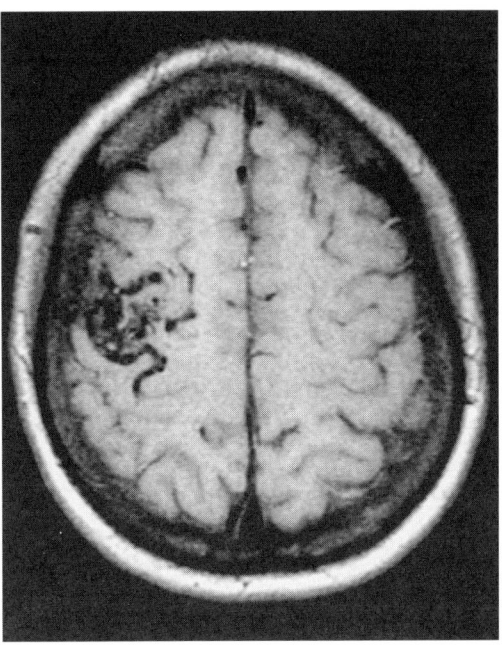

Figure 16: T_1 weighted axial MRI (SE 616/19) demonstrates characteristic serpiginous flow-voids from dilated venous drainage of an arteriovenous malformation.

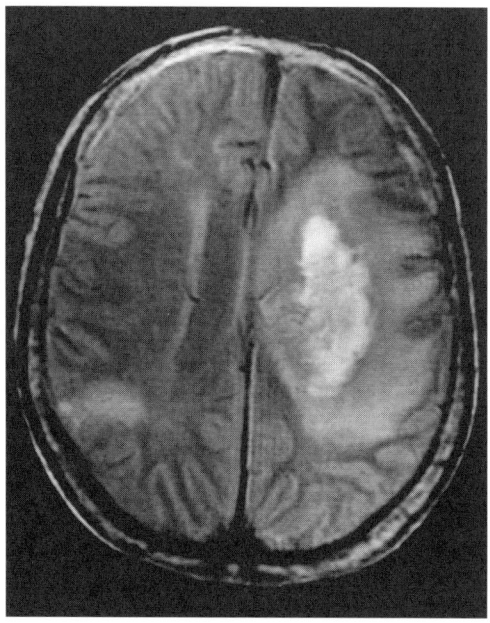

Figure 17: First echo of a T_2 weighted axial MRI (SE 2416/20) reveals a subacute left putaminal hemorrhage with surrounding edema. An incidental finding is an old right parietal infarction.

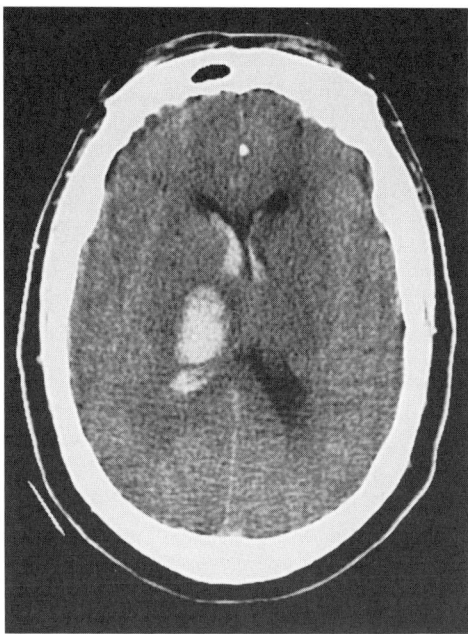

Figure 18: Axial noncontrast CT section demonstrates acute hemorrhage in the right thalamus with intraventricular blood in both lateral ventricular anterior horns. There is edema and mass effect associated with the thalamic hematoma.

follow-up is recommended due to the low diagnostic yield of angiography in hypertensives with ICH in these locations.[48]

MRI with Gd-DTPA and angiography should be performed in patients with a putaminal, thalamic, or caudate hematoma with no history of hypertension. If the MRI demonstrates a vascular malformation, the angiogram will define the feeding and draining vessels if it is an AVM. If a structural lesion is not identified by MRI, it may be obscured by the mass effect of the hematoma, emphasizing the value of angiography. If an angiogram already has identified an AVM, the MRI is useful in clarifying the architecture and geometry of the lesion as well as identifying if there has been previous hemorrhage.

Brainstem Hematoma

Younger patients (less than 45 years) with brainstem hematomas commonly have underlying vascular malformations (Figure 19). Consequently, both MRI and angiography are indicated in these patients for reasons similar

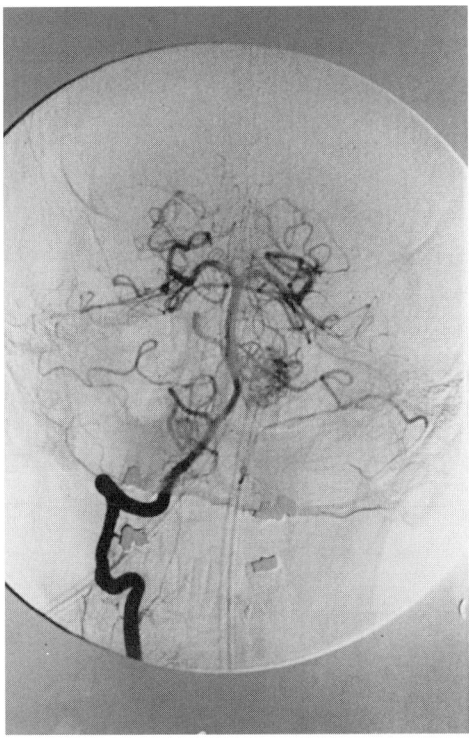

Figure 19: AP angiographic projection of the early arterial phase of a selective right vertebral artery injection reveals abnormal vasculature on the left side of the basilar artery corresponding to a pontine arteriovenous malformation.

to those discussed for hematomas in other regions when vascular malformation is an important diagnostic consideration.

Older patients with brainstem hematoma, particularly those with chronic hypertension, should have an MRI with Gd-DTPA. There are few indications for angiography in this subgroup unless the MRI demonstrates a lesion suggestive of a vascular malformation or other vasculopathy which may benefit from surgical intervention.

Cerebellar Hematoma

Cerebellar hematomas tend to involve the area surrounding the dentate nucleus, or less often the vermis (Figure 20). A large number of patients with cerebellar hematoma may have underlying structural lesions. However, the life-threatening nature of the problem and the dramatic benefit of emergent surgical intervention may not allow the luxury of preceding diagnostic investigations other than the initial blood work and CT.

Stable patients should have an MRI with Gd-DTPA. Angiography may be

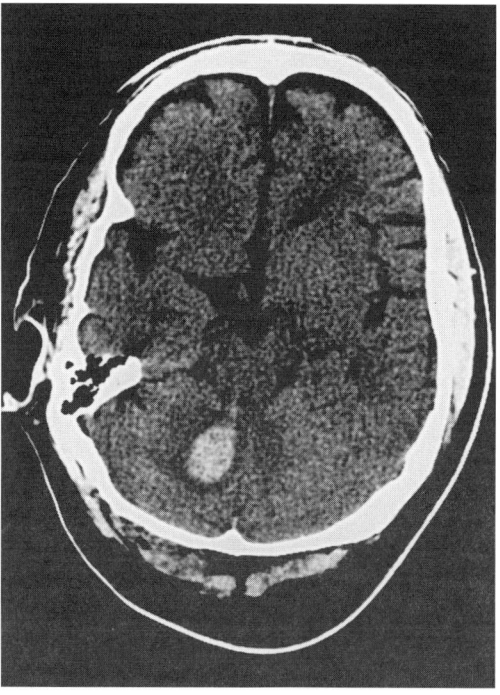

Figure 20: Axial noncontrast CT section in a 65-year-old man reveals an acute right cerebellar hematoma with surrounding edema.

necessary to search for and characterize any possible underlying structural lesion.

References

1. Kinkel WR, Jacobs L: Computerized axial tomography in cerebrovascular disease. *Neurology* 1976;26:924.
2. Scott WR, New PFJ, Davis KR, et al: Computerized axial tomography of intracerebral and intraventricular hemorrhage. *Radiology* 1974;112:73.
3. Weisberg L: Computerized tomography in intracranial hemorrhage. *Arch Neurol* 1979;36:422.
4. Huckman MS, Weinberg PE, Kim KS, et al: Angiographic and clinicopathologic correlates in basal ganglionic hemorrhage. *Radiology* 1970;95:79.
5. Bergstrom K, Lodin H: An angiographic observation in intracerebral haematoma. *Br J Radiol* 1967;4:228.
6. New PFJ: Computed tomography in the diagnosis of hemorrhagic stroke. In: Thompson RA, Green JR, eds: *Advances in Neurology,* Vol 16. New York: Raven Press, 1977:145.
7. Franke CL, van Swieten JC, van Gijn J: Residual lesions on computed tomography after intracerebral hemorrhage. *Stroke* 1991;22:1530.
8. Newell DW, LeRoux PD, Dacey RG Jr, et al: CT infusion scanning for detection of cerebral aneurysms. *J Neurosurg* 1989;71:175.
9. Fontaine S, de la Sayette V, Gianfelice D, et al: CT, MRI, and angiography of venous angiomas: a comparative study. *Can Assoc Radiol J* 1987;38:259.
10. Maiuri F, Gallicchio B, Iaconetta G, et al: Megadolichobasilar artery and acute cerebrovascular pathology. *Neurol Res* 1990;12:54.
11. Takahashi I, Sugimoto S, Nunomura M, et al: A case of cystic metastatic intracranial amelanotic melanoma—analysis of findings in CT and MRI. *No To Shinkei* 1990;42:1031.
12. Weisberg LA: Hemorrhagic primary intracranial neoplasms: clinical-computed tomographic correlations. *Comput Radiol* 1986;10:131.
13. Laster DW, Moody DM, Ball MR: Resolving intracerebral hematoma: alteration of the "ring sign" with steroids. *Am J Roentgenol* 1978;130:935.
14. Kasdon DL, Scott RM, Adelman LS, et al: Cerebellar hemorrhage with decreased absorption values on computed tomography: a case report. *Neuroradiology* 1977;13:265.
15. Chin D, Carney P: Acute cerebellar hemorrhage with brainstem compression in contrast with benign cerebellar hemorrhage. *Surg Neurol* 1983;19:406.
16. Komiyama M, Yasui T, Yagura H, et al: Computed tomographic evaluation of bleeding sites in primary pontine hemorrhages. *Stroke* 1991;22:1309.
17. Kushner MJ, Bressman SB: The clinical manifestations of pontine hemorrhage. *Neurology* 1985;35:637.

18. Muller HR, Wuthrich R, Wiggli U, et al: The contribution of computerized axial tomography to the diagnosis of cerebellar and pontine hematomas. *Stroke* 1975;6:467.
19. Weisberg LA: Cerebellar hemorrhage in adults. Clinical and computerized tomographic findings. *Comput Radiol* 1982;6:75.
20. Biller J, Gentry LR, Adams HP, et al: Spontaneous hemorrhage in the medulla oblongata: clinical MR correlations. *J Comput Assist Tomogr* 1986; 10:303.
21. Greenberg JO, Skubick DL: Unexpected brain hemorrhages and the value of computerized tomography. *Comput Tomogr* 1977;1:349.
22. Brott T, Broderick J, Barsan W, et al: Hyper-acute clot retraction in spontaneous intracerebral hemorrhage. *Stroke* 1992;23:8.
23. Broderick JP, Brott TG, Tomsick T, et al: Ultra-early evaluation of intracerebral hemorrhage. *J Neurosurg* 1990;72:195.
24. Chen ST, Chen SD, Hsu CY, et al: Progression of hypertensive intracerebral hemorrhage. *Neurology* 1989;39:1509.
25. Fehr MA, Anderson DC: Incidence of progression or rebleeding in hypertensive in intracerebral hemorrhage. *J Stroke Cerebrovasc Dis* 1991;1:111.
26. Bogousslavsky J, Regli F, Uske A, et al: Early spontaneous hematoma in cerebral infarct: is primary cerebral hemorrhage overdiagnosed? *Neurology* 1991;41:837.
27. Wakai S, Nagai M: "Nidus sparing sign" on computerized tomography in intracerebral hemorrhage due to a rupture of arteriovenous malformation. *Acta Neurochir* 1988;95:102.
28. Dolinskas CA, Bilaniuk LT, Zimmerman RA, et al: Computed tomography of intracerebral hematomas. I. Transmission CT observations of hematoma resolution. *Am J Roentgenol* 1977;129:681.
29. Livoni JP, McGahan JP: Intracranial fluid-blood levels in the anticoagulated patient. *Neuroradiology* 1983;25:335.
30. Lunsford LD, Martinez AJ, Latchaw RE: Stereotactic surgery with magnetic resonance and computerized tomography—compatible system. *J Neurosurg* 1986;64:872.
31. Matsumoto K, Hondo H: CT-guided stereotaxic evacuation of hypertensive intracerebral hematomas. *J Neurosurg* 1984;61:440.
32. Mohadjer M, Eggert R, May J, et al: CT-guided stereotactic fibrinolysis of spontaneous and hypertensive cerebellar hemorrhage: long-term results. *J Neurosurg* 1990;73:217.
33. Tanikawa T, Amano K, Kuwamura H, et al: CT-guided stereotactic surgery for evacuation of hypertensive intracerebral hematoma. *Appl Neurophysiol* 1985;48:431.
34. Tanizaki Y, Sugita K, Toriyama T, et al: New CT-guided stereotactic apparatus and clinical experience with intracerebral hematomas. *Appl Neurophysiol* 1985;48:11.
35. Andrews BT, Chiles BW, Olsen WL, et al: The effect of intracerebral hematoma location on the risk of brain-stem compression and on clinical outcome. *J Neurosurg* 1988;69:518.

36. Fieschi C, Carolei A, Fiorelli M, et al: Changing prognosis of primary intracerebral hemorrhage: results of a clinical and computed tomographic follow-up study of 104 patients. *Stroke* 1988;19:192.

37. Kitahama T, Takagi S, Suzuki H, et al: Prediction of outcome of conservatively treated thalamic hemorrhage. *Stroke* 1990;21(Suppl I):60.

38. Nath FP, Nicholls D, Fraser RJA: Prognosis in intracerebral hemorrhage. *Acta Neurochirurgica* 1983;67:29.

39. Portenoy RK, Lipton RB, Berger AR, et al: Intracerebral hemorrhage: a model for the prediction of outcome. *J Neurol Neurosurg Psychiatr* 1987; 50:976.

40. Steiner I, Gomori JM, Melamed E: The prognostic value of the CT scan in conservatively treated patients with intracerebral hematoma. *Stroke* 1984; 15:279.

41. Tuhrim S, Dambrosia JM, Price TR, et al: Prediction of intracerebral hemorrhage survival. *Ann Neurol* 1988;24:258.

42. Ropper AH: Lateral displacement of the brain and level of consciousness in patients with an acute hemispheral mass. *N Engl J Med* 1986;314:953.

43. DeLaPaz RL, New PFJ, Buonanno FS, et al: NMR imaging of intracranial hemorrhage. *J Comput Assist Tomogr* 1984;8:599.

44. Dooms GC, Brant-Zawadzki M, Kucharczyk W, et al: Spin-echo MR imaging of intracranial hemorrhage. *Neuroradiology* 1986;28:132.

45. Gomori JM, Grossman RI, Goldberg HI, et al: Intracranial hematomas: imaging by high-field MR. *Radiology* 1985;157:87.

46. Gomori JM, Grossman RI: Mechanisms responsible for the MR appearance and evolution of intracranial hemorrhage. *RadioGraphics* 1988;8:427.

47. Grossman RI, Gomori JM, Goldberg HI, et al: MR imaging of hemorrhagic conditions of the head and neck. *RadioGraphics* 1988;8:441.

48. Edelman RR, Johnson K, Buxton R, et al: MR of hemorrhage: a new approach. *AJNR* 1986;7:751.

49. Sipponen JT, Sipponen RE, Sivula A: Nuclear magnetic resonance (NMR) imaging of intracerebral hemorrhage in the acute and resolving phases. *J Comput Assist Tomogr* 1983;7:585.

50. Atlas SW, Mark AS, Grossman RI, et al: Intracranial hemorrhage: gradient-echo MR imaging at 1.5 T. Comparison with spin-echo imaging and clinical applications. *Radiology* 1988;168:803.

51. Di Chiro G, Brooks RA, Girton ME, et al: Sequential MR studies of intracerebral hematomas in monkeys. *AJNR* 1986;7:193.

52. Bydder GM, Pennock JM, Porteous R, et al: MRI of intracerebral haematoma at low field (0.15T) using T2 dependent partial saturation sequences. *Neuroradiology* 1988;30:367.

53. Miyashita K, Naritomi H, Nakamura M, et al: Old cerebral hemorrhages in cases of multiple lacunar infarction found by magnetic resonance imaging. *Cerebrovasc Dis* 1991;1:321.

54. Nakajima Y, Ohsuga H, Yamamoto M, et al: Asymptomatic cerebral hemorrhage detected by MRI. *Rinsho Shinkeigaku* 1991;31:270.

55. Davis DH, Kelly PJ: Stereotactic resection of occult vascular malformations. *J Neurosurg* 1990;72:698.

56. Lee BCP, Herzberg L, Zimmerman RD, et al: MR imaging of cerebral vascular malformations. *AJNR* 1985;6:863.

57. Lemme-Plaghos L, Kucharczyk W, Brant-Zawadski M, et al: MR imaging of angiographically occult vascular malformations. *AJNR* 1986;7:217.

58. Atlas SW, Grossman RI, Gomori JM, et al: Hemorrhagic intracranial malignant neoplasms: spin-echo MR imaging. *Radiology* 1987;164:71.

59. Forsting M, Bruckmann H, Thron A: How certain is the diagnosis of intracerebral tumor bleeding in magnetic resonance tomography? *ROFO Fortschr Geb Rontgenstr Nuklearmed* 1989;151:356.

60. Chambers SE, Hendry GMA, Wild SR: Real time ultrasound scanning of the head in neonates and infants, including correlation between ultrasound and computed tomography. *Pediatr Radiol* 1985;15:4.

61. Goldberg HI: Cerebral angiography. In: Barnett HJ, Mohr JP, Stein BM, et al: eds: *Stroke: Pathophysiology, Diagnosis, and Management.* New York: Churchill-Livingstone, 1986:221.

62. Earnest F IV, Forbes G, Sandok BA, et al: Complications of cerebral angiography: prospective assessment of risk. *AJNR* 1983;4:1191.

63. Kerber CW, Cromwell LD, Drayer BP, et al: Cerebral ischemia I. Current angiographic techniques, complications, and safety. *Am J Roentgenol* 1978; 130:1097.

64. Mani RL, Eisenberg RL, McDonald EJ: Complications of catheter cerebral arteriography: analysis of 5000 procedures. I. Criteria and incidence. *Am J Roentgenol* 1978;131:861.

65. Dion JE, Gates PC, Fox AJ, et al: Clinical events following neuroangiography: a prospective study. *Stroke* 1987;18:997.

66. Toffol GJ, Biller J, Adams HP, et al: The predictive value of arteriography in nontraumatic intracerebral hemorrhage. *Stroke* 1986;17:881.

67. Hiramatsu K, Utsumi S, Kyoi K, et al: Intracerebral hemorrhage in carotid cavernous fistulae. *Neuroradiology* 1991;33:67.

68. Lin TK, Chang CN, Wai YY: Spontaneous intracerebral hematoma from occult carotid-cavernous fistula during pregnancy and puerperium. *J Neurosurg* 1992;76:714.

69. Crane R, Kerr LD, Spiera H: Clinical analysis of isolated angiitis of the central nervous system. *Arch Intern Med* 1991;151:2290.

70. Kase CS, Foster TE, Reed JE, et al: Intracerebral hemorrhage and phenylpropanolamine use. *Neurology* 1987;37:399.

71. Maertens P, Lum G, Williams JP, et al: Intracranial hemorrhage and cerebral angiopathic changes in a suicidal phenylpropanolamine poisoning. *South Med J* 1987;80:1584.

72. Shibata S, Mori K, Sekine I, et al: Subarachnoid and intracerebral hemorrhage associated with necrotizing angiitis due to methamphetamine abuse—an autopsy case. *Neurol Med Chir* 1991;31:49.

73. Ries F, Buyenburg S, Jerusalem F: Cavernous angiomas in the differential

diagnosis of cerebrovascular malformations. *Fortschr Neurol Psychiatr* 1991;59:141.

74. Clifford-Jones RE, Love S, Gurusinghe N: Granulomatous angiitis of the central nervous system: a case with recurrent intracerebral hemorrhage. *J Neurol Neurosurg Psychiat* 1985;48:1054.

75. Weisberg LA: Clinical and computed tomographic findings in thrombosed and cryptic cerebrovascular malformations. *Comput Radiol* 1982;6:161.

76. Kuga Y, Waga S, Itoh H: Intracranial hemorrhage due to brain metastasis from hepatocellular carcinoma—case report. *Neurol Med Chir* 1990;30:768.

77. Halbach VV, Higashida RT, Yang P: Preoperative balloon occlusion of arteriovenous malformation. *Neurosurgery* 1988;22:301.

78. Kendall B: Survey of progress. Embolisation techniques in neuroradiology. *Neurology* 1986;233:323.

79. Halbach VV, Higashida RT, Hieshima GB: Interventional neuroradiology. *Neurology* 1986;233:323.

80. Gugliemi G, Viñuela F, Dion J: Special article. Electrothrombosis of saccular aneurysms via endovascular approach. Part 2: Preliminary clinical experience. *J Neurosurg* 1991;75:8.

81. Hashimoto M, Yakota A, Kajiwara H, et al: Repeated intracerebral hemorrhage associated with impaired platelet aggregation. Report of two cases. *Neurol Med Chir* 1992;32:13.

82. Biller J, Loftus CM, Moore SA, et al: Isolated central nervous system angiitis first presenting as spontaneous intracranial hemorrhage. *Neurosurgery* 1987;20:310.

83. Feldmann E, Tornabene: Diagnosis and treatment of cerebral amyloid angiopathy. *Clin Geriatr Med* 1991;7:617.

84. Greene GM, Godersky JC, Biller J, et al: Surgical experience with cerebral amyloid angiopathy. *Stroke* 1990;21:1545.

85. Inoue A, Sato K, Itagaki S, et al: A case of multiple cerebral hemorrhage related to cerebral amyloid angiopathy. *No Shinkei Geka* 1988;16:544.

86. Yong WH, Robert ME, Secor DL, et al: Cerebral hemorrhage with biopsy proved amyloid angiopathy. *Arch Neurol* 1992;49:51.

87. Glick R, Hoying J, Cerullo L, et al: Phenylpropanolamine: an over-the-counter drug causing central nervous system vasculitis and intracerebral hemorrhage. Case report and review. *Neurosurgery* 1987;20:969.

88. Lee MC, Heaney LM, Jacobsen RL: Cerebrospinal fluid in cerebral hemorrhage and infarction. *Stroke* 1975;6:638.

89. Merritt HH, Fremont-Smith F: *The Cerebrospinal Fluid*. Philadelphia: W.B. Saunders, 1938.

90. Sambrook MA, Hutchinson EC, Aber GM: Metabolic studies in subarachnoid hemorrhage and stroke. I. Serial changes in acid-base values in blood and cerebrospinal fluid. *Brain* 1973;96:171.

91. Sarnas R, Ostund H, Muller K: Cerebrospinal fluid cytology after stroke. *Arch Neurol* 1972;26:489.

92. Troost BJ, Walker JE, Cherington M: Hypoglycorrhachia associated with subarachnoid hemorrhage. *Arch Neurol* 1968;19:438.
93. Buruma OJS, Janson HLF, Den Bergh FAJTM, et al: Blood-stained cerebrospinal fluid: traumatic puncture or hemorrhage? *J Neurol Neurosurg Psychiatr* 1981;44:144.
94. Loes DJ, Smoker WRK, Biller J, et al: Nontraumatic lobar intracerebral hemorrhage: CT/angiographic correlation. *AJNR* 1987;8:1027.
95. Smith HJ, Strother CM, Kikuchi Y, et al: MR imaging in the management of supratentorial AVMs. *AJNR* 1988;9:225.

Part IV

Management of Intracerebral Hemorrhage

Chapter 13

Medical Therapy

Roger E. Kelley, MD

Basic Measures

The medical treatment of a patient with intracerebral hemorrhage (ICH) depends upon the neurologic status of the patient and the ultimate prognosis. Obviously, a moribund patient will require terminal conservative care, and it serves little purpose to delay an inevitable demise. A common dilemma is the patient who presents in a comatose state with impending herniation for whom little can be offered from either a surgical or medical standpoint. The aggressive management of increased intracranial pressure in such a patient can forestall mortality but promote morbidity. It is thus extremely important to determine prognosis to avoid what could be a prolonged and expensive course in an intensive care unit for a patient whose chances for a meaningful recovery are nil. It is hoped that the increased public awareness of advanced directives will prevent needless use of interventional therapy in such circumstances.

Factors associated with a poor prognosis in ICH include: (1) moribund condition on presentation, (2) rapidly deteriorating neurologic condition, (3) the size of the ICH,[1] (4) intraventricular extension of the hematoma with the finding of greater than 20 ccs of blood being associated with a very poor prognosis,[2] (5) hydrocephalus,[2] (6) homonymous hemianopsia in association with gaze paresis,[3] (7) active bleeding as demonstrated by serial brain scanning,[4] and (8) coexistent factors such as advanced age or unstable medical condition.

Survivors of ICH will benefit from early mobilization, a mainstay of stroke therapy in general. Early mobilization protects against the complications of prolonged bed confinement including decubitus ulceration, thrombophlebitis, pulmonary embolus, impaired pulmonary drainage, and infection. The development of deep venous thrombosis can be prevented by mobilization as well as by support stockings and pressure devices which are designed to promote venous return applied to the lower extremities. The use of low-dose subcutaneous heparin has become a routine means of preventing deep vein thrombosis following

From Feldmann E (ed). *Intracerebral Hemorrhage*. Armonk, NY: Futura Publishing Company, Inc., © 1994.

stroke.[5] There has been a legitimate concern about the use of subcutaneous low-dose heparin in hemorrhagic stroke, however. In a recent study which addressed this issue, early (day 2) low-dose heparin significantly lowered the risk of pulmonary embolism in spontaneous ICH, but was not associated with an increased risk of rebleeding.[6]

In a study of patients with severe stroke, including ICH, who required prolonged bed rest, we found that the use of a rotational bed significantly reduced the risk of complications of prolonged bed confinement.[7] Specifically, we found that the risk of infection, which was essentially universal for subjects who were confined to a routine hospital bed for 2 weeks or longer, was reduced by 50% with the use of a rotational bed. A summary of potential complications in ICH is provided in Table 1.

Other general measures are indicated for subjects with ICH who have a significant neurologic deficit. An adequate bowel program is mandatory, as constipation is a very common complication of stroke. A combination of a stool softener and bulk agent with cathartics, as necessary, is usually effective for this readily treatable condition.

Approximately one third of stroke patients suffer from a significant degree of depression.[8] This tends to be quite responsive to antidepressant medication[9] and will not only serve to improve the quality of life but also to enhance the effectiveness of rehabilitative therapy. A subject with persistent severe functional disability will also require proper attention to the emotional state. While antidepressant therapy can be quite effective in such a setting, psychological counseling and strong family support are also an important part of rehabilitation.

Typically, rehabilitative therapy involves an occupational therapist working with a paretic or ataxic upper extremity and a physical therapist working with the lower extremity and gait. Speech or swallowing impairment necessitates evaluation by a speech pathologist or speech therapist. The persistence of significant swallowing impairment will require a barium swallow to assess the nature and degree of the deficit.[10] Significant regurgitation, with the potential for aspiration, may well lead to a feeding gastrostomy to promote adequate

---

Table 1
Potential Complications of ICH

1. Transtentorial or tonsillar herniation
2. Obstructive or communicating hydrocephalus
3. Aspiration pneumonia
4. Infection—seen in up to 100% of subjects who are bed confined for 2 weeks or longer and who are not properly mobilized
5. Decubitus ulceration
6. Phlebothrombosis with the potential for pulmonary embolism
7. Seizures—seen in up to 15% to 20%
8. Depression—seen in up to one third of patients

Table 2
Basic Measures for the Medical Management of Patients with ICH

1. Early mobilization when possible
2. Adequate bowel program
3. Anti-embolism measures—which might include support stockings, intermittent leg pressure devices, as well as the judicious use of subcutaneous mini-dose heparin
4. Attention to pulmonary toilet with aspiration precautions
5. Prophylactic anticonvulsants in predisposed individuals
6. Antidepressant therapy when indicated
7. Rehabilitative therapy
8. Attention to social and emotional needs of the patient and family

nutrition. A summary of the basic measures for the management of the patient with acute ICH is provided in Table 2.

Blood Pressure Control in Hypertensive Intracerebral Hemorrhage

The mechanism of hypertensive ICH has been reevaluated in recent years. McCormick and Rosenfield[11] reported that hypertension explained only one quarter of their series of 144 patients with massive brain hemorrhage. In a retrospective study of 154 patients who had spontaneous ICH in Cincinnati, Ohio in 1982, only 45% of subjects had a well-documented history of hypertension, while another 12% had laboratory evidence of chronic hypertension.[12] This lack of a relationship between hypertension and spontaneous ICH in approximately 50% of subjects was also supported by a study of Bahemuka,[13] which examined heart weight as a marker of hypertension in subjects with primary ICH. Caplan[14] has recently emphasized that a sudden rise in blood pressure, with or without underlying chronic hypertension, is an important factor in ICH.

There remains little doubt, however, that severe hypertension, acute or chronic, is a major factor in the pathogenesis of ICH. The importance of poorly controlled hypertension at ICH onset and the occurrence of action bleeding by serial CT brain scan was underscored by Kelley et al.[4] Broderick et al[15] recorded a systolic blood pressure of 195 mm Hg or greater in 5 of 6 patients with a greater than 40% increase in the volume of hematoma by follow-up CT brain scan. In both series, there was a clear-cut relationship between active bleeding and neurologic deterioration. Mutlu et al[16] found a strong relationship between malignant hypertension at the time of presentation (systolic blood pressure of 280 to 300 mm Hg) and death within 14 hours. Other studies have not necessarily supported this relationship, although hypertensive individuals have a greater degree of persistent neurologic deficit, overall, than nonhypertensives.[17,18]

Meyer and Bauer[19] evaluated the effect of antihypertensive therapy on hypertensive ICH in a study published in 1962. The 167 patients were divided into three groups: adequate treatment (n = 40), inadequate treatment (n = 83) and no treatment (n = 44). Each group was further subcategorized into neurologically responsive and unresponsive at the time of presentation. The mortality rate for the treated group was 27% for the responsive and 76% for the unresponsive patients, for an overall mortality rate of 63%. For the inadequately treated group, the mortality rate was 45% for the responsive and 92% for the unresponsive patients, for an overall mortality rate of 82%. For the untreated group, the mortality rate was 67% for responsive and 100% for unresponsive patients, for an overall mortality of 98%. This study stands alone today as the guide for aggressive, immediate blood pressure control in hypertensive ICH.

The acute reduction of elevated blood pressure is most readily accomplished with rapidly acting, potent antihypertensive medication, along with effective control of increased intracranial pressure which exacerbates blood pressure elevation. An agent which can achieve both purposes, to some degree, is furosemide, a potent diuretic which can be administered intravenously. Diazoxide is a fast-acting benzothiadiazine derivative that reaches a maximal antihypertensive effect within 30 seconds of intravenous injection. Its method of action is relaxation of arteriolar smooth muscle and its duration of action approaches 12 hours. Its major drawback is a potential precipitous drop in blood pressure, which may promote cerebral, myocardial, or optic nerve infarction. The recommended dose is 1 to 3 mg/kg up to a maximum dose of 150 mg. Improved safety can be achieved with miniboluses of 1 to 3 mg/kg repeated at 5 to 15 minute intervals. Typically, the blood pressure declines within 5 minutes, to the maximal effect, and the response begins to wear off within 10 to 30 minutes.

Presently, the most commonly used agent for acute blood pressure management is sodium nitroprusside. This agent is administered intravenously in a 5% dextrose water solution. Its use mandates continuous arterial blood pressure monitoring via an arterial line to avoid significant hypotension. The average dose, by continuous infusion, is 3 μg/kg/min with a range of 0.5 to 10 μg/kg/min. If an effect is not seen within 10 minutes of starting a maximal infusion rate, the drug should be discontinued and an alternative agent administered.

Generally speaking, one is capable of achieving normotension with rapidly acting agents such as diazoxide or sodium nitroprusside. More chronic management is difficult, especially in the setting of a large intracerebral hematoma with significantly increased intracranial pressure. Agents which appear to be most effective for chronic management include labetalol, nifedipine, or clonidine. Minoxidil can be considered if the blood pressure elevation remains intractable.

Treatment of Increased Intracranial Pressure

A major question in the management of a patient with ICH is the nature of the associated brain swelling. A significant component of vasogenic edema[20] would imply that corticosteroids might provide protection against brain swell-

Table 3

Summary of Potential Medical Therapy for Increased Intracranial Pressure

1. Potent diuresis with an agent such as furosemide
2. Aggressive blood pressure control with an agent such as nitroprusside
3. Hyperventilation to maintain the PCO_2 in the 25 to 30 mm Hg range for the first 24 hours, and then as necessary
4. Antiedema agents such as mannitol or glycerol

ing. Cytotoxic edema,[21] on the other hand, would not necessarily be amenable to steroid therapy. Interstitial edema[22] might also play an important role in ICH when there is an associated acute obstructive hydrocephalus.

In experimental models, the increased intracranial pressure (ICP) associated with ICH was responsive to intravenous mannitol, steroids,[23] or glycerol,[24] but the use of corticosteriods in the clinical setting has been controversial. The ring of contrast enhancement observed with resolving intracerebral hematomas is diminished with steroids,[25] but this has not correlated with clinical improvement. In a controlled study, Poungvarin et al[26] randomized patients with supratentorial ICH to either dexamethasone or placebo. Dexamethasone provided no beneficial effect and led to a higher complication rate.

The hyperosmolar agent, mannitol, is an effective, rapidly acting antiedema agent. A major concern with mannitol is the potential for a rebound effect on the ICP. To effectively avoid this problem, titered doses with avoidance of relatively large boluses have been proposed.[27] Specifically, 100 cc boluses of 20% mannitol should be used. Regular mannitol use may necessitate a device to monitor ICP, which in the setting of ICH requires a careful approach. Unilateral mass lesions produce a differential in the ICP between the ipsilateral and contralateral sides.[28] In addition, the accuracy of the pressure monitoring devices varies. Subarachnoid catheters and ventricular drains appear to be superior to subarachnoid bolts.[29]

Some neurologists and neurosurgeons favor glycerol over mannitol, as it is less likely to promote ICP rebound. Favorable effects on cerebral hemodynamics in patients with ICH have been reported with intravenously administered 10% glycerol.[30] In a recent controlled clinical study of intravenous glycerol in acute ICH, however, no benefit was observed.[31]

Hyperventilation remains a primary means of acutely lowering the ICP, mainly by lowering the cerebral blood flow. Maintaining PCO_2 between 25 and 30 mm Hg serves as an effective therapy for high ICP for 24 hours. More prolonged cerebral blood flow reduction may have a long-term deleterious effect, however. After the first 24 hours of treatment, the patient can be ventilated only as necessary to lower periodic increases in ICP. The measures presently available for management of elevated ICP are summarized in Table 3.

Treatment of Intraventricular Hemorrhage

Obstructive hydrocephalus secondary to intraventricular extension of blood is most readily treated by ventricular drainage. Unfortunately, this rarely helps the patient. Todo et al[32] assessed the use of intraventricularly infused urokinase to treat ventricular cast formation. This thrombolytic agent resulted in clinical improvement in five of six patients with severe intraventricular hemorrhage.

Treatment of Secondary Seizures

The incidence of seizures complicating ICH is nearly 25%.[33] Not surprisingly, seizures that complicate ICH are most common when there is cortical extension,[34,35] but seizures have been reported in deep ICH.[36] Weisberg et al[37] reported that 15% of 222 consecutive patients with nontraumatic parenchymal brain hemorrhage had seizures. Of the 33 patients with seizures, 27 had seizures begin within 72 hours and 6 had seizures begin from 3 days to 4 months after ICH. None had an initial seizure beyond this time period. Of the 27 subjects who had seizures with 72 hours, 8 had an isolated seizure and 19 had recurrent seizures. Of the six subjects whose seizure activity developed between 2 and 4 months, all had recurrent seizures. Seizures were associated with frontal, parietal, or temporal lobe hemorrhage, and were less common in hypertensive or spontaneous ICH compared with ICH originating from aneurysm, angioma, or neoplasm.

The findings of Weisberg et al[37] are in apparent contradiction to those of Berger et al[38] who noted the typical development of seizures within minutes to hours of presentation. They found no late development of seizure activity in their 112 consecutive subjects with ICH. In addition, they found no relationship between seizures and hemorrhage size or ventricular extension, although they did report the obvious association with cortical involvement. Of note, roughly half of their 93 patients without seizures received prophylactic anticonvulsant therapy. The authors concluded that the routine use of prophylactic anticonvulsant therapy in ICH appeared to be unwarranted.

From a practical standpoint, one can derive certain guidelines from these studies. Seizures can occur in approximately 15% to 20% of patients with nontraumatic ICH. They are uncommon in the absence of cortical extension of blood. The majority of subjects will develop seizure activity within the first 72 hours of ictus. Therefore, a decision regarding anticonvulsant therapy will likely be predicated upon the clinical presentation and whether or not there is cortical involvement by the hematoma.

Correction of Coagulation Parameters in Hemorrhage Secondary to Bleeding Diathesis

The most common cause of intracranial hemorrhage promoted by bleeding diathesis is iatrogenic. The frequency of iatrogenic ICH can be expected to increase, as there are now clear-cut indications for chronic anticoagulant therapy in nonvalvular atrial fibrillation.[39-41] The risk of ICH is 11-fold higher for subjects on oral anticoagulants than for those not on anticoagulants.[42] Neurologic abnormalities often progress for several hours,[43] which presumably reflects persistent bleeding.

Sodium warfarin interferes with the extrinsic coagulation system by interfering with the vitamin K-dependent factors II, VII, IX, and X, and by reducing the level of fibrinogen. Treatment with vitamin K requires 8 to 24 hours to correct an elevated prothrombin time, and precious time can be lost in this interval. The administration of fresh frozen plasma immediately restores diminished clotting factors and thus is the treatment of choice in the emergency setting.

Heparin interferes with the intrinsic coagulation system. Neurologists typically terminate heparin infusion in the setting of potential ICH, but protamine sulfate injection remains the treatment of choice for reversal of the heparin effect. Intravenous doses of up to 50 mg at 10 minute intervals are administered. In the emergency setting, no more than 100 mg are administered immediately because of its anticoagulant effect. This potential side effect must be balanced by requirements for the drug, as each 1 mg of protamine reduces approximately 100 units of heparin.

Hemophilia A affects approximately 1 in 10,000 males and is commonly associated with ICH. The traditional treatment since the 1960s had been factor VIII (antihemophiliac factor) concentrates.[44] In view of increasing concerns about viral transmission in factor VIII concentrates, recombinant DNA-derived antihemophiliac factor has been reported to be both safe and effective for the treatment of hemophilia A.[45]

Thrombocytopenia has a number of possible etiologies, any of which predisposes toward ICH. Figure 1A illustrates the CT of a woman with severe thrombocytopenia following liver transplantation who developed a right thalamic hematoma with intraventricular extension. A follow-up study 1 day later reveals enlargement of the thalamic hematoma despite platelet transfusions (Figure 1B).

Typically, the platelet count should drop below 30,000/mm^3 in order to see a significant bleeding tendency. Thrombotic thrombocytopenic purpura can be associated with a severe thrombocytopenia and secondary hemorrhage. Once considered an extremely malignant process, this disease responds to both plasma infusion and plasma exchange, with the latter being more effective.[46] Idiopathic (autoimmune) thrombocytopenic purpura carries the greatest risk of ICH within the first 2 weeks of disease onset.[47] Therapy is dependent upon the potential for spontaneous remission of the primary platelet disorder. Most adults will require a combination of prednisone, at a dose of 1 to 2 mg/kg/day, and splenectomy. Alternative therapy in patients unresponsive to this regimen includes intravenous immunoglobulin therapy, danazol, or immunosuppressive agents. Platelet transfusion is to be avoided unless life-threatening active hemorrhage is present.

Disseminated intravascular coagulation (DIC) can result in ICH.[48] Typically,

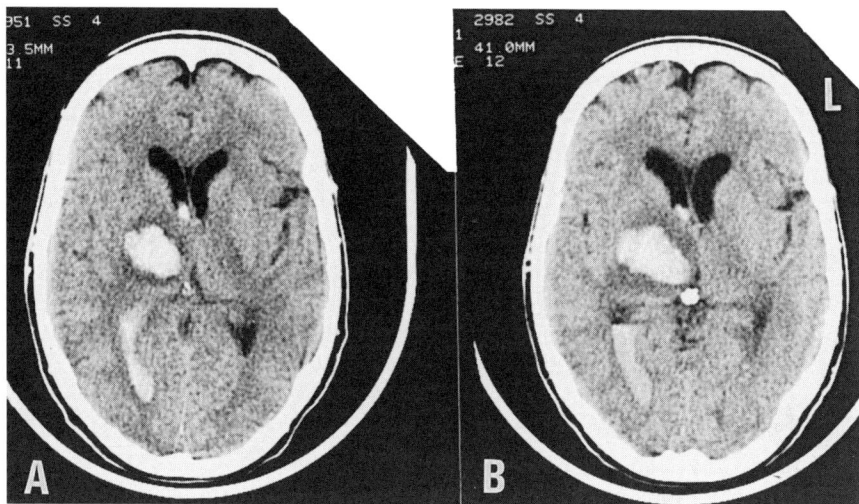

Figure 1: A: Noncontrast CT brain scan that demonstrates a right thalamic hematoma with intraventricular extension. **B:** A follow-up CT brain scan performed 24 hours later. There is enlargement of the hematoma despite platelet transfusions.

laboratory studies reveal hypofibrinogenemia, thrombocytopenia, fibrin degradation products, and a prolonged prothrombin time. The major therapeutic goal is to treat the underlying illness. In select circumstances, platelet transfusion is indicated to maintain the platelet count above 50,000/mm^3. A severe hypofibrinogenemia may require infusion of cryoprecipitate. A severe deficiency of coagulation factors may necessitate transfusion of fresh frozen plasma.

Management of Rare Causes of Intracranial Hemorrhage

The connective tissue disorders, specifically polyarteritis nodosa (PAN) and systemic lupus erythematosus (SLE), can result in ICH. PAN is characterized by acute, necrotizing inflammation of small to medium size arteries. Secondary aneurysmal dilatation can result in rupture of the artery with secondary hemorrhage. PAN is often a fulminating disease, although it is variably responsive to high-dose corticosteriods and immunosuppressive therapy with an agent such as cyclophosphamide. SLE can promote similar vasculitic changes with secondary arterial rupture.[49]

There is an increasing body of literature[50,51] describing the relationship between illicit drug ingestion and ICH. A number of mechanisms are possible, including a sudden rise in the blood pressure with secondary rupture of a pre-existing vascular anomaly,[52] as well as promotion of a vasculitis pathologically similar to PAN.[53,54] The vasculitic-type process appears to be a self-limited reaction to the offending agent. Immunosuppressive therapy does not appear to be justified unless there is clinical evidence of a progressive vasculitic process.

References

1. Hier DP, Davis KR, Richardson EP Jr, et al: Hypertensive: putaminal hemorrhage. *Ann Neurol* 1977;1:152.
2. Young WB, Lee KP, Pessin MS, et al: Prognostic significance of ventricular blood in supratentorial hemorrhage: a volumetric study. *Neurology* 1990; 40:616.
3. Kelley RE, Kovacs AG: Horizontal gaze paresis in hemispheric stroke. *Stroke* 1986;17:1030.
4. Kelley RE, Berger JR, Scheinberg P, et al: Active bleeding in hypertensive intracerebral hemorrhage: computed tomography. *Neurology* 1982;32:852.
5. McCarthy ST, Turner JJ, Robertson D, et al: Low-dose heparin as a prophylaxis against deep vein thrombosis after acute stroke. *Lancet* 1977;2:800.
6. Boeer A, Voth E, Henze Th, et al: Early heparin therapy in patients with spontaneous intracerebral hemorrhage. *J Neurol Neurosurg Psychiat* 1991; 54:466.
7. Kelley RE, Vibulsresth S, Bell L, et al: Evaluation of Kinetic therapy in the prevention of complications of prolonged bedrest secondary to stroke. *Stroke* 1987;18:638.
8. Robinson RG, Price TR: Post-stroke depressive disorders: a follow-up study of 103 patients. *Stroke* 1982;13:635.
9. Reding MJ, Orto LA, Winter SW, et al: Antidepressant therapy after stroke: a double-blind trial. *Arch Neurol* 1986;43:763.
10. Horner J, Massey EW: Silent aspiration following stroke. *Neurology* 1988; 38:317.
11. McCormick WF, Rosenfield DB: Massive brain hemorrhage: a review of 144 cases and an examination of their causes. *Stroke* 1973;4:946.
12. Brott T, Thalinger K, Hertzberg V: Hypertension as a risk factor for spontaneous intracerebral hemorrhage. *Stroke* 1986;17:1078.
13. Bahemuka M: Primary intracerebral hemorrhage and heart weight: a clinicopathologic case-control review of 218 patients. *Stroke* 1987;18:531.
14. Caplan L: Intracerebral hemorrhage revisited. *Neurology* 1988;38:624.
15. Broderick JP, Brott TG, Tomsick T, et al: Ultra-early evaluation of intracerebral hemorrhage. *J Neurosurg* 1990;72:195.
16. Mutlu N, Berry RG, Alpers BJ: Massive cerebral hemorrhage. *Arch Neurol* 1963;8:644.
17. Luyendijk W, Schoen JHR: Intracerebral hematomas. A clinical study of 40 surgical cases. *Psychiat Neurol Neurochir* 1964;67:445.
18. Luyendijk W: Intracerebral hematoma. In: Vinken PJ, Bruyn GW, eds: *Handbook of Clinical Neurology*. New York: Elsevier Publishing Co., 1972: 660.

19. Meyer JS, Bauer RB: Medical treatment of spontaneous intracranial hemorrhage by the use of hypotensive drugs. *Neurology* 1962;12:36.

20. Wahl M, Unterberg A, Baethman A, et al: Mediators of blood-brain barrier dysfunction and formation of vasogenic brain edema. *J Cereb Blood Flow Metabol* 1987;8:621.

21. Klatzo I: Pathophysiological aspects of brain edema. *Acta Neuropathol* 1987;72:236.

22. Fishman RA: Brain edema. *N Engl J Med* 1975;293:706.

23. Hooshmand H, Dove J, Houff, et al: Effects of diuretics and steroids on CSF pressure. A comparative study. *Arch Neurol* 1969;21:499.

24. Guisado R, Arieff AI, Massry SG: Effects of glycerol administration on experimental cerebral edema. *Neurology* 1976;26:69.

25. Lester DW, Moody DM, Ball MR: Resolving intracerebral hematoma: alteration of the "Ring Sign" with steroids. *AJR* 1978;130:935.

26. Poungvarin N, Bhoopat W, Viriyavejakul A, et al: Effects of dexamethasone in primary supratentorial hemorrhage. *N Engl J Med* 1987;316:1229.

27. McGraw CP, Alexander E, Howard G: Effect of dose and dose schedule on the response of ICP to mannitol. *Surg Neurol* 1978;10:127.

28. Weaver DD, Winn HR, Jane JA: Differential intracranial pressure in patients with unilateral mass lesions. *J Neurosurg* 1982;56:660.

29. Mollman HD, Rockswold GL, Ford SE: A clinical comparison of subarachnoid catheters to ventriculostomy and subarachnoid bolts: a prospective study. *J Neurosug* 1988;68:737.

30. Takashima S, Gotoh F, Fukuuchi Y, et al: The hemodynamic effect of intravenous glycerol infusion in patients with intracerebral hemorrhage (abstract). *Stroke* 1990;21(Suppl I):I-63.

31. Yu YL, Kumana CR, Lauder IJ, et al: Treatment of acute cerebral hemorrhage with intravenous glycerol: a double-blind, placebo-controlled, randomized trial. *Stroke* 1992;23:967.

32. Todo T, Usui M, Takakura K: Treatment of severe intraventricular hemorrhage by intraventricular infusion of urokinase. *J Neurosurg* 1991;74:81.

33. Faught E, Peters D, Bartolucci A, et al: Seizures after primary intracerebral hemorrhage. *Neurology* 1989;39:1089.

34. Olsen TS, Hogenhaven H, Thage O: Epilepsy after stroke. *Neurology* 1987;37:1209.

35. Richardson EP Jr, Dodge PR: Epilepsy in cerebral vascular disease: a study of the incidence and nature of seizures in 104 consecutive autopsy proven cases of cerebral infarction and hemorrhage. *Epilepsia* 1954;3:49.

36. Weisberg LA: Computerized tomography in intracranial hemorrhage. *Arch Neurol* 1979;36:422.

37. Weisberg LA, Shamsnia M, Elliott D: Seizures caused by nontraumatic parenchymal brain hemorrhages. *Neurology* 1991;41:1197.

38. Berger AR, Lipton RB, Lesser ML, et al: Early seizures following intracerebral hemorrhage. *Neurology* 1988;38:1363.

39. Boston Area Anticoagulation Trial for Atrial Fibrillation Investigators: The

effect of low-dose warfarin on the risk of stroke in patients with nonrheumatic atrial fibrillation. *N Engl J Med* 1990;323:1505.

40. Peterson P, Boysen G, Godtfredson J, et al: Placebo-controlled, randomized trial of warfarin and aspirin for prevention of thromboembolic complications in chronic atrial fibrillation. *Lancet* 1989;1:175.

41. Stroke Prevention in Atrial Fibrillation Study Group Investigators: Preliminary report of the Stroke Prevention in Atrial Fibrillation Study. *N Engl J Med* 1990;322:863.

42. Wintzen AR, de Jonge H, Loeliger EA, et al: The risk of intracerebral hemorrhage during oral anticoagulant treatment: a population study. *Ann Neurol* 1984;16:553.

43. Case CS, Robinson RK, Stein RW, et al: Anticoagulant-related intracerebral hemorrhage. *Neurology* 1985;35:943.

44. Levine PH: Efficacy of self-therapy in hemophilia: a study of 72 patients with hemophilia A and B. *N Engl J Med* 1974;291:1381.

45. Schwartz RS, Abildgaard CF, Aledort LM, et al, and the Recombinant Factor VIII Study Group: Human recombinant DNA-derived antihemophilic factor (factor VIII) in the treatment of hemophilia A. *N Engl J Med* 1990;323:1800.

46. Rock GA, Shumak KH, Buskard NA, et al, and the Canadian Apheresis Study Group: Comparison of plasma exchange with plasma infusion in the treatment of thrombotic thrombocytopenic purpura. *N Engl J Med* 1991;325:393.

47. Adams Jr HP, Biller J: Hemorrhagic intracranial vascular disease. In: Joynt RJ, ed: *Clinical Neurology*. Philadelphia: J.B. Lippincott Co., 1991:36.

48. Schwartzman RJ, Hill JB: Neurologic complications of disseminated intravascular coagulation. *Neurology* 1982;32:791.

49. Kelley RE, Stokes W, Reyes P, et al: Cerebral transmural angiitis and ruptured aneurysm. A complication of systemic lupus erythematosus. *Arch Neurol* 1980;37:526.

50. Sloan MA, Kittner SJ, Rigamonti D, et al: Occurrence of stroke associated with use/abuse of drugs. *Neurology* 1991;41:1358.

51. Levine SR, Brust JCM, Futrell N, et al: A comparative study of the cerebrovascular complications of cocaine: alkaloidal versus hydrochloride — a review. *Neurology* 1991;41:1173.

52. Wojak JC, Flamm JS: Intracranial hemorrhage and cocaine use. *Stroke* 1987;18:712.

53. Kessler JT, Jortner BS, Adapon BD: Cerebral vasculitis in a drug abuser. *J Clin Psychiat* 1978;39:559.

54. Fallis RJ, Fisher M: Cerebral vasculitis and hemorrhage associated with phenylpropanolamine. *Neurology* 1985;35:405.

Chapter 14

Surgical Therapy

Jeffrey L. Saver, MD

More than a century after the first surgical treatment of intracerebral hemorrhage (ICH),[1] the indications for and optimal timing of operative evacuation of parenchymal brain hematoma continue to engender controversy. In selected cases, surgery clearly can be lifesaving. Few would dispute that evacuation benefits patients with cerebellar or lobar hemorrhage exhibiting delayed deterioration secondary to mass effect. In other settings, experience with surgical treatment has been uniformly dismal. Elderly patients with deep coma, fluctuating vital signs, and massive dominant hemisphere basal ganglionic hemorrhage are unlikely to benefit from operative intervention. Between such extremes, firm guidelines for surgical management have not been established.

The rationale for surgical treatment is compelling. Brain hemorrhages produce injury both by direct destruction of local tissue and by dissection through and displacement of surrounding brain parenchyma, especially white matter. Physiologically, decreased cerebral blood flow, disruption of autoregulation, and breakdown of the blood-brain barrier in perilesional areas are observed.[2,3] Pathologic examination demonstrates edema, ischemic necrosis, and small petechial hemorrhages in perilesional tissue.[4] Surgery can, in principle, ameliorate several mechanisms leading to damage of secondary tissue. By reducing elevated compartmental pressures, clot removal may prevent reductions in blood flow perfusion pressure.[5] Compartmental decompression also prevents cerebral herniation. Hematoma evacuation may prevent the accumulation of peroxidases and other toxic blood products injurious to surrounding tissue.[6,7] An open procedure may allow the identification and obliteration of the source of bleeding. In cases of obstructed CSF pathways, ventricular drainage will relieve generalized increases in intracranial pressure.

For several reasons, however, caution regarding surgical therapy must be maintained. Primary destruction of brain tissue will not be reversed by clot removal. Even without surgery, continued bleeding or spontaneous rebleeding with delayed hematoma enlargement is rare. The surgical procedure may re-

From Feldmann E (ed). *Intracerebral Hemorrhage*. Armonk, NY: Futura Publishing Company, Inc., © 1994.

quire minor injury of intact brain tissue. Small hematomas that displace rather than destroy tissue will spontaneously be reabsorbed and leave minimal clinical abnormalities. In some animal models, hematoma evacuation has not been demonstrated to reduce brain edema effectively.[8]

With opposing theoretical viewpoints, the efficacy of surgical management needs to be established by empirical clinical observation. Over 100 series of surgically and conservatively treated ICH patients have been published in the CT scan era. These studies have demonstrated that important prognostic factors predictive of outcome in both medically and surgically treated patients include level of consciousness on admission, hematoma size, hematoma site, and the presence or absence of intraventricular extension of blood.[9-16] However, there has been a paucity of well-controlled, randomized clinical trials directly comparing medical and surgical management. As a result, the indications for surgery remain ill defined. Contributing to this uncertainty is the steady stream of innovations in surgical technique over the past 15 years which prevent settled conclusions from being reached regarding the costs and benefits of operative intervention. A useful approach to the topic is to review the few randomized studies that have been carried out, describe conventional and innovative surgical techniques, consider the varying indications for surgery at different hematoma locations, and discuss the way vascular malformations, amyloid angiopathy, coagulopathies, and other special clinical issues should influence surgical management.

Randomized Trials

In a pioneering pre-CT scan era study, McKissock et al[17] randomized 180 consecutive patients with suspected supratentorial hemorrhage to receive either craniotomy and hematoma evacuation or medical therapy (Table 1). The overall mortality was 65% in the surgically treated group and 51% among the

Table 1
Randomized Trials of Surgery versus Medical Therapy for ICH

Trial	Surgical Therapy			Medical Therapy			Risk Reduction	Relative Risk of Death, with 95% CI
	Deaths	N	%	Deaths	N	%		Surgical Therapy Better / Medical Therapy Better
McKissock '61	58	89	65%	46	91	51%	−30%	
Auer '89	21	50	42%	35	50	70%	+93%	
Juvela '89	12	26	46%	10	26	38%	−12%	
Batjer '90*	4	8	50%	7	9	77%	+125%	

* Outcome in published study only available as deaths plus vegetative state at 6 months

medically treated patients. The authors could not demonstrate any benefit from surgery in regard either to mortality or morbidity.

More recent CT scan era studies have achieved improved surgical mortality and morbidity rates, but have still failed to indicate unequivocally the superiority of medical or surgical therapy. Juvela et al[18] assigned 52 patients with CT confirmed spontaneous supratentorial ICH who were unconscious or exhibited severe focal neurologic deficits to medical therapy or craniotomy and clot evacuation. Despite randomization, the groups were not strictly comparable at entry. The surgical group presented with an overall lower Glasgow Coma Score and more frequent intraventricular extension of hemorrhage than the medical patients. Overall mortality at 6 months was 38% in the nonsurgically treated group and 46% in the operative group. After stratification for the prognostic variables differing between the groups, a statistically significant improved rate of survival with surgery was found for a subgroup of patients with Glasgow Coma Scale scores of 7 to 10. However, all surviving patients in this group were severely disabled.

Batjer et al[19] designed a study to distribute 60 patients with hypertensive putaminal hemorrhage among three treatment arms: medical management, medical management plus intracranial pressure (ICP) monitoring, or surgical evacuation. The study was halted early, after entry of only 21 patients, due to lower than expected recruitment rates and poor outcome in all treatment arms. Seven of nine medical therapy patients, four of four medical therapy plus ICP monitoring patients, and four of eight surgical patients were dead or vegetative at 6 months. The groups were too small to allow statistically valid conclusions to be drawn regarding outcome differences between groups.

Auer et al[20] randomized 100 patients with spontaneous supratentorial hemorrhage of greater than 10 cc to medical treatment or endoscopic evacuation. Randomization produced treatment groups fairly well matched for several important prognostic factors including level of consciousness, hematoma size, and hematoma site, but the surgical group had younger patients. The 6-month mortality was 42% in the surgical group and 70% in the medical group, a statistically significant benefit. Functional outcome was also superior among the surgical patients. However, subgroup analysis revealed that lower mortality and better quality of survival were confined to patients younger than 60 years of age with small lobar hemorrhages. In addition, outcome assessment was not blinded.

A formal, statistical meta-analysis of all randomized trials of medical versus surgical therapy shows no difference in overall mortality between treatment arms (Table 2). When the analysis is confined to CT scan era series, surgery appears beneficial in averting death in studied patients. However, this analysis is largely influenced by one study[20] which also found severe morbidity among surgical survivors in most subgroups.

Prospective, randomized trials have thus failed to define firm indications for surgical intervention in parenchymal brain hemorrhage. The decision to operate must therefore be tailored to the individual clinical setting, taking into account the age and physiologic status of the patient, and drawing upon

Table 2
Meta-analysis of Randomized Trials of Surgery versus Medical Therapy for ICH

Trial Analyzed	Number of Trials	Surgical Deaths/ Patients	Medical Deaths/ Patients	O − E	Variance	Odds Ratio 95% C.L.** Surgical Therapy Better	Medical Therapy Better
All randomized	4	95/173	98/176	−.60	21.5		
CT era randomized	3	37/84	52/85	−7.18	10.5		

* For full statistical methods, see Antiplatelet Trialists' Collaboration, 1988.[134] O − E: Observed minus expected deaths. For each trial of N patients, n of whom were treated and d of whom died, O is the observed number of deaths in the treatment arm, and E is the expected number of deaths in the treatment arm if the treatment were wholly without effect. E may be calculated by the formula, $E = n \cdot d/N$. O − E from each independent trial is added for grand total O − E. Variance: variance for the grand total O − E is obtained by adding the variance of each trial. Within each trial variance for O − E is calculated by $V = E(1 - n/N)(N - d)/N - 1$.
** C.L. = confidence limits

experience in the above trials and the many additional series of surgically and medically treated patients that have been reported.

Surgical Techniques

Craniotomy

The standard surgical approach is a craniotomy with careful evacuation of the hematoma through a cortical incision. Preoperatively, a radial arterial line is established for continuous monitoring of blood pressure and periodic blood gas assessments. A Foley catheter is placed, anesthesia induced, and intubation carried out. The patient is hyperventilated and a 50 to 100 gm dose of mannitol is administered intravenously. For supratentorial hemorrhages, the patient is generally placed in a supine or semilateral position with the head rotated so that the affected hemisphere is superior. In cases of cerebellar hemorrhage, the patient is positioned prone with the head moderately flexed

A 2 to 3 cm cortical incision is performed at a site that provides the most direct access to the hematoma cavity yet spares eloquent and motor cortex and major blood vessels (Figure 1). For frontal hematomas, the superior frontal gyrus is incised; for parieto-occipital lesions, the superior parietal lobule; and for temporal clots, the anterior superior temporal gyrus. A vermian approach is employed for midline cerebellar lesions, a paramedian approach for lateral cerebellar clots. For putaminal hemorrhages, two strategies are commonly employed. In the transcortical procedure, an initial incision is made in the anterior superior temporal gyrus and a second incision in the underlying insula. Suzuki

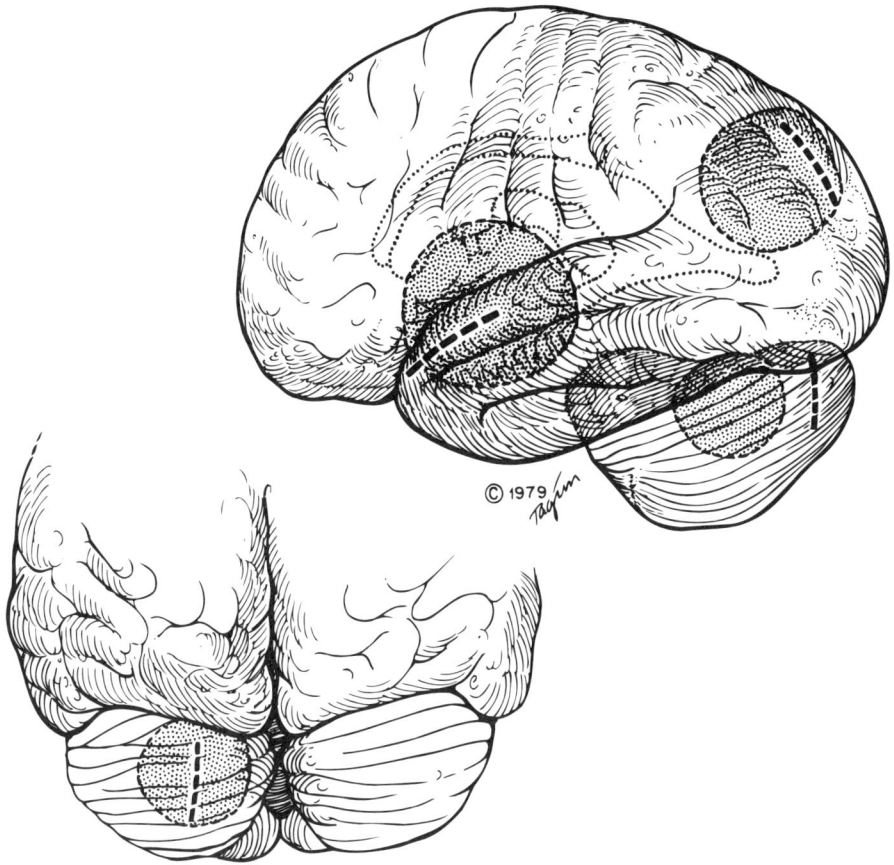

Figure 1: Open surgical evacuation of ICHs. Dashed lines indicate cortical incision sites often employed when approaching the most common surgically treated hematomas: lobar, putaminal, and cerebellar. These incisions provide satisfactory access to the hematoma cavities with minimal trauma to intact brain tissue and vessels. Reproduced with permission from Crowell and Ojemann, 1981.[133]

and Sato described a transsylvian approach employing only one incision but also requiring greater maneuvering among the important peri-Sylvian vessels.[21]

The magnification and illumination of an operating microscope aids visualization when operating through a small cortical incision or splitting the Sylvian fissure. Careful dissection through intervening brain tissue allows exposure of the ICH. The hematoma is evacuated with gentle suction, irrigation, and forceps, employing microsurgical technique. The hematoma is removed to the greatest extent feasible, but portions of clot adherent to the walls are left undisturbed to avoid injury to adjacent brain and bleeding from the fragile, edematous walls of the cavity. Bleeding is controlled with bipolar cautery. Infrequently, clips are required. Diffuse bleeding from cavity walls is arrested by applying cottonoid patties and hemostatic gelatin sponge, gauze, or fibrillar collagen. A careful search is conducted to identify the source of the original bleed. If an occult vascular malformation, tumor, or suspicious appearing brain tissue is identified, a biopsy is taken for careful histologic examination. If the biopsy is positive, consideration should be given to immediate resection of the underlying lesion. In less stable patients, definitive resection may be deferred to a second, delayed operation. Irrigating the cavity with a gentle saline lavage will uncover persistent bleeding sites. Once hemostasis is achieved, the hematoma cavity is lined with surgicel. Some authors suggest raising blood pressure briefly to 145 to 150 mm Hg to confirm hemostasis.[22]

After removal of larger hematomas, warm saline or artificial cerebrospinal fluid may need to be instilled to avert a residual depressed brain cavity. Tight closure of the dura prevents subcutaneous leakage of spinal fluid and decreases the risk of subsequent infection. Intraparenchymal drainage is generally not employed. In cases of cerebellar hemorrhage with hydrocephalus, an intraventricular drain may be left in place for a few days.

Postoperative care is initially maintained in an intensive care unit setting. Blood pressure control must be meticulous. Elevated mean arterial pressures increase the risk of recurrent hemorrhage and promote edema. Careful fluid management and corticosteriods are also of benefit in diminishing brain swelling. Neurologic deterioration may reflect rebleeding, which tends to occur early, or hydrocephalus, which more often occurs after a delay. A CT scan should be obtained promptly to distinguish between the two. Seizures and infection are additional complications which may be seen in the postoperative period.

Stereotactic Aspiration

Two major stumbling blocks impeded early attempts to aspirate deep hematomas through a burr hole and avoid the rigors of open operative evacuation: targeting the clot and heterogeneity of clot consistency.[23,24] With the advent of stereotactic techniques solving the problem of clot localization, and the development over the past decade of an imaginative array of mechanical aspiration devices and fibrinolytics improving the degree of achievable clot extraction, aspiration procedures are now the subject of active investigation and widening clinical use.

Stereotaxy facilitates accurate penetration of deep hematoma cavities. With the patient placed in a stereotactic frame, CT or, rarely, MR images are obtained to locate the hematoma site, assess its size, and determine its three-dimensional coordinates (Figure 2). Trajectories for accessing the target may then be calculated automatically by computer. A number of such stereotactic systems are commercially available. When an approach along the long axis of a large hematoma is not feasible, two targets may be plotted and separate "double track" aspirations performed at anterior and posterior sites within the cavity.[25]

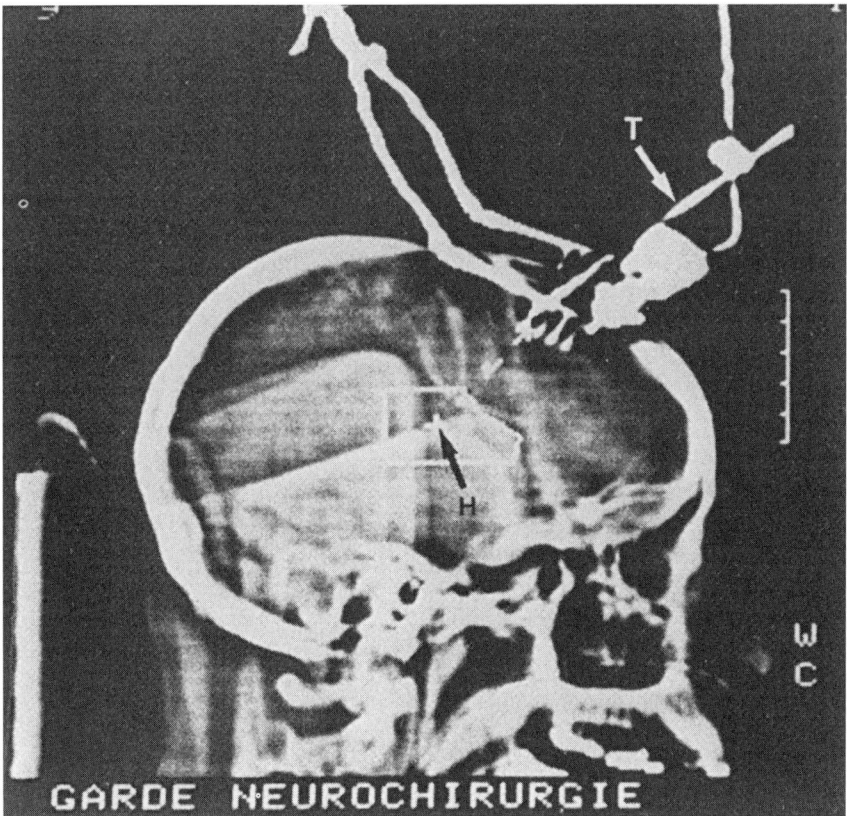

Figure 2: Stereotactic aspiration of ICH. Sagittal CT image shows target hematoma (H) and needle tip placed over the brain surface (T). The needle trajectory is adjusted according to CT coordinates, providing access to the center of the hematoma. Reproduced with permission from Nguyen JP, Gaston A, Brugieres P, et al, 1991.[27]

Aspirations are carried out under local anesthesia. A needle cannula is advanced through a burr hole to pierce the hematoma. Several techniques have been developed that enable monitoring of, and adjustments for changes in, target position as lesions are manipulated. In operating suites equipped with scanners, intraoperative CT images may be obtained.[26-28] Intraoperative ultrasound can also be quite helpful in localizing the hemorrhage cavity, identifying liquid and solid components of the hematoma and ascertaining the degree of clot extraction at any given point in time (Figure 3).[29]

Mechanical Devices

Within a few hours of the onset of intracerebral bleeding, the hematoma consists of about one-fourth liquid blood and three-fourths denser clot by vol-

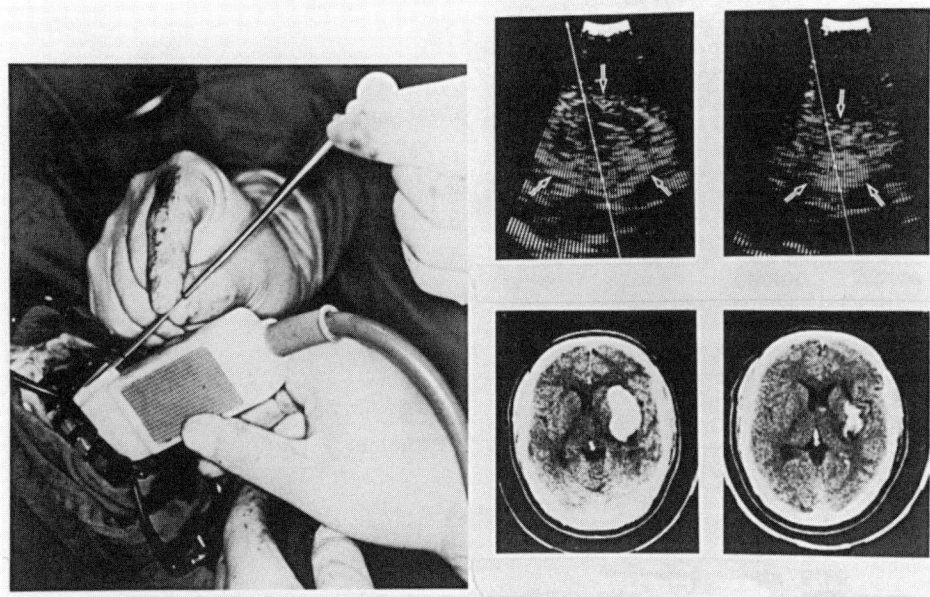

Figure 3: Ultrasound-guided stereotactic aspiration. **A.** Intraoperative ultrasound allows observation of the efficacy of aspiration in real-time. **B.** Pre- and postoperative sonography demonstrates reduction in size of hematoma with hypoechoic and hyperechoic components. Pre- and postoperative CT scans demonstrate 90% reduction in hematoma volume. Modified from Kanaya and Kuroda, 1992.[29]

ume.[30,31] Simple manual aspiration through a cannula often results in insufficient decompression due to difficulty in removing solidified hematoma material. A variety of instruments have been developed to fragment and collect this consolidated clot and increase the volumetric yield of aspiration.

Backlund and von Holst pioneered the first such device in 1978.[32] They developed a 4 mm cannula containing an Archimedes screw which the surgeon rotates manually. The application of suction draws hematoma material into the cannula where the whirling screw morcellates dense clot. Small clot fragments are then aspirated through the cannula into the bottle. Subsequent surgeons have introduced several modifications of the original device. The addition of a tubular vent along the cannula allows saline irrigation, instillation of contrast, and maintenance of vacuum if the cannula lumen becomes occluded by clot.[33] A further refinement of the system employs a thinner screw propelled by an electric motor and recessed a short distance from the cannula tip, as well as a shorter tube, a straight line of aspiration, and adjustable vacuum.[30,34] With this device, the incidence of clogging is reduced and the effectiveness of aspiration is increased.

In addition to Archimedes screw instruments, several additional types of mechanical aspirators have been developed. One apparatus employs a high-pressure water jet, with irrigation pressures of 8 to 15 kg/cm^2, to break up dense clot. In initial studies in 14 patients, this instrument removed 87.2% of hematoma volume.[35] Another device utilizes an ultrasonic aspirator to fragment dense clot and has been demonstrated to increase the effectiveness of aspiration of hypertensive hemorrhages in the acute stage.[26,36,37]

Laser-Assisted Endoscopy

One of the drawbacks of aspiration procedures is difficulty controlling bleeding sites in the hematoma cavity. To overcome this problem, Auer and colleagues developed a stereotactic neuroendoscope with built-in video camera and Nd Yag microlaser. The fiberoptic video system enables the surgeon to identify visually bleeding locations in the cavity wall; the laser tube is then introduced through a channel in the probe and activated to coagulate the leaking vessels. Additional channels in the instrument allow the introduction of irrigation-suction systems and an ultrasound generator for clot fragmentation. With this system, near total evacuation of hematomas was achieved in one third of patients and greater than 50% evacuation in over one half of patients.[38] As noted above, a prospective, randomized trial comparing neuroendoscopic surgical evacuation with medical therapy in spontaneous intracerebral hematoma suggested a benefit from surgery in the subgroup of patients with lobar hemorrhage under 60 years of age.[20]

Fibrinolytics

A different strategy to maximize the effectiveness of aspiration procedures that has been widely investigated over the past decade is chemical lysis of dense elements of clot through the instillation of thrombolytic agents (Figure 4).[28,39,40] Urokinase is most commonly employed. Tissue plasminogen activator is also actively being studied.[41] Stereotactic placement of a cannula and initial aspiration of the hematoma are carried out in the usual fashion. A silicone catheter is then positioned in the hematoma cavity. Five to six thousand units of urokinase in saline is injected, allowed to remain in the cavity for several hours, and then drained. Thereafter, protocols vary. Most commonly the catheter is left in place for a few days, and bedside urokinase infusion and drainage repeated at 6- to 24-hour intervals until repeat scanning shows minimal remaining blood. Intracerebral and intraventricular injections of fibrinolytics do not appreciably increase the risk of systemic bleeding. In one recent large series, 175 patients with putaminal hemorrhage underwent stereotactic aspiration. In 43%, more than four fifths of the hematoma volume was aspirated at the initial operation. With daily urokinase administration for up to 8 days, greater than 80% reduction in volume was attained in an additional 39% of patients.[42]

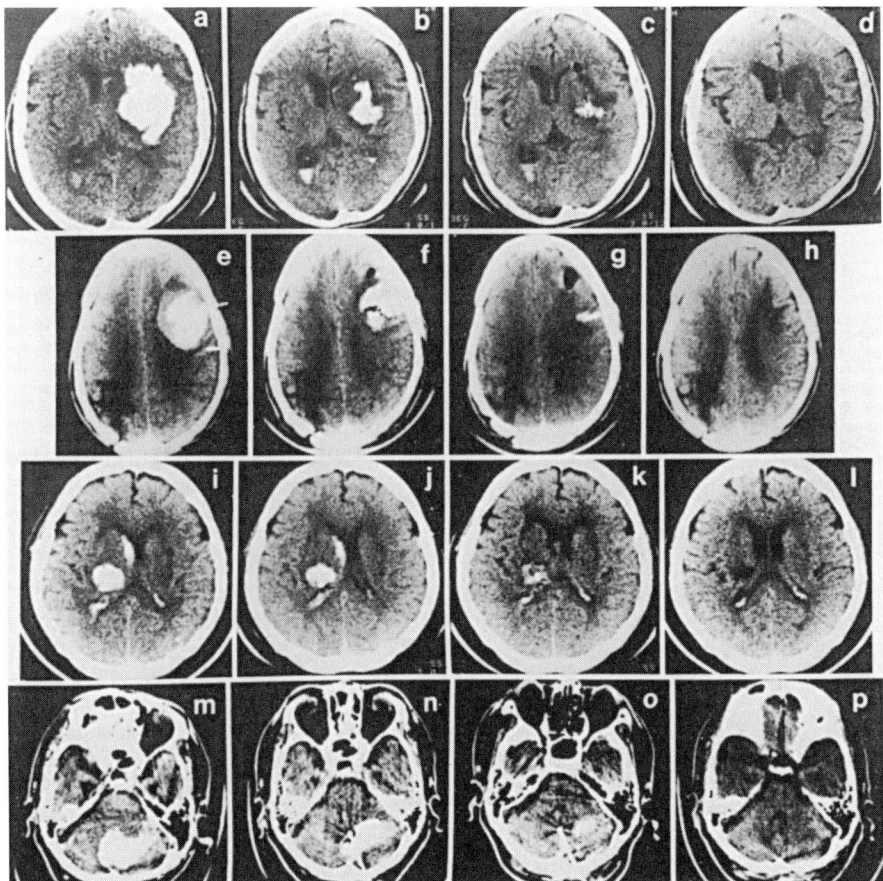

Figure 4: Stereotactic aspiration and fibrinolysis of hematomas at common sites within the brain. After initial manual aspiration, a drain was placed, urokinase infused, and aspiration repeated at 6 to 12 hour intervals over several days until CT revealed minimal residual hematoma. First row: Putaminal hemorrhage. **a**) preoperative scan, **b**) postoperative scan, **c**) day 5, **d**) day 15. Second row: Subcortical lobar hemorrhage. **e**) preoperative scan, **f**) postoperative scan, **g**) day 4, **h**) day 30. Third row: Thalamic hemorrhage. **i**) preoperative scan, **j**) postoperative scan, **k**) day 3, **l**) day 7. Fourth row: Cerebellar hemorrhage. **m**) preoperative scan, **n**) postoperative scan, **o**) day 4, **p**) day 9. Reproduced with permission from Matsumoto and Hondo, 1984.[39]

Management of Hematomas by Location

The decision to operate, and other aspects of surgical management, are strongly influenced by hemorrhage size and location within the brain. Approximately 75% of primary ICHs are supratentorial, with 30% situated in the putamen, 15% in the thalamus, and 25% lobar. The remainder arise in the posterior fossa and intraventricularly, most frequently in the pons (11%) and cerebellum (8%).[43]

Putaminal Hemorrhage

Hemorrhages in the putamen are common, widely variable in severity, and of intermediate surgical accessibility. As a consequence, they have occasioned a great deal of controversy regarding indications for surgical management. However, among several series that have retrospectively compared medical with surgical treatment, a pattern emerges.[44–49] Patients with small putaminal hemorrhages (less than 25 ml) and no or minimal impairment of consciousness of presentation have superior functional outcome when treated conservatively. Patients with large putaminal hematomas (80 ml or greater) and deep coma at presentation have decreased mortality with surgery, but functional outcome among survivors is quite poor, failing to clearly justify surgical intervention. In intermediate grades of putaminal hemorrhage, surgery may improve both mortality and quality of life among survivors. Data from nonrandomized, retrospective treatment series, however, must be interpreted with great caution, and some authors have failed to find a benefit of surgery in any subgroup.[50]

By far the largest nonrandomized study comes from the Japanese cooperative group,[46,51] where 7,010 patients with putaminal hemorrhages were collected from 339 centers. Of these, 3,635 received medical treatment, 3,375 surgical treatment, and outcome 3 months postictus was assessed. Overall mortality was 24.7% in the medical group and 21.9% in the surgical group. To allow analysis of cases stratified by important prognostic factors, detailed clinical and CT classification schemes divided patients into five neurologic grades and hemorrhages into five anatomic subgroups. Among patients alert or with minimal impairment of consciousness at presentation, medical therapy was superior. Good functional recovery (full-time work or minimal disability) was observed in 58% with medical treatment and 23% with surgical treatment. In patients with stupor or coma, surgery reduced mortality, 35% versus 72%, but did not increase the proportion of patients attaining a good functional outcome (Table 3). Heterogeneity of the surgical treatments performed complicate interpretation of this study. Open craniotomy, CT-guided aspiration, and echo-guided aspiration were variously employed at different centers, and timing of

Table 3
Results of Japan Cooperative Study of Surgical Therapy for Putaminal Hemorrhage[55,60]

Neurologic Grade at Presenation	Treatment	Number of Patients	Full Work or Minimal Disability	Partial Disability	Total Disability or Vegetative	Death
Alert or somnolent	Medical	2577	62%	28%	4%	6%
	Surgical	1725	24%	58%	8%	10%
Stupor or coma	Medical	1005	6%	12%	9%	72%
	Surgical	1602	5%	41%	18%	35%

operation ranged from within 6 hours of onset to greater than 7 days post-ictus. Outcome assessments were not blinded, and the choice to employ medical or surgical treatment was at the discretion of the treating physicians.

Most surgeons will forego evacuation of small putaminal hemorrhages in alert patients and massive putaminal hemorrhages in deeply comatose patients. When patients with hematomas of intermediate grade develop progressive neurologic deficit or impairment of consciousness, surgical intervention should be entertained.

Thalamic Hemorrhage

Due to their deep location within the brain, most thalamic hemorrhages are not evacuated lest additional damage be produced through surgical invasion of brain parenchyma. Accepted treatment consists of medical therapy. Occasionally, continuous ventricular drainage is undertaken. Several reports have associated ventricular dilatation with poor outcome.[52,53] Ventricular drainage may restore consciousness when coma results from secondary hydrocephalus rather than direct destruction or compression of the brainstem by the hematoma.[52,54] MRI scanning may be helpful in distinguishing these conditions.

As stereotactic aspiration techniques have advanced, allowing deep hematomas to be removed with minimal trauma to intact brain tissue, interest in surgical evacuation of thalamic hematomas has been renewed.[26,55,56] One group performed a single aspiration 2 weeks after onset in 17 patients.[55] Compared with similar medically treated patients, operated patients who had hematomas less than 25 mm in diameter were reported to have improved functional recovery. In contrast, another center carried out CT-guided aspiration, supplemented by urokinase infusion for large hematomas in 75 patients.[56] The operations were often performed within the first 48 hours post-ictus. Mortality at 6 months was 7%, but patients with coma or herniation were not operated on. Contrasted with a comparable medically treated group, functional outcome was better in patients with surgical treatment when hematomas exceeded a diameter of 32 mm. As these opposing results suggest, indications for surgical aspiration of thalamic hemorrhages are not yet defined.

Lobar Subcortical Hemorrhages

Lobar hemorrhages have more diverse etiologies than bleeds at other sites. When CT, MRI, and angiogram identify an underlying neoplastic or vascular lesion, surgery is indicated to evacuate the hematoma and prevent further bleeding by removing the causative pathologic condition. Criteria for surgery in patients without known lesions are less well defined.[57] In selected patients in whom preoperative workup is unrevealing, intraoperative biopsy of the walls of the hematoma cavity may provide a specific etiologic diagnosis. In one report, tissue was obtained in 54 cases of intracerebral hemorrhage of unknown etiology, and a specific diagnosis was made in 14 patients, all with lobar hemorrhages.[58] Neoplasm was found in 7 cases, amyloid angiopathy in 6, and abscess in 1. The extent of the preoperative workup was not described. In another study, biopsy and histopathologic examination provided a specific diagnosis in 7 of 14 patients with lobar or cerebellar hemorrhage who had no angiographic evidence of the cause of bleeding.[59] Five arteriovenous malformations and two cases of amyloid angiopathy were found. In the remaining seven patients, a potential bleeding source, microaneurysms, was definitely identified in five. Further studies with more extensive preoperative neuroimaging are required to define the diagnostic role of surgery in lobar hemorrhage, as detection of amyloid angiopathy and microaneurysms will not lead to curative therapy, and preoperative CT and MRI imaging may detect treatable etiologies (vascular malformation, neoplasm, abscess) more frequently than angiography alone.

A generally accepted indication for operative intervention at lobar sites is progression of deficits despite maximal medical therapy. Size, site, and shift are additional variables that influence the decision to operate. One retrospective study suggested that surgery improves outcome in lobar hemorrhages between 25 ml and 80 ml in size. Smaller bleeds will do well without evacuation, while larger bleeds will fare poorly irrespective of the treatment pursued.[60] Temporal hematomas warrant a lower threshold for surgical intervention, as they are more likely to cause herniation and brainstem compression than bleeds at other lobar locations.[61] Mass effect with midline shift in excess of 6 to 7 mm or CT evidence of basal cistern effacement should also prompt consideration for surgery.[43]

Cerebellar Hemorrhages

Intracerebellar hemorrhages can rapidly be fatal. Bleeding usually erupts in the medial aspect of the cerebellar hemisphere, near the dentate nucleus. Because of the small size of the posterior fossa, the acute onset of the space occupying lesion may quickly lead to direct brainstem compression, or obliteration of the fourth ventricle or aqueduct and resulting hydrocephalus. Penetration of blood into the ventricular system, as occurs in 70% to 80% of cerebellar hemorrhages, may also produce hydrocephalus.[40] For these reasons, it has been widely agreed that surgical decompression of larger cerebellar hemorrhages can be lifesaving, though this consensus has never been substantiated by a well-controlled trial.

Level of consciousness, size of hematoma, and CT evidence of cisternal compression or hydrocephalus are important determinants of outcome.[62-64] Several authors have suggested that 3 cm transverse diameter is the critical size for cerebellar hemorrhages, recommending that all hematomas greater than 3 cm should be evacuated immediately, as deterioration can be unpredictable and rapid, while smaller hematomas may initially be managed medically.[63,65–67] However, when there is no ventricular extension and the mass effect is limited, unoperated patients with hemorrhages that exceed 3 cm may have a benign outcome.[68–70] Moreover, hydrocephalus may occur with lesions under 3 cm in size, appearing in 29% in one large series of 155 cerebellar hemorrhages.[71] An alternative approach is to operate immediately on any patient who has impairment of consciousness, signs of ambient cistern or brainstem compression, or hydrocephalus, while monitoring closely all patients who are awake without CT signs of herniation irregardless of hematoma size.[64,70–73] Once a patient's alertness begins to deteriorate, the need for surgery is urgent. When the patient is still arousable, the mortality ranges from 0% to 27% in various series. In patients who are comatose before operation, the mortality averages 72%, and functional outcome in survivors may be poor.[74] Pessimism, but not nihilism, guides the decision to operate on patients in coma, as a minority may make satisfactory functional recoveries, especially if the interval between the development of coma and surgery is brief.[64,67,75,76]

Overall, surgical mortality in CT scan era surgical series is about 35%.[74] The standard operative procedure is ventriculostomy to relieve hydrocephalus, followed immediately by suboccipital craniotomy and hematoma evacuation to avert or relieve direct brainstem compression. A minority of patients with small, strategically placed hemorrhages producing hydrocephalus may be treated with ventricular drainage alone.[77–79] However, isolated ventricular drainage without removal of the posterior fossa lesion may suddenly reverse the pressure gradient between the infratentorial and supratentorial compartments, causing upward herniation of the cerebellum.[80] Stereotactic aspiration and fibrinolysis of cerebellar hemorrhages is the subject of active investigation.[28,81] In one report, 13 of 14 patients undergoing CT-guided evacuation with urokinase showed good or very good functional outcome at 6 months, and 1 died (7% mortality).[40] However, no patients in a preoperative comatose state were subjected to surgery.

Pontine Hemorrhages

The pons is the most common site of spontaneous brainstem hemorrhage, accounting for 85% of cases.[43] Formerly regarded as "a neurologic delight for diagnosis, and neurosurgical despair for therapeusis,"[82] pontine hematomas successfully treated by surgical evacuation are being reported more frequently in the literature, but indications for surgery remain poorly defined.[83–88]

Several authors have divided pontine hemorrhages into two classes.[86,89] Diffuse tegmentobasilar hemorrhages are more frequent, are associated with hypertension, and generally occur in older patients. When large, their course is often fulminating, with rapid onset of coma and a 90% mortality rate regardless of treatment modality.[71] Smaller hemorrhages have a better prognosis, but it is unclear if conventional surgical techniques improve outcomes obtained with medical therapy. The advent of stereotactic aspiration may improve operative results. Twenty patients underwent CT-guided stereotactic aspiration in one recent series.[87] There were no deaths and 65% attained good or fair recovery of activity. When the aspiration group was contrasted with medically treated patients with hemorrhages of comparable size, but unmatched in other respects, surgical benefits were restricted to patients with hematomas 5 to 10 ml in volume. Patients with hematomas less than 5 ml fared well, with greater than 10 ml faired poorly, in both treatment arms.

Subependymal or tegmental hematomas most commonly appear in younger patients as the result of bleeding from a cryptic brainstem vascular malformation. The focal lesion is generally limited by the ependyma of the floor of the fourth ventricle, and is more likely to displace than destroy brain tissues. Bleeding can recur, and the clinical presentation may be variable, including inexorable progression suggesting neoplasm, relapse, and remission mimicking multiple sclerosis and subacute onset consonant with an infectious process or stroke.[82,86,90–93] Subependymal hemorrhages are disproportionately represented in surgical series of pontine hematomas. Surgery reduces the compressive effect of space-occupying hematomas in patients with progressive neurologic deterioration, and preempts further bleeding by excising the underlying lesion in patients who harbor a vascular malformation. The most common microsurgical procedure is to take a posterior approach through the inferior vermis, expose the lesion through the floor of the fourth ventricle, drain the hematoma, and explore the cavity wall to identify and, if possible, remove a vascular anomaly.[94] Konovalov et al reported good outcomes in 15 of 15 surgical cases, confirming the feasibility of surgery in carefully selected patients.[84] Direct comparison has not been made with the alternative therapeutic strategies of initial medical management or stereotactic aspiration, followed by radiotherapy with a linear accelerator or a gamma knife for MRI-delineated vascular malformations.

Intraventricular Hemorrhage

Primary ventricular hemorrhage from arteriovenous malformation, aneurysm, choroid hemangioma, or other abnormal vessels within the ventricular walls may produce hydrocephalus if blood occludes cerebrospinal fluid pathways.[43,95] Delayed hydrocephalus is also a major complication when intraparenchymal hematomas extend through ependymal walls to produce secondary intraventricular hemorrhage. Ventricular enlargement may decrease spontaneously, but neurologic deterioration or advancing ventricular dilatation is an indication for drainage. Initial experience suggests that intraventricular infusion of urokinase in cases of severe hemorrhage with casting of the ventricles produces immediate reduction of clot volume, and may allow faster removal of the drain or conversion to a ventricular shunt.[96,97]

Special Clinical Conditions

Hemorrhage Due to Tumor

Brain neoplasms are responsible for 5% to 10% of all spontaneous intracerebral hemorrhages.[98,99] Bleeding most commonly occurs into malignant tumors, such as glioblastoma multiforme or metastases from systemic cancers, particularly melanoma or bronchogenic carcinoma. When clinical and neuroimaging findings raise suspicion of peritumoral ICH, the hemorrhage should be removed via craniotomy and the walls of the hematoma cavity carefully explored and biopsied. If histopathologic exam confirms the diagnosis of neoplasm, and the patient is able to tolerate further surgery, immediate resection of gliomas or lone metastases should be pursued to avoid the burden of another operation.[100–102]

Arteriovascular Malformations and Aneurysms

The most common symptomatic presentation of arteriovascular malformations (AVMs) is intracranial bleeding, and over half of these hemorrhages are intracerebral. Early rebleeding is infrequent in patients with ruptured AVMs. Accordingly, the indications for urgent hematoma evacuation are essentially the same as those for other types of spontaneous intraparenchymal hemorrhage.[22] If feasible, the malformation may be excised at the time of clot removal. If the AVM is not immediately accessible or requires extensive surgery, extirpation may be deferred for several weeks until brain edema decreases. Small hemorrhages should initially be managed medically, with definitive resection of the AVM after an interval of several weeks.[103]

Bleeding into brain parenchyma accompanies subarachnoid hemorrhage (SAH) in 20% of cerebral aneurysms that present with rupture, and the presence of ICH clearly worsens the prognosis in these patients.[104,105] While the relative merits of early versus late surgical repair of aneurysms in patients with SAH in poor condition at presentation remains controversial, patients with ICH may comprise a distinct subgroup in whom early operation is indicated. In one report, 47 patients with aneurysmal ICH operated on early were contrasted with 149 treated under a delayed surgery policy. Overall mortality in the two groups did not differ significantly (62% early, 70% late), but patients in Hunt's grade IV (56% good or fair outcome early, 17% late) and V (15% good or fair outcome early, 2% late) did appear to benefit from early intervention. However, patients were not prospectively randomized or stratified for important prognostic factors, and several of the clots were subdural rather than intraparenchymal.

Aneurysm-related ICHs most frequently appear in the temporal lobe, arising from middle cerebral artery aneurysm rupture. Compared with patients with aneurysmal ICH at other sites, such as frontal hematomas from anterior communicating artery aneurysms, patients with aneurysmal temporal ICH may especially benefit from early surgery.[106-110] Hematoma evacuation reduces the risk of temporal lobe herniation, and aneurysm clipping prevents postoperative rebleeds.

Chronic Encapsulated Hematomas

Most nonoperated ICHs are gradually reabsorbed, leaving a small residual scar or cyst. Recently there have been several case reports of chronic, encapsulated hematomas that steadily expand.[111-113] The clinical presentation generally simulates tumor, with gradual onset of a slowly progressive neurologic deficit and, frequently, seizures. The lesions may occur in children, more often in adults, and generally arise at a lobar site. Only a minority are associated with an AVM or other underlying vascular anomaly. Further complicating the diagnostic differentiation from tumor, the CT appearance may closely resemble neoplasm, with peripheral edema and ring-like enhancement encircling a hypodense or mixed density core (Figure 5). At surgery, a thick fibrous capsule is found, surrounding central clots in varying stages of resolution. Pathologically,

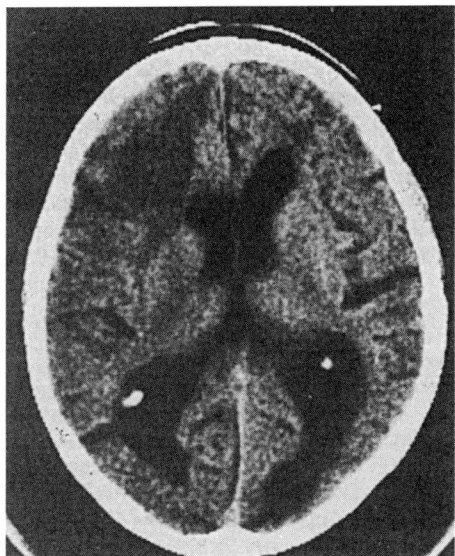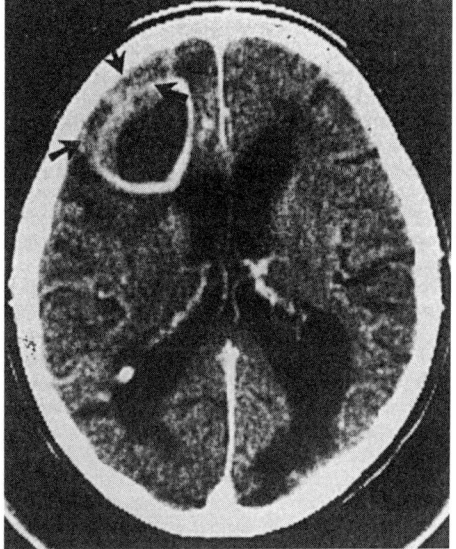

Figure 5: Chronic encapsulated hematoma. **Left:** CT scan without contrast demonstrates hypodense lesion with edema and mass effect in the right frontal lobe. **Right:** After injection of contrast, ring enhancement appears encircling hypodense core. (Also noted on both scans is an old hypodense area in left occipital lobe). Reproduced with permission from Fiumara, Gambacorta, D'Angelo et al, 1989.[112]

the capsule consists of an outer layer of thick collagenous tissue and an inner layer of fibroblastic granulation tissue rich in neovascular channels. Recurrent bleeding or exudation from capillaries in the granulation tissue is the likely mechanism of hematoma self-perpetuation and growth.[114]

Chronic encapsulated hematomas need to be distinguished from chronic nonencapsulated hematomas, which are liquid in composition, not surrounded by a fibrous covering, and likely to resolve spontaneously over time. If the patient's clinical condition is stable, serial CT scans may be obtained. Disappearance of ring-like enhancement and decrease in attenuation and size of the lesion are consistent with a resolving hematoma, and permit continued medical management.[115] MRI scanning may also be useful. Neuroimaging evidence of an underlying vascular malformation, or of continuing expansion consistent with encapsulation, should prompt surgical resection.

Amyloid Angiopathy

Cerebral amyloid angiopathy (CAA) accounts for 10% to 17% of ICHs.[116,117] The incidence rises sharply with age,[118] and amyloid angiopathy is the leading diagnosis in normotensive patients with lobar hemorrhage over age 60. Cerebral amyloid angiopathy rarely produces deep hemorrhages. Bleeding likely occurs through small leptomeningeal and cortical vessels weakened by amyloid deposits in the media and adventitia.[119] The underlying vasculopathy is widespread, and subsequent episodes of hemorrhage in the same or new locations occur in 10% of cases.[120] Nonsurgical management of ICH in amyloid angiopathy patients has been recommended because of concern that vessel fragility would lead to difficulty in controlling intraoperative bleeding and frequent postoperative hemorrhages. Greene et al, however, reported 11 CAA patients undergoing intracranial surgery, evacuation of hematoma in 9, and biopsy for dementia in 2, none of whom experienced abnormal intraoperative bleeding or recurrent hemorrhage.[121] Surgical mortality was 22% among the patients subjected to hematoma removal. The authors suggested that surgery may be pursued safely in patients requiring hematoma evacuation due to progressive deterioration secondary to mass effect.

Coagulation Disorders

Hemophilia

Hemophilia is due to a congenital deficiency of clotting factors of the first stage of the coagulation cascade. The largest proportion of patients are deficient in factor VIII, 10% to 20% in factor IX, and rare patients are deficient in factor XI. Approximately 2% to 3% of hemophiliacs develop hemorrhages in the cen-

Table 4
Indications for Surgical Evacuation of ICHs

Most firmly established	Cerebellar hemorrhage with progressive deterioration secondary to mass effect
	Lobar hemorrhage with progressive deterioration secondary to mass effect
	Expanding chronic encapsulated hematoma
	Preoperative neuroimaging suggests hemorrhage due to brain neoplasm
Less firmly established	Putaminal hemorrhage of intermediate size (~25 to 80 ml) or any putaminal hemorrhage with progressive deterioration secondary to mass effect, when patient and/or family are willing to accept increased risk of moderate to severe postoperative morbidity
	Lobar hemorrhage in young patient with unrevealing CT, MRI, and angiographic studies (to detect or rule out underlying tumor or vascular malformation)
	Subependymal pontine hemorrhage associated with vascular malformation
	Aneurysm-related ICH, especially in temporal lobe (with aneurysm clipping performed simultaneously)
Not firmly established	Thalamic hemorrhage
	Tegmentobasilar pontine hemorrhage

tral nervous system, often associated with mild trauma, but apparently spontaneous in half.[122,123] In general, indications for surgical evacuation of ICH in hemophiliacs are the same as in other patients (Table 4). In addition, as intermittent continued bleeding despite adequate factor replacement therapy may occur, hemophiliac patients with ICH who do not respond to medical management after a few hours should undergo surgical evacuation.[124] Concentrate transfusions to achieve a level of 50% to 100% of the deficient factor are given immediately prior to surgery to prevent intraoperative or postoperative bleeding, and one continued until the incision is healed.[22,124,125]

Thrombocytopenia

Insufficient number or impaired qualitative function of platelets may produce a bleeding diathesis. Thrombocytopenia results from either diminished platelet production due to bone marrow suppression (drugs, radiation) or replacement (leukemia, metastatic tumor), or accelerated platelet destruction or sequestration (autoimmune reactions, splenomegaly). Thrombocytopenia regularly prolongs the bleeding time when platelet counts fall below 75,000/mm. Intracerebral hemorrhage has been reported in idiopathic thrombocytopenic purpura and several secondary thrombocytopenias.[126] Indications for surgery are the same as in other conditions. It is essential that a satisfactory hemostatic level be achieved by platelet transfusions before surgery proceeds. While platelet counts as low as 50,000 may pose only a minimal hazard, maintaining counts above 100,000 for the duration of the procedure and immediate postoperative period is optimal.[125,127]

Conventional Anticoagulation

About 1% of patients on oral anticoagulation develop intracranial hemorrhage, an 8- to 11-fold increase in incidence compared with nonanticoagulated patients with similar bleeding risk factors.[99] Together, heparin- and warfarin-associated bleeding account for up to 9% of ICH.[98] Patients with anticoagulant-related ICH may present with a distinctive course of gradual progression of focal deficits over long periods, up to 72 hours.[128] Guidelines for surgical intervention are the same as those for spontaneous brain hemorrhage. In patients taking warfarin, preoperative transfusion of fresh frozen plasma immediately reverses anticoagulation. Vitamin K is administered parenterally to hasten long-term restoration of normal coagulation. Because of its short half-life, heparin is generally undetectable in a patient's plasma within hours of discontinuation of therapy. When the need for surgery is urgent, protamine sulfate may be infused to reverse anticoagulation more rapidly. Overall mortality in anticoagulant-related hemorrhages regardless of treatment is in the range of 65%.[128,129]

Thrombolytic Therapy

The incidence of ICH in patients receiving thrombolytic therapy with tissue plasminogen activator, streptokinase, or urokinase for acute myocardial infarction is approximately 1%. The hematomas generally appear in lobar locations, and 75% are associated with major morbidity or mortality.[130,131] Supervening cerebral hemorrhages have also been observed in clinical trials of thrombolytic agents for the treatment of acute cerebral ischemia. Two to 4 hours may elapse after streptokinase or urokinase is discontinued before fibrinolysis and coagulation normalize. Eleff and colleagues have recommended an aggressive "shotgun" approach to perioperative management when thrombolysis-related ICH is life-threatening and neurosurgical intervention cannot be delayed.[132] Fibrinolytic agents are immediately held. Σ-aminocaproic acid and cryoprecipitate are administered to reverse the inhibition of the fibrinolytic system. Protamine is given slowly intravenously if heparin has been employed. During the surgical procedure, fresh frozen plasma is infused continuously, and blood transfusions are given as needed to maintain oxygen-carrying capacity. Thrombolytic agent-related hemorrhage is likely to become increasingly common. Further studies are needed to clarify optimal surgical management.

Acknowledgments: I thank Steven L. Denlinger, MD, for his thoughtful review and suggestions.

References

1. MacEwen W: An address on the surgery of the brain and spinal cord. *Br Med J* 1888;2:302.

2. Kawakami H, Kutsuzawa T, Uemura K, et al: Regional cerebral blood flow in patients with hypertensive intracerebral hemorrhage. *Stroke* 1974;5: 207.

3. Ropper A, Zervas NT: Cerebral blood flow after experimental basal ganglia hemorrhage. *Ann Neurol* 1980;11:266.

4. Blackwood W: Vascular disease of the central nervous system. In: Greenfield JG, ed: *Neuropathology*. London: Arnold, 1958;113.

5. Tanizaki Y: Improvement of cerebral blood flow following stereotactic surgery in patients with putaminal hemorrhage. *Acta Neurochir* 1988;90: 103.

6. Jenkins A, Mendelow AD, Graham DI, et al: Experimental intracranial haematoma: the role of blood constituents in early ischaemia. *Br J Neurosurg* 1990;4:45.

7. Suzuki J, Ebina T: Sequential changes in tissue surrounding ICH. In: Pia H, Langmaid C, Zierski J, eds: *Spontaneous Intracerebral Hematomas*. Berlin: Springer-Verlag, 1980;121.

8. Hatashita S, Koike J, Ishii S: Effect of surgery on brain edema associated with intracerebral hematoma and arterial hypertension. *Neurol Med Chir* 1987;27:11.

9. Garde A, Bohmer G, Selden B, et al: One hundred cases of spontaneous intracerebral hematoma. *Eur Neurol* 1983;22:161.

10. Helweg-Larsen S, Sommer W, et al: Prognosis for patients treated conservatively for spontaneous intracerebral hematomas. *Stroke* 1984;15:1045.

11. Hungerbuhler JP, Regli F, Van Melle DG, et al: Spontaneous intracerebral hemorrhages. Clinical and CT features; immediate evaluation of prognosis. *Arch Suisses Neurol Neurochir Psychiatr* 1983;132:13.

12. Nath FP, Nicholls D, Fraser RJA: Prognosis in intracerebral hemorrhage. *Acta Neurochir* 1983;67:29.

13. Portenoy RK, Lipton RB, Berger AR, et al: Intracerebral hemorrhage: a model for the prediction of outcome. *J Neurol Neurosurg Psychiatr* 1987; 50:976.

14. Tuhrim S, Dambrosia JM, Price TR, et al: Prediction of intracerebral hemorrhage survival. *Ann Neurol* 1988;24:258.

15. Turtas S, Perria C, Orunesu G, et al: The value of some clinical and computer tomographic parameters in the prognosis of surgically treated patients with intracerebral hematoma. *Zent bl Neurochir* 1990;51:190.

16. Volpin L, Cervellini P, Colombo F, et al: Spontaneous intracerebral hematomas: a new proposal about the usefulness and limits of surgical treatment. *Neurosurgery* 1984;15:663.

17. McKissock W, Richardson A, Taylor J: Primary intracerebral hemorrhage. A controlled trial of surgical and conservative treatment in 180 unselected cases. *Lancet* 1961;2:221.

18. Juvela S, Heiskanen O, Poranen A, et al: The treatment of spontaneous intracerebral hemorrhage: a prospective randomized trial of surgical and conservative treatment. *J Neurosurg* 1989;70:755.

19. Batjer HH, Reisch JS, Allen BC, et al: Failure of surgery to improve outcome in hypertensive putaminal hemorrhage. *Arch Neurol* 1990;47:1103.

20. Auer LM, Deinsberger W, Niederkorn K, et al: Endoscopic surgery versus medical treatment for spontaneous intracerebral hematoma: a randomized study. *J Neurosurg* 1989;70:530.

21. Suzuki J, Sato S: The new transsylvian approach to the hypertensive intracerebral hematoma. *Jpn J Surg* 1972;2:47.

22. Ojemann RG, Heros RC, Crowell RM: *Surgical Management of Cerebrovascular Disease*. Williams and Wilkins, 1987:435.

23. Browder EJ, Cooradini EW: Surgical treatment of intracerebral hematomas. *Arch Neurol Psychiatr* 1951;65:112.

24. Lazorthes G: Surgery of cerebral hemorrhage. Report on the result of 52 surgically treated cases. *J Neurosurg* 1959;16:355.

25. Niizuma H, Suzuki J: Stereotactic aspiration of putaminal hemorrhage using a double track aspiration technique. *Neurosurgery* 1988;22:432.

26. Hondo H, Uno M, Sasaki K, et al: Computer tomography controlled aspiration surgery for hypertensive intracerebral hemorrhage. *Stereotact Funct Neurosurg* 1990;54:432.

27. Nguyen JP, Gaston A, Brugieres P, et al: Hematomes intracerebraux operes sous controle scanographique a l'aide du trocart de Backlund. *Neurochir* 1991;37:50.

28. Niizuma H, Suzuki J: Computed tomography-guided stereotactic aspiration of posterior fossa hematomas: a supine lateral retromastoid approach. *Neurosurgery* 1987;21:422.

29. Kanaya H, Kuroda K: Development in neurosurgical approaches to hypertensive intracerebral hemorrhage in Japan. In: Kaufman HH, ed: *Intracerebral Hematomas*. New York: Raven Press, 1992:197.

30. Kandel EI, Peresedov VV: Stereotaxic evacuation of spontaneous intracerebral hematomas. *J Neurosurg* 1985;62:206.

31. Mohadjer M, Ruh E, Hiltl DM: CT-stereotactic evacuation and fibrinolysis of hypertensive intracranial hematoma. *Fibrinolysis* 1988;2:43.

32. Backlund E-O, von Holst H: Controlled subtotal evacuation of intracerebral hematomas by stereotactic technique. *Surg Neurol* 1978;9:99.

33. Higgins AC, Nashold BSJ: Stereotactic evacuation of large intracerebral hematomas. *Appl Neurophysiol* 1980;43:96.

34. Kandel EI, Peresedov VV: Stereotactic evacuation of intracerebral hematomas. In: Schmidek HH, Sweet WH, eds: *Operative Neurosurgical Techniques*. Grune & Stratton, 1988:889.

35. Ito H, Muka H, Kitamura A: Stereotactic aqua stream and aspirator for removal of intracerebral hematoma. *Stereotact Funct Neurosurg* 1990; 54–55:457.

36. Iseki H, Amano K, Kawamura H, et al: A new apparatus using the micro ultrasonic (MUSA) system for microneurosurgery. *No Shinkei Gekka-Neurol Surg* 1989;17:835.

37. Matsumoto K, Hondo H, Tomida K: Aspiration surgery for hypertensive

brain hemorrhage in the acute stage. In: Suzuki J, ed: *Advances in Surgery for Cerebral Stroke*. Tokyo: Springer, 1988:433.

38. Auer LM, Holzer P, Ascher PW, et al: Endoscopic neurosurgery. *Acta Neurochir* 1988;90:1.

39. Matsumoto K, Hondo H: CT-guided stereotactic evacuation of hypertensive intracerebral hematomas. *J Neurosurg* 1984;61:440.

40. Mohadjer M, Eggert R, May J, et al: CT-guided stereotactic fibrinolysis of spontaneous and hypertensive cerebellar hemorrhage: long-term resutls. *J Neurosurg* 1990;73:217.

41. Kaufmann HH, Schochet S, Koss W, et al: Efficacy and safety of tissue plasminogen activator. *Neurosurgery* 1987;20:403.

42. Niizuma H, Shimizu Y, Yonemitsu T, et al: Results of stereotactic aspiration in 175 cases of putaminal hemorrhage. *Neurosurgery* 1989;24:814.

43. Weisberg LA, Stazio A, Shamsnia M, et al: Nontraumatic parenchymal brain hemorrhages. *Medicine* 1990;69:277.

44. Fujitsu K, Muramoto M, Ikeda Y, et al: Indications for surgical treatment of putaminal hemorrhage. *J Neurosurg* 1990;73:518.

45. Hondo H, Matsumoto K, Tomida K, et al: CT-controlled stereotactic aspiration in hypertensive brain hemorrhage. *Appl Neurophysiol* 1987;50:233.

46. Kanaya H: All Japan co-cooperative study on the treatment of hypertensive intracerebral hemorrhage. *Jpn J Stroke* 1990;12:509.

47. Kanaya H, Saiki I, Ohuchi T, et al: Hypertensive intracerebral hemorrhage in Japan: Update on surgical treatment. In: Mizukami M, Kanaya H, Kogure K, et al, eds: *Hypertensive Intracerebral Hemorrhage*. New York: Raven Press, 1981:147.

48. Kanno T, Sano H, Shinomiya Y, et al: Role of surgery in hypertensive intracerebral hematoma. *J Neurosurg* 1984;61:1091.

49. Yamanaka R, Satoh S: Comparison of stereotactic aspiration, craniotomy, and conservative treatment for putaminal hemorrhage. *Neurol Med Chir* 1988;28:986.

50. Waga S, Miyazaki M, Okada M, et al: Hypertenisve putaminal hemorrhage: analysis of 182 patients. *Surg Neurol* 1986;26:159.

51. Kanno T, Nagata J, Nonomura K, et al: Treatment of hypertensive intracerebral hemorrhage: new approaches. 18th Princeton Conference: Rochester Hills, MI: 1992.

52. Kwak R, Kadoya S, Suzuki T: Factors affecting the prognosis in thalamic hemorrhage. *Stroke* 1983;14:493.

53. Walshe TM, Davis KR, Fisher CM: Thalamic hemorrhage: a computed tomographic-clinical correlation. *Neurology* 1977;27:217.

54. Kagawa Y, Kanno T, Sano H, et al: Thalamic hemorrhage. Clinical classification based on the CT findings and its surgical treatment. *Neurol Med Chir* 1977;17:243.

55. Honda E, Hayashi T, Shimamoto H, et al: A comparison between stereotaxic operation and conservative therapy for thalamic hemorrhage. *Kurume Med J* 1987;34:9.

56. Niizuma H, Yonemitsu T, Hidehumi J, et al: Stereotactic aspiration of thalamic hematoma. *Stereotact Funct Neurosurg* 1990;54–55:438.

57. Masdeu JC, Rubino FA: Management of lobar intracerebral hemorrhage: medical or surgical. *Neurology* 1984;34:381.

58. Hinton DR, Dolan E, Sima AAF: The value of histopathological examination of surgically removed blood clot in determining the etiology of spontaneous intracerebral hemorrhage. *Stroke* 1984;15:517.

59. Wakai S, Nagai M. Histological verification of microaneurysms as a cause of cerebral haemorrhage in surgical specimens. *J Neurol Neurosurg Psychiatr* 1989;52:595.

60. Maiuir F, Corriero G, Passarelli F, et al: CT indications for surgery and evaluation of prognosis in patients with spontaneous intracerebral hematomas. *Br J Neurosurg* 1990;4:155.

61. Andrews BT, Chiles BW, Olsen WL, et al: The effect of intracerebral hematoma location on the risk of brain-stem compression and on clinical outcome. *J Neurosurg* 1988;69:518.

62. Kobayashi S, Miyata A, Serizawa T, et al: Treatment of cerebellar hemorrhage—surgical or conservative. *Stroke* 1990;21(Suppl 1):62.

63. Little JR, Tubman DE, Ethier R: Cerebellar hemorrhage in adults. *J Neurosurg* 1978;48:575.

64. Taneda M, Hayakawa T, Mogami H: Primary cerebellar hemorrhage. Quadrigeminal cistern obliteration on CT scans as a predictor of outcome. *J Neurosurg* 1987;67:545.

65. Acompora S, Guarnieri L, Troisi F: Spontaneous intracerebellar haematoma. *Acta Neurochir* 1982;66:83.

66. Donauer E, Faubert C: Management of spontaneous intracerebral and cerebellar hemorrhage. In: Kaufman HH, ed: *Intracerebral Hematomas.* New York: Raven Press, 1992:211.

67. Lui T-N, Fairholm DJ, Shu T-F, et al: Surgical treatment of spontaneous cerebellar hemorrhage. *Surg Neurol* 1985;23:555.

68. Bogousslavsky J, Regli F, Jeanrenaud X: Benign outcome in unoperated large cerebellar haemorrhage. *Acta Neurochir* 1984;73:59.

69. Melamed N, Satya-Murti S: Cerebellar hemorrhage. A review and reappraisal of benign cases. *Arch Neurol* 1984;41:425.

70. van der Hoop RG, Vermeulen M, van Gijn J: Cerebellar hemorrhage: diagnosis and treatment. *Surg Neurol* 1988;29:6.

71. Da Pian R, Bazzan A, Pasqualin A: Surgical versus medical treatment of spontaneous posterior fossa haematomas: a cooperative study on 205 cases. *Neurol Res* 1984;6:145.

72. Auer LM, Auer T, Sayama I: Indications for surgical treatment of cerebellar hemorrhage and infarction. *Acta Neurochir* 1986;79:74.

73. Etou A, Mohadjer M, Braus D, et al: Stereotactic evacuation and fibrinolysis of cerebellar hematomas. *Stereotact Funct Neurosurg* 1990;54–55, 445.

74. Sypert GW. Posterior fossa hematomas. In: Fein J, Flamm E, eds: *Cerebrovascular Surgery.* New York: Springer-Verlag, 1985:1283.

75. Heros RC: Cerebellar hemorrhage and infarction. *Stroke* 1982;13:106.

76. Ott KH, Kase CS, Ojemann RG, et al: Cerebellar hemorrhage: diagnosis and treatment. A review of 56 cases. *Arch Neurol* 1974;31:160.

77. Seelig JM, Selhorst JB, Young HF, et al: Ventriculostomy for hydrocephalus in cerebellar hemorrhage. *Neurology* 1981;31:1537.

78. Shenkin HA, Zavala M: Cerebellar strokes: mortality, surgical indications, and results of ventricular drainage. *Lancet* 1982;2:429.

79. Waidhauser E, Hamburger C, Marguth F: Neurosurgical management of cerebellar hemorrhage. *Neurosurg Rev* 1990;13:211.

80. Cuneo RA, Caronna JJ, Pitts L, et al: Upward transtentorial herniation: seven cases and a review of the literature. *Arch Neurol* 1979;36:618.

81. Mohadjer M, Eggert R, Johannes M, et al: CT-guided stereotactic fibrinolysis of spontaneous and hypertensive cerebellar hemorrhage: long-term results. *J Neurosurg* 1990;73:217.

82. Teilmann K: Hemangiomas of the pons. *Arch Neurol Psychiatr* 1953;69:208.

83. Beatty RM, Zervas NT: Stereotactic aspiration of a brain stem hematoma. *Neurosurgery* 1983;13:204.

84. Konovalov AN, Spallone AS, Makhmudov UB, et al: Surgical management of hematomas of the brain stem. *J Neurosurg* 1990;73:181.

85. O'Laoire SA, Crockard HA, Thomas DCT: Brainstem hematoma. A report of six surgically treated cases, *J Neurosurg* 1982;56:222.

86. Mangiardi JR, Epstein FJ: Brainstem haematomas: review of the literature and presentation of five new cases. *J Neurol Neurosurg Psychiatr* 1988;51:966.

87. Shitamichi M, Nakamura J, Sasaki T, et al: Computer tomography guided stereotactic aspiration of pontine hemorrhages. *Stereotact Funct Neurosurg* 1990;54–55:453.

88. Thomas DGT, Nouby RM: Experience in 300 cases of CT-directed stereotactic surgery for lesion biopsy and aspiration of haematoma. *Br J Neurosurg* 1989;3:321.

89. Goto N, Kaneko M, Hosaka Y, et al: Primary pontine hemorrhage: clinicopathologic correlations. *Stroke* 1980;11:84.

90. Abroms IF, Yessayan L, Shillito J, et al: Spontaneous intracerebral haemorrhage in patients suspected of multiple sclerosis. *J Neurol Neursurg Psychiatr* 1971;34:157.

91. Kashiwagi S, Van Laveren RH, Tew JM, et al: Diagnosis and treatment of vascular brain stem malformations. *J Neurosurg* 1990;72:27.

92. Pouyanne M, Got M, Julien J, et al: Deux cas d'hématome intraprotubérantiels opérés. Etude critique. *Soc Neurochir* 1967;13:738.

93. Tung H, Giannotta SL, Chandrasoma PT, et al: Recurrent intraparenchymal hemorrhages from angiographically occult vascular malformations. *J Neurosurg* 1990;73:174.

94. Colak A, Bertan V, Benli K, et al: Pontine hematoma. A report of three surgically treated cases. *Zent bl Neurochir* 1991;52:33.

95. Little JR, Blomquist GA, Ethier R: Intraventricular hemorrhage in adults. *Surg Neurol* 1977;8:143.

96. Shen P-H, Matsuoka Y, Kawajiri K, et al: Treatment of intraventricular hemorrhage using urokinase. *Neurol Med Chir* 1990;30:329.

97. Todo T, Usui M, Takakura K: Treatment of severe intraventricular hemorrhage by intraventricular infusion of urokinase. *Stroke* 1990;21(suppl 1):61.

98. Feldmann E: Intracerebral hemorrhage. *Stroke* 1991;22:684.

99. Kase CS: Intracerebral hemorrhage: non-hypertensive causes. *Stroke* 1986;17:590.

100. Bitoh S, Hasegawa H, Othsuki H: Cerebral neoplasms initially presenting with massive intracerebral hemorrhage. *Surg Neurol* 1984;22:57.

101. Little JR, Dail B, Belanger G, et al: Brain hemorrhage from intracranial tumor. *Stroke* 1979;10:283.

102. Wakai S, Yamakawa K, Manaka S, et al: Spontaneous intracerebral hemorrhage caused by brain tumor. Its incidence and clinical significance. *Neurosurgery* 1982;10:437.

103. Gentleman D, Bullock R: Management of life-threatening acute intracerebral haematomas due to vascular lesions. *J Neurol Neurosurg Psychiatr* 1992;55:518.

104. Hijdra A, Van Gijn J: Early death from rupture of an intracranial aneurysm. *J Neurosurg* 1982;13:177.

105. Weisberg LA: Computed tomography in aneurysmal subarachnoid hemorrhage. *Neurology* 1979;29:802.

106. Anonymous: Intracerebral haematoma from aneurysm rupture: operation in moribund patients? *Lancet* 1987;2:1186.

107. Auer LM: The comatose patient at the acute stage—a surgical taboo? In: Auer LM, ed: *Timing of Aneurysm Surgery.* Berlin: Walter de Gruyter, 1985.

108. Brandt L, Sonesson B, Ljunggren B, et al: Ruptured middle cerebral artery aneurysm with intracerebral hemorrhage in younger patients appearing moribund: emergency operation? *Neurosurgery* 1987;20:925.

109. Page RD, Richardson PL: Emergency surgery for haematoma-forming aneurysmal haemorrhage. *Br J Neurosurg* 1990;4:199.

110. Papo I, Badosi M, Doczi T: Intracerebral haematomas from aneurysm rupture: their clinical significance. *Acta Neurochir* 1987;89:100.

111. Andres JML, Rieger SJ, Torrella EJV, et al: Chronic intracerebral haematoma. *Br J Neurosurg* 1989;3:513.

112. Fiumara E, Gambacorta M, D'Angelo V, et al: Chronic encapsulated intracerebral haematoma: pathogenetic and diagnostic considerations. *J Neurol Neurosurg Psychiatr* 1989;52:1296.

113. Pozzati E, Giuliani G, Gaist G, et al: Chronic expanding intracerebral hematoma. *J Neurosurg* 1986;65:611.

114. Reid JD, Kommaredi S, Lankerani M, et al: Chonic expanding hematomas. A clinicopathologic entity. *JAMA* 1980;244:2441.

115. Zimmerman RD, Leeds NE, Naidich TP: Ring blush associated with intracerebral hematoma. *Radiology* 1977;122:707.

116. Kalyan-Raman UP, Kalyan-Raman K: Cerebral amyloid angiopathy causing intracranial hemorrhage. *Ann Neurol* 1984;16:321.

117. Feldman E, Tornabene J: Diagnosis and treatment of cerebral amyloid angiopathy. *Clin Geriat Med* 1991;7:617.
118. Vinters HV, Gilbert JJ: Cerebral amyloid angiopathy: incidence and complications in the aging brain. II. The distribution of amyloid vascular changes. *Stroke* 1983;14:924.
119. Maruyama K, Ikeda S, Ishihara T, et al: Immunohistochemical characterization of cerebrovascular amyloid in 46 autopsied cases using antibodies to β-protein and cystatin C. *Stroke* 1990;21:397.
120. Gilles C, Brucher JM, Khoubesserian P, et al: Cerebral amyloid angiopathy as a cause of multiple intracerebral hemorrhages. *Neurology* 1984; 34:730.
121. Greene GM, Godersky JC, Biller J, et al: Surgical experience with cerebral amyloid angiopathy. *Stroke* 1990;21:1545.
122. Raish RJ, Hoak JC: Coagulopathy and stroke. In: Barnett H, Mohr J, Stein B, et al, eds: *Stroke, Pathophysiology, Diagnosis and Management.* New York: Churchill Livingstone, 1985:887.
123. Eyster ME, Gill FM, Blatt PM, et al: Central nervous system bleeding in hemophiliacs. *Blood* 1978;51:1179.
124. Martinowitz U, Heim M, Tadmor R, et al: Intracranial hemorrhage in patients with hemophilia. *Neurosurgery* 1986;18:538.
125. Fellin F, Murphy S: Hematologic problems in the preoperative patient. *Med Clin North Am* 1987;71:477.
126. Almaani WS, Awidi AS: Spontaneous intracranial bleeding in hemorrhagic diathesis. *Surg Neurol* 1981;17:137.
127. Chan K-H, Mann KS, Chan TK: The significance of thrombocytopenia in the development of postoperative intracranial hematoma. *J Neurosurg* 1989;71:38.
128. Kase CS, Robinson RK, Stein RW, et al: Anticoagulant-related intracerebral hemorrhage. *Neurology* 1985;35:943.
129. Wintzen AR, de Jonge H, Loeliger EA, et al: The risk of intracerebral hemorrhage during oral anticoagulant treatment: a population study. *Ann Neurol* 1984;16:553.
130. Fennerty AG, Levine MN, Hirsh J: Hemorrhagic complications of thrombolytic therapy in the treatment of myocardial infarction and venous thromboembolism. *Chest* 1989;9:88S.
131. Sloan MA, Price TR, Randall AM, et al: Intracerebral hemorrhage after rTPA and heparin for acute myocardial infarction: the TIMI II pilot and randomized trial experience. *Stroke* 1990;21:182.
132. Eleff SM, Borel C, Bell WR, et al: Acute management of intracranial hemorrhage in patients receiving thrombolytic therapy: case reports. *Neurosurgery* 190;26:867.
133. Crowell RM, Ojemann RG: Surgery for brain hemorrhage. In: Mossy J, Reinmuth OM, eds: *Cerebrovascular Disease.* New York: Raven Press, 1981.
134. Antiplatelet Trialists' Collaboration: Secondary prevention of vascular disease by prolonged antiplatelet treatment. *Br Med J* 1988;296:320.

Part V

Prognosis

Chapter 15

Prognosis

Stanley Tuhrim, MD

Over the past 30 years, both the reported incidence and case fatality rate for primary intracerebral hemorrhage (ICH) have declined. The incidence of ICH parallels the decline in cerebral infarction, largely due to aggressive treatment of hypertension, the primary modifiable risk factor for stroke. The decline in hypertensive hemorrhage has more than offset the increasing number of anticoagulant-related hemorrhages following the advent of widespread anticoagulation in the 1950s. For example, in a population-based study of residents of Rochester, Minnesota, the age-adjusted incidence of nontraumatic ICH fell from 15.7 per 100,000 in the years 1945–1952, to 9.3 in 1961–1968, to 6.0 in 1969–1976.[1] This progressive decline apparently reversed in the latter half of the 1970s when the rate returned to 9 per 100,000.[2] This apparent reversal can be attributed to a second major medical development — the advent of computerized tomography (CT). Previously, ICH was either diagnosed at autopsy or on the basis of clinical criteria that required profound neurologic compromise. When scanning acute stroke patients became routine, smaller hemorrhages with milder symptoms which had been erroneously diagnosed as infarctions were correctly classified. This had the dual effect of increasing the apparent incidence of ICH and decreasing the case fatality rate, since most patients with these smaller hemorrhages survived.

Elimination of other sources of bias and advances in management of critically ill patients also contributed to a dramatic drop in the case fatality rate for ICH in the same time period. For example, in another population-based study of Rochester, Minnesota, Drury et al reported an 8% 30-day survival rate for the period 1945–1974, but a 44% rate in 1975–1979.[2] More recent studies report an overall 30-day survival of approximately 70%.[3–9]

Reliable localization of hemorrhages during life by CT has allowed more accurate correlation of specific lesion location and outcome for patients who survive. In one approach, outcome for specific lesion sites, such as thalamus or cerebellum, has been described as a function of presenting clinical character-

From Feldmann E (ed). *Intracerebral Hemorrhage*. Armonk, NY: Futura Publishing Company, Inc., © 1994.

istics. While these series contain too few patients for the application of sophisticated statistical techniques, they provide a wealth of information regarding specific clinical situations. Another approach seeks to generate meaningful observations regarding ICH in more heterogenous, but larger, groups of patients, such as those with supratentorial hemorrhage. Powerful statistical techniques have been applied in these kinds of studies, enabling inferences to be drawn about the joint effects of isolated factors identified in smaller groups of patients. Unfortunately, examining aggregate data may not lead to inferences based upon clinical signs found in individual patients. The sections that follow review the information provided by these complementary approaches. We first examine outcome correlates for specific lesion sites, then present analyses of aggregate data. Most studies discuss survival as the primary endpoint, but data pertaining to the prognosis of longer term outcome are also presented. The final section discusses anticoagulant related hemorrhages.

Prognosis by Specific Lesion Site

Putaminal Hemorrhage

Intracerebral hemorrhage occurs primarily in the deep portions of the cerebral hemispheres. The putamen is the most common site, accounting for approximately 40% of ICH. The clinical spectrum of putaminal hemorrhage is extremely broad, ranging from very small, asymptomatic lesions[10] to "massive," invariably fatal ones. The overall mortality for putaminal hemorrhage is comparable to that of ICH in general.

Shortly after the advent of CT scanning, Hier et al studied 24 cases of putaminal hemorrhage. Pupillary abnormalities, disturbance in extraocular movements, and bilateral Babinski signs were associated with larger hematomas and a poor chance for survival, while preserved higher cortical function and partial sparing of motor function were associated with good outcome. The four patients with absent extraocular movements had massive hemorrhages and fatal outcomes. Age, sex, size of lesion, and admission blood pressure were unrelated to outcome.[11] Predictive CT scan findings included large hemorrhage size and presence of intraventricular blood. Mizukhami et al suggested that if the hematoma is confined to the region below the level of the lateral ventricle on CT scans performed parallel to the orbitomeatal line, the prognosis for recovery of motor function is much better than if the hemorrhage extends upward. In the latter case, destruction of the posterior limb of the internal capsule is virtually assured, making recovery of motor function improbable.[12] Kanaya, on the basis of extensive experience with medically and surgically treated patients, developed a classification schema that incorporates this principle. He reports that lesions involving only the anterior limb of the internal capsule (grades I and II) fare much better than those involving the posterior limb (grades III and IV) or thalamus (grade V).[13]

Caudate Hemorrhage

Although the caudate is supplied by deep penetrating branches of large superficial cerebral vessels, similar to branch vessels supplying putamen and thalamus, hemorrhage originating in the caudate is rare, accounting for only 5% to 7% of all ICH. Stein et al suggest that patients with caudate hemorrhage can be divided into two groups. One group mimics subarachnoid hemorrhage (SAH) with meningismus, vomiting, headache, and changes in level of consciousness and behavior. Intraventricular blood is always present and frequently accompanied by hydrocephalus. This group of patients generally makes a full recovery. A second group, in addition to the manifestations described above, has hemiparesis and conjugate gaze paresis indicating compression of the internal capsule. These patients also experience complete recovery, though they frequently take longer to do so. For example, in the series of Stein et al four patients had transient hemipareses, while the remaining three patients took several weeks to return to normal.[14] The consistently good outcome, despite intraventricular hemorrhage in these patients, is in sharp contradistinction to putaminal hemorrhage, where such extension is invariably associated with a fatal outcome in the series of Hier et al.[11] The significance of intraventricular extension of hemorrhage will be discussed in detail below.

Thalamic Hemorrhage

Thalamic hemorrhage represents 10% to 15% of ICH. While overall survival in thalamic hemorrhage appears comparable to putaminal hemorrhage, little consensus exists regarding prognostic factors. Fisher, in an early detailed description of the clinical findings in thalamic hemorrhage, commented that large lesions are "well tolerated."[15] However, in the earliest CT scan era report, Walshe, Davis, and Fisher reported that in 18 hypertensive thalamic hemorrhages, all those with a maximum diameter greater than 3.3 cm were fatal, while the overall mortality rate was 50%.[16] Piepgras and Rieger, however, reported that 2 of their 7 patients with hemorrhages larger than this survived, while 5 of 14 patients with smaller hemorrhages died.[17] Barraquer-Bordas et al confirmed Walshe's view by finding that 9 of 23 patients with thalamic hemorrhage succumbed, all with lesions larger than 3.3 cm. None of their patients with larger lesions survived.[18] Kwak et al, in a study of 29 patients, identified 3 cm as distinguishing patients with good prognosis from those likely to die.[19] Finally, in the largest series to date, Weisberg found a strong correlation between hematoma size and recovery, noting that no patients whose hematoma had a maximum diameter of less than 2.5 cm died, while all those with hematomas larger than 3 cm had ventricular extension, became comatose, and died. While a precise hematoma size inconsistent with survival has not been defined, it is apparent that hematoma size correlates with prognosis and that patients with lesions greater than 3 cm in diameter rarely survive. Ventricular extension occurs in most thalamic hemorrhages and carries a variable prognosis, but hydrocephalus, presumably secondary to intraventricular hemorrhage, is associated with a high mortality rate.[20]

The clinical findings associated with thalamic hemorrhage have been well described,[15-20] but only the level of consciousness is consistently related to survival. For example, Walsh et al reported that 4 of 5 patients admitted in coma died, whereas the overall mortality rate in their series of 18 thalamic hemorrhages was 50%.[16] Similarly, Piepgras and Rieger reported that six of seven patients admitted in coma died, while five of six with an initially clear sensorium survived.[17] However, posterior thalamic lesions rarely result in significant permanent deficit.[20,21] Hirose et al describe a syndrome of posterior thalamic hemorrhage consisting of ipsilateral ptosis and miosis, contralateral sensory neglect and hemiparesis, defective pursuit toward the lesion, and hypometric saccades away from the lesion in which five of six patients survived with little or no deficit. Similarly, the aphasia seen with left-sided thalamic hemorrhage is usually transient, and the deficits seen with less than 0.8 cm diameter hematomas may be so transient as to be confused with transient ischemic attacks.[20]

Lobar Hemorrhage

Lobar hemorrhages differ from other supratentorial hemorrhages in that a history of hypertension is found less frequently, occurring in only about one third of cases.[22-25] Patients without a history of hypertension have a substantially better prognosis. In a series of 50 patients reported by Weisberg, all normotensive patients survived and two thirds had little or no residual disability. Among patients with a hypertensive history, 50% worsened in hospital, 28% died, and 77% of survivors had significant neurologic disability.[25] It should be noted that half the hypertensive, but only 6% of the normotensive patients had hematomas larger than 4.0 cm, so that a history of hypertension and hematoma size were interdependent in these patients. Lobar hemorrhage may carry a lower mortality risk than ICH in other locations. Reported mortality rates range from 9% to 32%, substantially less than other sites. Level of consciousness, hemorrhage size, intraventricular extension and degree of midline shift have been identified as important prognostic variables.[22-25] For example, Kase et al found that 11 of 12 patients with hematoma volumes of 40 cc or less survived, while 6 of 10 with larger hematomas died, as did 5 of 8 with intraventricular extension, 4 of whom had hemorrhages larger than 40 cc.[23]

Pontine Hemorrhage

Pontine hemorrhage accounts for approximately 5% of ICH.[26] Previously, this lesion was believed to be almost universally fatal. When pontine hemorrhage involves the paramedian area bilaterally and ruptures into the ventricular system, most patients die. Those who survive are neurologically devastated. CT scanning, however, has demonstrated small hemorrhages limited to the pontine tegmentum or encompassing a small portion of the basis pontis whose signs and symptoms sometimes mimic those of lacunes, producing an ataxic hemiparesis or dysarthria-clumsy hand syndrome.[27] The prognosis in these small hemorrhages is excellent, with full recovery reported.[28-30] The milder, generally laterally placed lesions are more closely associated with vascular malformations of the brainstem than more medial lesions.[31]

Cerebellar Hemorrhage

Cerebellar hemorrhage accounts for approximately 10% of ICH. Most cerebellar hemorrhages occur in the cerebellar hemispheres. The clinical course is highly variable, but certain prognostic signs have been identified. Patients who remain alert fare far better than those who become stuporous or comatose, regardless of whether they undergo evacuation of the hematoma. When patients are operated while still arousable, the reported mortality rate is less than 30%, but evacuation of a cerebellar hematoma after the onset of coma is associated with at least a 72% mortality rate.[32,33] Clinical findings at presentation other than level of consciousness have not been found to be reliable predictors of outcome, but CT scan findings may be more informative. Hemorrhage diameter greater than 3 cm, obstructive hydrocephalus, and intraventricular hemorrhage are associated with a decreased level of consciousness and a high mortality rate.[33] Overall, the survival rate for cerebellar hemorrhage is higher than for other ICH locations. For example, in the NINDS Stroke Data Bank series, over 80% of cerebellar hemorrhage patients survived at least 30 days. Patients who survive frequently make excellent recoveries.[33,34] This is in sharp contrast to the pre-CT era, when cerebellar hemorrhage was believed to be fatal and surgery was believed to be a lifesaving measure for those few fortunate enough to be diagnosed during life.[34]

Although the neurologic signs and CT scan findings associated with short-term survival differ among lesion sites, the overall survival rates for most sites are comparable. Supratentorial hemorrhages currently appear to have a 75% survival rate, with some studies reporting slightly better rates for lobar than deep hemorrhages. Posterior fossa hematomas carry the same prognosis as supratentorial lesions, but lesions confined to the cerebellum have a survival rate that surpasses other categories.

General Prognostic Features

The information in the preceding section regarding specific hemorrhage locations is based on observation of small groups of patients. Another approach

Table 1

Author	Age	EKG Abn	Heme Size	GCS/ Loc	IVH	Location	Pulse Pressure	Midline Shift
Daverat[35]			X	X	X			X
Dixon[36]		X	X	X	X	X		
Fieschi[3]	X		X	X				
Garde[4]			X	X		X		
Helweg-Larsen[8]			X	X				
Mayr[7]	X			X				
Nath[6]			X		X			X
Portenoy[37]			X	X	X			
Senant[38]	X		X	X	X			
Steiner[5]			X	X		X		
Tuhrim '88[39]			X	X			X	
Tuhrim '91[9]			X	X	X		X	

Heme size = hemorrhage size; GCS/Loc = Glascow Coma Scale score or level of consciousness: IVH = Intraventricular hemorrhage.

assesses outcome in larger, heterogeneous groups, such as all patients with supratentorial hemorrhage, with the potential advantage of applying more powerful statistical techniques. This approach may lose information applicable to small subgroups.

Several studies have attempted to identify characteristics of supratentorial hemorrhages that allow clinicians to predict prognosis. Table 1 summarizes the findings.

The early studies[3-8] performed only univariate analysis of factors associated with outcome. Age, lesion location, electrocardiographic abnormalities, and hypertensive history were inconsistently associated with prognosis. Shift of midline structures, only considered in two studies, was associated with fatal outcome. Ropper associated changes in level of consciousness with degree of horizontal displacement of the pineal body in acute hemispheral mass lesions, mainly ICHs.[40] Level of consciousness, in turn, is the clinical sign most consistently associated with ICH prognosis. The consistent importance of hemorrhage size, level of consciousness or Glasgow Coma Scale score, and intraventricular hemorrhage extension, mirror the prominent role these factors played in the previous discussion of specific hemorrhage types.

Univariate studies are limited to studying the relationship between one factor and outcome. With large groups of patients it is possible to apply multivariate techniques to determine if several factors, taken together, contribute to outcome. Alternatively, two separate factors apparently predictive of outcome may be found on multivariate analysis to be dependent on one another, such that only one factor independently predicts outcome. For example, although hemorrhage size and level of consciousness are important predictors of outcome, it is possible that impaired consciousness is related pathophysiologically and statistically to the size of the hematoma. Therefore, measuring hemorrhage size may not contribute substantially to the prediction of outcome in a patient with impaired consciousness.

The six studies listed in Table 1 employing multivariate analysis[9,35-39] produce fairly consistent results despite minor variations in patient selection, variables assessed, and statistical methods. Hemorrhage size, intraventricular extension of blood, and Glasgow Coma Scale score or level of consciousness emerge as consistent, independent predictors of survival. Midline shift, oxygen saturation, pulse pressure, electrocardiographic abnormalities, and age may be included in some models. Tuhrim et al attempted to validate a logistic regression model, developed with data from one group of patients, on data from an independent group of patients.[9] The initial model contained three factors — hemorrhage size, Glasgow Coma Scale score, and pulse pressure — and correctly categorized 92% of patients in the original data set as alive or dead at 30 days.[39] Application of this model to all patients with complete information in the NINDS Stroke Data Bank resulted in 90% correct prediction.[9] This original model did not include intraventricular hemorrhage extension because it was not in the original data set. When this factor was considered, it was possible to classify 94% of the supratentorial ICH patients in the Stroke Data Bank as alive or dead at 30 days. This second model also indicated that Glasgow Coma Scale score and intraventricular hemorrhage interacted additively. A patient who had impaired consciousness and extension of blood into the ventricular system fared more poorly than would be expected by the presence of either factor alone. The presence of both intraventricular hemorrhage and hemorrhage size in this model implies that each factor independently contributes to morbidity. Pulse pressure is probably a marker for increased intracranial pressure, which was not directly measured in this study but was shown previously to be an indicator of poor outcome.[41]

The information contained in this logistic regression model may be used by clinicians to calculate directly the probability for a given patient outcome by using the equation:

$$P \text{ (outcome)} = e^{BX}/1 + e^{BX}$$

where BX is defined as: $-3.3349 + (.9716)$ PP $+ (.5936)$ GCS $+ (.7008)$ H-Size $+ (.4287)$ IVH $+ (2.4958)$ IVH-GCS for PP (pulse pressure) $= 0$ (< 85 mm Hg), 1 (> 85 mm Hg); GCS (Glasgow Coma Scale score) $= 0$ (> 8), 1 (< 8); IVH (intraventricular hemorrhage extension) $= 0$ (no), 1 (yes); H-Size (hemorrhage size) $= 0$ (small, < 27 cc), 1 (moderate, 27 to 72 cc), 2 (large, > 72 cc); IVH-GCS (interaction term) $= 1$ if IVH $= 1$ and GCS $= 1$, and 0 otherwise.

The investigators in the study from which this equation is derived measured hemorrhage size by drawing the hemorrhage on a CT grid composed of rectangles whose areas were known. Hemorrhage size can be measured more easily at the CT console by using the algorithms provided in most modern scanners for measuring areas traced on each slice, multiplying by slice thickness, and summing the volumes computed. Alternatively, the experienced observer can correctly categorize most lesions by inspection of the printed scan.

The use of this equation can be illustrated by considering the example of a patient admitted with a pulse pressure of 60, a GCS score of 6, intraventricular hemorrhage, and a 40 cc (moderate) ICH. The probability of the patient dying could be calculated as slightly greater than 70%: BX = $-3.3349 + (.9716)(0) + (.5936)(1) + (.4287)(1) + (.7008)(1) + (2.4958)(1) = 0.884$ P (outcome) $= e^{0.884}/1 + e^{0.884} = 0.7076$.

Long-Term Prognosis

Long-term outcome has been studied less frequently than early mortality for several reasons. Initially, there appeared to be relatively few survivors of ICH. Also, obtaining information at appropriate intervals postdischarge is more difficult than collecting in-hospital mortality figures. Finally, while death is an easily defined endpoint, it is more difficult to measure recovery or functional capacity. Those long-term stroke outcome studies do not separate ICH from infarction. Most that do are based on relatively few patients. The results of several of the larger studies are summarized below.

Garde et al reported 100 consecutive patients with spontaneous ICH, of whom 63 survived the first month and were followed for an average of 13.3 months. Of these, 34 remained paretic (11 plegic), although only 5 were not ambulatory. Thirty-five returned to work and only 6 remained institutionalized, the rest having returned home. Return to functional status was largely independent of hemorrhage location but was related to original hematoma size and coma scale score.[4]

Fieschi et al followed 69 survivors from a series of 104 nonoperated ICH patients for 1 year. At 1 year, 51 made a good to excellent recovery. The 18 patients who had persistent severe neurologic deficits and had significantly larger hemorrhages, were older (mean age 65 versus 58), and twice as likely to have had intraventricular hemorrhage. None of the patients rebled during the follow-up period.[3]

Douglas et al followed 42 survivors from a series of 70 ICH patients for an average of 29 months. An additional seven died during the follow-up period, none of vascular disease. No recurrent hemorrhages occurred, but five patients suffered seizures. Only 5 of the 35 surviving patients returned to work, 19 were independently ambulatory, and 13 ambulated with assistance. The authors noted that most patients remained functionally the same during the follow-up period as at discharge.[42]

Daverat et al used the Glasgow Outcome Scale to assess functional status following ICH in a cohort 166 ICH patients, of whom 95 survived 6 months. Of these 95 patients, 78% functioned independently at 6 months. Again, large hemorrhage size and ventricular hemorrhage were related to poor outcome, as were the severity of limb paresis and communication disorders. Age was believed to be the single most important determinant of functional recovery, although initial survival was unrelated to age.[35]

Tuhrim et al used factors predictive of 30-day survival to devise a model predicting long-term outcome. The model correctly classified 95% of patients as having a good (defined as alive, Barthel's Index of Activities of Daily Living (ADL) > 60) or poor outcome (defined as death or Barthel's Index < 60) at 1 year. This study made no attempt to determine if age or premorbid level of function related to long-term outcome.[9]

Helweg-Larsen et al, with the longest median follow-up of 4.5 years, found that 28% of 29 patients had returned to work and 30% had normal neurologic examinations. Only 17% were incapacitated, and none had recurrent hemorrhages.[8]

Although the data are limited, the same factors that determine early mortality are predictive of poor long-term functional outcome. This is not surprising, since patients with these factors who unexpectedly survive are more devastated than those without them. Age may play a greater role in determining functional outcome than in predicting initial survival. Recurrent hemorrhage appears to be a rare event, except in nonhypertensive hemorrhages. Several authors suggest that long-term functional recovery is better for ICH survivors than for those who suffer infarctions, but this has not been rigorously studied.

Anticoagulant-Related Hemorrhage

Two recent reports focused on prognosis in anticoagulant-related hemorrhage. Forsting et al reported that 20 of 40 patients did not survive, but 18 of 20 survivors recovered completely. Five patients suffered concomitant subdural hematomas, but no patients had multiple ICHs.[43] Radberg et al found that 28 of a series of 200 patients with ICH had been taking warfarin at the time of the hemorrhage. The mortality of the entire group was 30%, but 57% of those with anticoagulant-related hemorrhages died. The anticoagulant-related hemorrhages were also larger on average.[44] Anticoagulant-related hemorrhages tend to be larger, with a poorer prognosis. Hemorrhage size, intraventricular hemorrhage, and level of consciousness or GCS score continue to predict outcome accurately in these patients, as they do for most patients with ICH. Patients with anticoagulant-related ICH do not appear to differ in degree of recovery, frequently returning to a high level of functioning.

References

1. Furlan AJ, Whisnant JP, Elveback LR: The decreasing incidence of primary intracerebral hemorrhage: a population study. *Ann Neurol* 1979;5: 367.
2. Drury I, Whisnant JP, Garraway WM: Primary intracerebral hemorrhage: impact of CT on incidence. *Neurology* 1984;34:653.
3. Fieschi C, Carolei A, Fiorelli M, et al: Changing prognosis of primary intra-

cerebral hemorrhage: results of a clinical and computed tomographic follow-up study of 104 patients. *Stroke* 1988;19:192.

4. Garde A, Bohmer G, Selden B, et al: 100 cases of spontaneous intracerebral hematoma. *Eur Neurol* 1983;22:161.

5. Steiner I, Gomori JM, Melamed E: The prognostic value of the CT scan in conservatively treated patients with intracerebral hematoma. *Stroke* 1984; 15:279.

6. Nath FP, Nicholls D, Fraser RJA: Prognosis in intracerebral hemorrhage. *Acta Neurochirurgia* 1983;67:29.

7. Mayr U, Bauer P, Fischer J: Non-traumatic intracerebral hemorrhage. *Neurochirurgica* 1983;26:36.

8. Helweg-Larsen S, Sommer W, Stange P, et al: Prognosis for patients treated conservatively for spontaneous intracerebral hematomas. *Stroke* 1984;15:1045.

9. Tuhrim S, Dambrosia JM, Price TR, et al: Intracerebral hemorrhage: external validation and extension of a model for prediction of 30-day survival. *Ann Neurol* 1991;29:658.

10. Rudick RA: Asymptomatic intracerebral hematoma as an incidental finding. *Arch Neurol* 1981;38:396.

11. Hier DB, Davis KR, Richardson EP, et al: Hypertensive putaminal hemorrhage. *Ann Neurol* 1977;1:152.

12. Mizukhami M, Nishijima M, Kin H: Computed tomographic findings of good prognosis for hemiplegia in hypertensive putaminal hemorrhage. *Stroke* 1981;648.

13. Kanaya H: Results of conservative and surgical treatment in hypertensive intracerebral hemorrhage — co-operative study in Japan. *Jpn J Stroke* 1990;12:509.

14. Stein RW, Kase CS, Hier DB, et al: Caudate hemorrhage. *Neurology* 1984; 34:1549.

15. Fisher CM: The pathologic and clinical aspects of thalamic hemorrhage. *Trans Amer Neurol Assoc* 1959;84:56.

16. Walshe TM, Davis KR, Fisher CM: Thalamic hemorrhage: a computed tomographic-clinical correlation. *Neurology* 1977;27:217.

17. Piepgras U, Rieger P: Thalamic bleeding. *Neuroradiology* 1981;22:85.

18. Barraquer-Bordas L, Illa I, Escartin A, et al: Thalamic hemorrhage. A study of 23 patients with diagnosis by computed tomography. *Stroke* 1981; 12:524.

19. Kwak R, Kadoya S, Suzuki T: Factors affecting the prognosis in thalamic hemorrhage. *Stroke* 1983;14:493.

20. Weisberg LA: Thalamic hemorrhage: clinical-CT correlations. *Neurology* 1986;36:1382.

21. Hirose G, Kosoegawa H, Saeki M, et al: The syndrome of posterior thalamic hemorrhage. *Neurology* 1985;35:998.

22. Ropper AH, Davis KR: Lobar cerebral hemorrhages: acute clinical syndromes in 26 cases. *Ann Neurol* 1980;8:141.

23. Kase CS, Williams JP, Wyatt DH, et al: Lobar intracerebral hematomas: clinical and CT analysis of 22 cases. *Neurology* 1982;32:1146.

24. Tanaka Y, Furuse M, Iwasa H, et al: Lobar intracerebral hemorrhage: etiology and long-term follow-up study of 32 patients. *Stroke* 1986;17:51.

25. Weisberg LA: Subcortical lobar intracerebral hemorrhage: clinical-computed tomographic correlations. *J Neurol Neurosurg Psychiatry* 1985;48: 1078.

26. Silverstein A: Primary pontine hemorrhage. *Confin Neurol* 1967;29:33.

27. Tuhrim S, Yang WC, Rubinowitz H, et al: Primary pontine hemorrhage and the dysarthria-clumsy hand syndrome. *Neurology* 1982;32:1027.

28. Burns J, Lisak R, Schut L, et al: Recovery following brainstem hemorrhage. *Ann Neurol* 1980;7:183.

29. Payne HA, Maravilla KR, Levinstone A, et al: Recovery from primary pontine hemorrhage. *Ann Neurol* 1978;4:556.

30. Weisberg LA: Primary pontine hemorrhage: clinical and computed tomographic correlations. *J Neurol Neurosurg Psychiatry* 1986;49:346.

31. Kilpatrick TJ, Davis SM, Tress BM, et al: Lateral tegmental haemorrhage due to vascular malformations. *Cerebrovasc Res* 1991;1:108.

32. Ott KH, Kase CS, Ojemann RG, et al: Cerebellar hemorrhage: diagnosis and treatment. *Arch Neurol* 1974;31:160.

33. Little JR, Tubman DE, Ethier R: Cerebellar hemorrhage in adults: diagnosis by computerized tomography. *J Neurosurg* 1978;48:575.

34. Fisher CM, Picard ED, Polak A, et al: Acute hypertensive cerebellar hemorrhage: diagnosis and treatment. *Arch Neurol* 1974;31:160.

35. Daverat P, Castel JP, Dartigues JF, et al: Death and functional outcome after spontaneous intracerebral hemorrhage: a prospective study of 166 cases using multivariate analysis. *Stroke* 1991;22:1.

36. Dixon AA, Holness RO, Howes WJ, et al: Spontaneous intracerebral hemorrhage: an analysis of factors affecting prognosis. *Can J Neurol Sci* 1985; 12:267.

37. Portenoy RK, Lipton RB, Berger AR, et al: Intracerebral hemorrhage: a model for the prediction of outcome. *J Neurol Neurosurg Psychiatry* 1987; 50:976.

38. Senant J, Samson M, Proust B, et al: Approche multi-factorielle du pronostic vital des hematomas intra-cerebraux spontanes. *Rev Neurol* 1988;144: 279.

39. Tuhrim S, Dambrosia JM, Price TR, et al: Prediction of intracerebral hemorrhage survival. *Ann Neurol* 1988;24:258.

40. Ropper AH: Lateral displacement of the brain and level of consciousness in patients with an acute hemispheral mass. *N Engl J Med* 1986;314:953.

41. Ropper AH, King RB: Intracranial pressure monitoring in comatose patients with cerebral hemorrhage. *Arch Neurol* 1984;41:725.

42. Douglas MA, Haerer AF: Long-term prognosis of hypertensive intracerebral hemorrhage. *Stroke* 1982;13:488.

43. Forsting M, Mattle HP, Huber P: Anticoagulation-related intracerebral hemorrhage. *Cerebrovasc Dis* 1991;1:97.

44. Radberg JA, Olsson JE, Radberg CT: Prognostic parameters in spontaneous intracerebral hematomas with special reference to anticoagulant treatment. *Stroke* 1991;22:571.

Index